Publishing Your Medical Research

SECOND EDITION

Publishing Your Medical Research

SECOND EDITION

Daniel W. Byrne

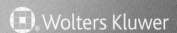

Philadelphia · Baltimore · New York · London
Buenos Aires · Hong Kong · Sydney · Tokyo

Acquisitions Editor: Kel McGowan
Development Editor: Kristina Oberle
Production Project Manager: David Saltzberg
Design Coordinator: Steve Druding
Marketing Manager: Rachel Mante Leung
Senior Manufacturing Coordinator: Beth Welsh
Prepress Vendor: Absolute Service, Inc.

© 2017 by Wolters Kluwer

First edition © 1998 by Lippincott Williams & Wilkins

IBM, the IBM logo, ibm.com, and SPSS are trademarks or registered trademarks of **International Business Machines Corporation**, registered in many jurisdictions worldwide. Other product and service names might be trademarks of IBM or other companies. A current list of IBM trademarks is available on the Web at "IBM Copyright and trademark information" at www.ibm.com/legal/copytrade.shtml.

9 8 7 6 5 4 3 2 1

Printed in China

Library of Congress Cataloging-in-Publication Data

Names: Byrne, Daniel W., author.
Title: Publishing your medical research / Daniel W. Byrne.
Description: Second edition. | Philadelphia : Wolters Kluwer Health, [2017] |
   Includes bibliographical references and index.
Identifiers: LCCN 2016028215 | ISBN 9781496353863
Subjects: | MESH: Medical Writing | Publishing | Biomedical Research
Classification: LCC R119 | NLM WZ 345 | DDC 808/.06661—dc23 LC record available at
https://lccn.loc.gov/2016028215

LWW.com

In memory of Art Wheeler

Contents

PLANNING

OBSERVING

WRITING

EDITING

REVISING

APPENDIXES

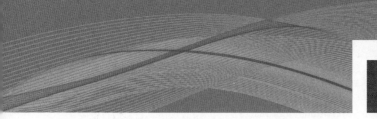

List of Tables

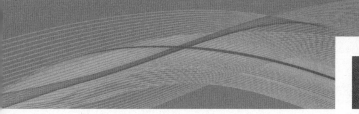

List of Figures

"Worship the spirit of criticism," Pasteur advised his fellow scientists. Today, most scientists recognize the importance of this advice, but nearly all prefer the spirit of praise from one particular group: peer reviewers. The bad news is that each year, reviewers reject hundreds of thousands of medical manuscripts. The good news is that many are rejected for common flaws that can be avoided.

Numerous books have described how to write a scientific paper, notably those by Day and Gastel (2011), Huth (1999), Browner (2012), and Hall (2012). My goal in writing *Publishing Your Medical Research* was to explain how to anticipate and avoid the problems typically encountered in designing a research study and writing a publishable paper.

Many common reviewer criticisms can be avoided simply by understanding the research and publishing processes and by following certain fundamental principles. This book presents more than 200 principles in five sequential phases: Planning, Observing, Writing, Editing, and Revising. Applying these POWER principles will increase the likelihood that your research will be accepted for publication. The information in this book will also help you critically assess new medical information and extract what you need to know.

As background research for this book, I surveyed a number of experts, including editors-in-chief of prominent medical journals, peer reviewers, and Nobel Laureates. I conducted this survey for the first edition and then again recently for the second edition. Additionally, I analyzed hundreds of actual reviews to identify common themes and distilled specific comments into positive guidance. These ideas are arranged into principles presented in an easy-to-read format, with short examples of actual peer review critiques. To protect the privacy of those involved, some of these comments are paraphrased or generalized.

Publishing Your Medical Research is designed to help researchers work effectively with epidemiologists, informatics experts, biostatisticians, technical writers, graphic artists, and other methodologists. It provides an organized collection of solutions to help you publish your medical research paper. For those who manage a research team, these solutions will help you stretch your research funds. Although this book focuses on clinical research, most of the principles can also be applied to nonclinical biomedical research, which is increasingly requiring more of these principles. This book is a guide, not a cookbook, and therefore does not attempt to explain everything you need to know about statistical analysis, epidemiology, or writing. For more complex problems, a suitable modern reference or resource is recommended.

Academic publishing requires time, dedication, practice, and, above all, persistence. If you can muster these resources, you will be rewarded with seeing your article in print and knowing that your work has made a difference. As the clinical psychologist and educator Anne Roe said, "Nothing in science has any value to society if it is not communicated."

—**Daniel W. Byrne**

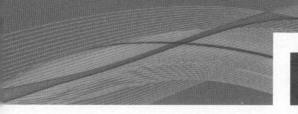

Acknowledgments

All published work and quotations are referenced as accurately as possible. As promised, the survey responses were kept anonymous, but I am nonetheless grateful to the reviewers and editors who completed and returned my questionnaires.

Gertrude Elion and Robert Jacoby were kind enough to read and find something nice to say about early drafts of the first edition of this book. I continue to be grateful to all of the people who helped with the first edition, including Paul van Niewerburgh, Jane Petro, Harold Horowitz, Jean Morgan, Albert Lowenfels, Chris Hunter, Lawrence Wexler, Luis Bracero, P.D. Reddy, Evan Jones, Michael Blumenfield, Elizabeth Nieginski, Julie Scardiglia, Karla Schroeder, Rosanne Hallowell, Beth Goldner, and Jacqueline Jenks.

For the second edition, I would like to thank David Robertson, Bob Dittus, Hank Domenico, Li Wang, Rachel Walden, Art Wheeler, Gordon Bernard, Kel McGowan, Kristina Oberle, Jim Ware, Tom Hazinski, Nancy Brown, Alp Ikizler, Mike Stein, Alastair Wood, Yu Shyr, Bill Dupont, Ayumi Shintani, Virginia Byrne, Brenda Minor, Paul Harris, and Vivian Siegel. Over the past 16 years, the trainees in Vanderbilt's Master of Science in Clinical Investigation program courses that I taught have provided me with valuable feedback on most of the material in this book. I am grateful for this feedback and honored to teach in this program.

Finally, but most of all, a special thanks to my wife, Loretta, for her insightful editing and almost endless patience.

Overview: Twenty Key Principles

Success in publishing your medical research paper will largely depend on how well you follow these twenty key principles. Study these points before moving on to the more detailed principles and periodically review these during your research project.

> *"You have to learn the rules of the game. And then you have to play better than anyone else."*
>
> —ALBERT EINSTEIN

PRINCIPLE 1 • Educate yourself in an aggressive and continuous way regarding clinical trials, study design, bias, and biostatistics.

There are no shortcuts to publishing papers. Clinical trials, in particular, have become a science, and there are plenty of pitfalls for those who are not experts in this science. Table 1.1 provides a reading list that will provide a preliminary plan for this self-education. A formal training program in medical research is also extremely valuable in learning how to write publishable papers, for example, a master of public health (MPH) or a master of science in clinical investigation (MSCI) program.

PRINCIPLE 2 • Select a clinically important problem to solve that will result in a high-impact paper.

Focus on answering questions that are important to improving patient-centered outcomes and avoid projects related to trivial correlations or meaningless interactions. Write one polished sentence that clearly defines the precise problem that your study addresses. This problem must describe the specific shape of the niche in the literature that your paper will fill—not a vague background statement, such as "There is an obesity epidemic in this country." A strong problem statement would be "It is unclear from the current medical literature whether an online diabetes prevention program would be as effective as an in-person program with regards to attendance and weight loss." Translate this problem into a testable null hypothesis to include in the Methods, for example, "The 1-year weight loss is no different between participants randomized to an in-person diabetes prevention program and those in an online program."

PRINCIPLE 3 • Invest ample time and money in planning.

"JUST DO IT" was a successful slogan for selling sneakers, but it is a poor approach to conducting medical research. You need both an experienced research team and an extensive understanding of the literature to avoid the common problems encountered in planning the study, designing the measures of outcome, creating the data collection forms, and performing the statistical analysis. An experienced and successful mentor is your best resource for understanding exactly how much time needs to be dedicated to the planning phase of a project.

TABLE 1.1   **A Self-Education Reading List for Medical Researchers**

Designing Clinical Research by Hulley et al. (2013)

Fundamentals of Clinical Trials by Friedman et al. (2015)

Evaluating Clinical and Public Health Interventions: A Practical Guide to Study Design and Statistics by Katz (2010)

Basic Statistics for the Health Sciences by Kuzma and Bohnenblust (2004)

How to Write a Lot: A Practical Guide to Productive Academic Writing by Silvia (2007)

Medical Uses of Statistics by Bailar and Hoaglin (2009)

Statistics with Confidence: Confidence Intervals and Statistical Guidelines by Altman et al. (2000)

How to Report Statistics in Medicine: Annotated Guidelines for Authors, Editors, and Reviewers by Lang and Secic (2006)

The Man Who Discovered Quality: How W. Edwards Deming Brought the Quality Revolution to America—The Stories of FORD, XEROX, and GM by Gabor (1992)

Epidemiology by Gordis (2013)

Essentials of Medical Statistics by Kirkwood and Sterne (2003)

Clinical and Translational Science: Principles of Human Research by Robertson and Williams (2016)

Statistical Modeling for Biomedical Researchers: A Simple Introduction to the Analysis of Complex Data by Dupont (2009)

Modern Epidemiology by Rothman et al. (2012)

Clinical Prediction Models: A Practical Approach to Development, Validation, and Updating by Steyerberg (2010)

Encyclopedia of Biostatistics: 8-Volume Set by Armitage and Colton (2005)

Essentials of Writing Biomedical Research Papers by Zeiger (1999)

Statistical Issues in Drug Development by Senn (2008)

Experimental Design for Biologists by Glass (2014)

Experimental Design for the Life Sciences by Ruxton and Colegrave (2010)

Thinking, Fast and Slow by Kahneman (2013)

PRINCIPLE 4 • Develop a robust study design and document it completely in the Methods (and Appendix).

It takes a lot of thought to plan a study carefully. Remember, a good paper is not about the prose, it is about both the prose and the science—and for the science you need crisp thinking in the planning phase. Develop a long-term collaboration with an experienced biostatistician and create good open communication at all phases of the research. Poor methodology annoys reviewers and must be avoided at all costs.

PRINCIPLE 5 • Write a detailed study protocol to create reproducible research.

The study protocol is the written plan for your research project. A good protocol provides direction, focus, and structure. An analogy is a cake recipe that includes an appropriate level of detail with ingredients, amounts, duration, and temperature. As you conduct your study, follow this plan and document all decisions and developments. This approach allows you to monitor and describe the accuracy and appropriateness of your methods. Keep the protocol and all documents related to the study organized into files and folders labeled carefully so that anyone on your research team could retrieve and use those files years later.

For examples of modern, professional medical research protocols, see the protocols posted on the journal's website, for example, at The New England Journal of Medicine's website, these can be found under Supplementary Material for each paper.

http://www.nejm.org/toc/nejm/medical-journal

Standard Protocol Items: Recommendations for Interventional Trials (SPIRIT) is "an international initiative that aims to improve the quality of clinical trial protocols by defining an evidence-based set of items to address in a protocol." The SPIRIT Statement provides protocol recommendations and a checklist.

http://www.spirit-statement.org/spirit-statement/

Another resource is Protocol Exchange, which is an open repository for sharing scientific protocols.

http://www.nature.com/protocolexchange/

PRINCIPLE 6 • Prespecify the analysis and interim monitoring plan in your protocol and register it before you start the study.

This plan must include a definition of the primary end point and only a very limited number of secondary end points. Any subgroup analysis must also be clearly predefined to avoid the appearance of a fishing expedition—or digging out post hoc subgroups. All projects, even observational studies and animal experiments, should have a detailed prespecified analysis plan. Registration systems vary by country: In the United States, clinical trials should be registered on the website http://www.ClinicalTrials.gov. Failing to register your trial properly may make it impossible to publish your paper in a high-profile journal. For more information, see

http://www.nlm.nih.gov/services/ctwhatis.html

If a trial is registered in more than one registry, it must be cross-referenced. See the International Clinical Trials Registry Platform (ICTRP):

http://www.who.int/ictrp/trial_reg/en/index.html

PRINCIPLE 7 • Build a complete, unbiased, high-quality data set.

Demonstrate that the way you gathered the data is unbiased. Measure a comprehensive set of important variables at baseline and regular intervals rather than assuming perfect compliance with the protocol, blinding, etc. These variables must include covariates, potential confounders, and measures of intermediate efficacy (to understand the mechanism and the mediation model).

PRINCIPLE 8 • Aim to keep the manuscript short, especially the Introduction and Discussion—clarity with brevity.

Plan to submit a paper that is 10% shorter in word count than the maximum limit for the target journal. This will help you avoid the inefficiency of writing and deleting superfluous text. Check the total length of the paper, the length of each section, and the number of references. Having said that, it is sometimes prudent to include slightly more tables and figures than average; reviewers appreciate tables and figures—and your first goal is to keep them happy. Use the appendix to include additional figures, tables, and detail about the methods.

PRINCIPLE 9 • Describe your methods thoroughly for reproducible research.

To show that your findings can be applied to larger populations, clearly describe your study design. Readers and reviewers will scrutinize your methods before they accept your conclusions. Be sure that you can reproduce your own analysis. Save your statistical coding/syntax in the Appendix of your paper.

PRINCIPLE 10 • Describe the rationale for the size of your sample.

Explain how and why you chose to study the specified number of patients. Discuss the implications and statistical power of your decision. Help the reader understand your logic in selecting this group of patients for the study.

PRINCIPLE 11 • Construct tables that are informative and transparent.

The tables should present an honest and complete account of all positive and negative outcomes, complications, and side effects. Provide 95% confidence intervals around important point estimates. Add extensive footnotes to every table to explain which statistical test was used for each P value and provide additional detail to make each table stand alone.

PRINCIPLE 12 • Create modern professional graphs/figures that illustrate the conclusions in an honest fashion.

The graphs should stand alone, with everything needed for interpretation self-contained in the figure itself (or in the figure legend). Conduct internal prereviews to test whether others can understand your graphs and then edit for clarity before submitting. For randomized clinical trials, include a carefully constructed CONSORT flow diagram showing the number of participants at each stage of the trial.

> http://www.consort-statement.org/consort-statement/flow-diagram0/

PRINCIPLE 13 • Explain for the editor what is new, interesting, and useful about your results.

What do your findings contribute to the medical literature? Explain the importance of the research problem and your findings for both physicians and patients. The editors' mantra is "What's new? And why should I care?" Answer these questions head-on and in a forceful way. Define the knowledge gap and show how you filled it to advance the field sufficiently.

PRINCIPLE 14 • Elaborate further to answer the reviewers' questions: "So what?" and "Who cares?"

Emphasize the points that distinguish your study from other research. Your paper must contain sections anticipating negative reactions from skeptical reviewers. To be accepted, your subject must interest most of your target journal's readers—so tell a story.

PRINCIPLE 15 • Describe the limitations of the study.

Do not force the editors and reviewers to ask for this. Anticipate several areas that reviewers will point out as drawbacks and demonstrate that you thought long and hard about these—and that the conclusions are still valid despite these apparent weaknesses. The 'Limitations' section of the Discussion should be of this form: "Here are all the things that could be wrong with what I just told you. As you can see from our Results, we investigated each of these and found that the conclusions are still supported by the data."

PRINCIPLE 16 • Follow the guidelines and format of the target journal precisely.

Consult the information for authors and several recent issues of the target journal. Be sure that your submission meets the journal's definition of a complete manuscript. Also consider the timeliness of the subject from the perspective of the readers.

One reviewer described the following common problems:

"Being sent manuscripts that are not in compliance with journal guidelines—usually manuscripts that greatly exceed limits. Being sent manuscripts that are clearly not suitable for consideration in the journal due to poor content, offensive tone, or not in line with journal priorities."

PRINCIPLE 17 • Edit ruthlessly to eliminate jargon, poor grammar, and poor writing.

Ask experienced colleagues to read your paper objectively. Continue to revise your manuscript until it is both clear and polished. Write an Introduction that captures the reader's attention, and rewrite the remaining text as necessary to flow smoothly and maintain that interest.

PRINCIPLE 18 • Write and polish a crisp Abstract in the target journal's format that demonstrates that you have new and important findings.

The Abstract is much more important than most people realize. Spend more time with your Abstract. Edit until it is easy for the reader to see what you are trying to do—and why. Make sure your Abstract shows that you have a solid study design and a high-quality data set. Polish the conclusions until they are appropriate for <u>your</u> results. The editor will be looking to see that your study will result in a high-impact paper that will be of interest to that journal's audience and will be referenced by other authors.

PRINCIPLE 19 • Write conclusions that are objective, conservative, perceptive, and supported by the results presented.

Be modest and do not overreach with your conclusions. Every sentence must be supported by the facts. If the results are negative, accept it—do not put a spin on it. Do not repurpose a "negative" study into a noninferiority design. Ensure that your tone is objective and unbiased, not overly enthusiastic or angry. End with your specific take-home message but avoid the vague "More research is needed." Was there a possibility that you could have ended the need for all research?

PRINCIPLE 20 • Revise the conclusions to tighten up the logic and writing.

Devote the necessary time and effort to fine-tune and tone down your conclusions to match your data. Avoid an overinterpretation of the data. Your conclusions must be insightful and clearly justified. They should include a smooth, logical transition from your results and end with a bang! Finally, carefully reflect on the question: "What might be wrong with what I just concluded?"

PLANNING

Key Questions to Answer in the Planning Phase:

- What is the specific research problem that this study will address?
- What is the plan to study this problem?
- How will the data be analyzed?
- What are the plans for study oversight, interim analysis, and stopping rules?
- How can this research improve the health outcomes of patients?
- How can this information be translated into a measurable impact on society?
- How can patients and other stakeholders be involved in a meaningful way?
- Will the study provide information that will enable clinicians and patients to make more informed decisions to improve patient outcomes?
- If the study is "positive," what is the plan to make your findings sustainable?
- If the study is "negative," will there be sufficient information to tell a publishable story?

Laying the Groundwork

> *"A good paper moves science upwards, not sideways."*
> —ANONYMOUS

CHOOSING A TOPIC

PRINCIPLE 21 • Choose a topic that is timely, important, and interesting.

The 20 key principles discussed in Chapter 1 outline the process of writing an article for publication, but the remaining chapters provide the all-important details, starting with Principle 21. Obviously, the first step in planning is to select a worthwhile research topic.

How do you select a topic for study? Your interest in and passion for a research topic should be the prime motivators. Because, however, you are also planning to publish your results, you must understand how the journal publishing process works and consider where your topic fits in.

First, you must consider the target audience. You can begin by asking yourself three questions:

1. Is my primary research question interesting to enough readers and important to patients?
2. Has this specific question been adequately answered previously in the literature?
3. Do I have the resources to answer this question?

A research project demands a significant investment of time, so you must be genuinely interested in the topic and internally motivated to complete the project. The key to getting your study published is, however, the importance of the topic. A common reason for rejection is simply a lack of importance. For this reason, choose a topic that has clinical interest, but keep your study design as straightforward and focused as possible. When you find an interesting problem, focus on studying and presenting a solution, particularly one that is pragmatic and sustainable. In this way, the focus of your study will be on the solution, not the problem. A research project that goes the extra mile to document improved patient outcomes in a randomized controlled trial is much more valuable than just another paper describing factors associated with poor outcomes.

If you are a novice at writing papers, seek advice from an experienced investigator, mentor, or department chairperson who can help you select a worthwhile research project with a publishable slant. The paper should also put you in a better position to obtain future grant funding (e.g., see Maron et al., 2011) and should fit into your 5-year strategic career plan.

Design your study so that you can write a paper whether the final results are negative or positive. Often, you can do this by identifying the important question that needs to be answered and collecting a comprehensive amount of data around that question.

VITAL POINT

Early in your project, solicit opinions of other researchers and experienced methodologists. They can help you avoid many pitfalls. A classic mistake of the inexperienced researcher is waiting until the study is nearly complete to ask for help. You will hear the advice, "You should consult a biostatistician early." A more successful approach is to develop a long-term continuous collaboration with a biostatistician who is part of your research team and funded for a good portion of his or her time ($\geq 10\%$) on your research grant or by your department.

> *"To consult the statistician after an experiment is finished is often merely to ask him to conduct a postmortem examination. He can perhaps say what the experiment died of."*
> —R. A. FISHER

FOR MORE INFORMATION

See *Designing Clinical Research* by Hulley et al. (2013) and Healthy People 2020 (U.S. Department of Health and Human Services, http://www.healthypeople.gov), which provides a detailed account of the U.S. government's health goals for the year 2020. Also, the Agency for Healthcare Research and Quality's (AHRQ) Effective Health Care Program has a list of suggested topics for research.

http://www.effectivehealthcare.ahrq.gov/index.cfm/submit-a-suggestion-for -research/read-suggested-topics-for-research/

CONDUCTING A LITERATURE SEARCH TO IDENTIFY THE GAP IN KNOWLEDGE

When you review the literature, do not be intimidated by the work that has been published. Much of the medical literature is flawed, underpowered, or outdated—so be skeptical. By studying the literature carefully, you often can design a study that is superior to those already published. Although your work should not duplicate published reports, do not hesitate to continue your research if someone has published a paper that initially looks like a barrier to your progress, because many publications are not as strong as they initially appear. An experienced mentor can teach you more about this.

Reviewers from my survey pointed out the following problems with literature searches:

"Incomplete review of prior literature (especially older papers)"
"Selective reviewing of the literature, i.e. US researchers tend to only include other US research (even if there is international research that is relevant)"
"Excessive citation of authors' previous publications"

REDUNDANT AND MULTIPLE PUBLICATIONS

One important principle to keep in mind in the early planning stage is never to submit a paper that is a redundant publication or a duplicate publication. A duplicate/redundant paper is basically the same as one of your previous publications but with minor changes such as the title and abstract. As one editor warned, "Avoid cutting a single study into a large number of small parts." In other words, do not stretch one natural paper into several trivial papers with overlapping results. Another said, "Multiple manuscripts that could have been submitted as one manuscript were not received well by the editor or the reviewers, and if the papers were not rejected outright, the authors were requested to combine the manuscripts into one concise manuscript." One reviewer advised, *"Make a contribution to mankind, not just to your curriculum vitae."*

To be efficient, it is wise to plan a study that will enable your research team to write multiple important papers that could not be written as one. A little planning and extra data can provide you with the information needed to write several papers. For example, you might obtain permission and record multiple methods of contacting the patients in 5 years to write a paper about long-term outcomes. Having patients complete a comprehensive health risk assessment will not only provide for an additional paper but will also provide you with the ability to adjust for confounding factors. Finally, collecting data and obtaining permission for genetic analysis will provide one more dimension.

FOR MORE INFORMATION

See the following sections in Appendix A: "Duplicate Submission" (section III.D.1) and "Acceptable Secondary Publication" (section III.D.3).

PRINCIPLE 22 • Understand what reviewers consider a "good" article.

You can increase the likelihood that your paper will be accepted by learning what reviewers look for in submissions.

Table 2.1 shows the responses of reviewers who were asked to define a good article.

TABLE 2.1 | **Reviewers' Responses to the Question: "What Is Your Definition of a Good Article?"**[a]

- One that makes the reader wonder: "Why didn't I think of that?"
- Short and with simple experiments and easily interpreted results
- Well written, thoughtful, follows the objective of the paper, and referenced appropriately to support the findings provided
- Everything builds and integrates with the prior section: Introduction, Methods, Results, Discussion including implications.
- Clearly written article describing a well-designed experiment
- Important questions, focused study, presented so that it can be understood by as many readers as possible
- Tackles a topical issue, uses novel methods
  [Note: A topical issue is of immediate relevance, interest, or importance owing to its relation to current news or events.]
- Concise Introduction setting up the problem, readable and appropriate Methods, data presentation that flows well, standalone tables, acknowledgment of (and approach to reducing) limitations, thoughtful Discussion
- One that has a clear hypothesis, that has tested it carefully, and that presents the Methods, Results, and Discussion clearly
- Innovative idea, well-conceived study to test this idea, crisp and focused presentation of the data followed by a succinct Discussion
- Short, clear, important topic, appropriate study design, clearly presented Results, appropriate interpretation
- Well-defined Methods and statistical analysis

(continued)

TABLE 2.1	**Reviewers' Responses to the Question: "What Is Your Definition of a Good Article?"[a]** *(continued)*

- Well written, good methodology, conclusions supported by data
- An article that is well written and provides a solid scientific rationale for the study. The methodology should be appropriate to test hypotheses and answer research questions. Presentation of results should be clear and concise. Discussion should frame the current study within the context of previous research, reiterate the importance of the study findings, and tell the reader what the broader takeaway message is.
- Focused clinical question that does not overreach with the analysis or conclusion
- Clean, tight, focused, crisp writing, simple question with a simple methodologic approach, no longer than it needs to be to describe what was done and found
- Clearly written, with a well-formulated and tested hypothesis on a new or high-impact question, with conclusions based on the results
- Brief, to the point, focused, clear, simple, clear tables, nice illustrations if possible, great language
- Novel hypothesis and creative treatment with appropriate design, sufficient data with careful analysis and conservative interpretation
- Deals with an important, interesting, and contemporary topic; the aim is clearly stated; the methodology is correct; the study is well presented and has a concise, interesting discussion.
- Relevant to the audience and clinical practice
- Results should be reproducible.
- Good design of experiments to answer a specific question that has not already been answered in the literature
- Adequate discussion of the shortcomings of the design and conclusion
- Tight, clear organization
- Clear, easy-to-read communication that teaches or stimulates ideas in the reader
- Omits irrelevant points
- An article that honestly reports the answer to a good question with adequate Methods even if the Results are not particularly exciting
- A paper that addresses an interesting and important question; that presents the context, Methods, and Results clearly; and that reasons to the conclusion with consideration of alternative explanations
- Novel/innovative, concise, clear outcomes, appropriate analyses, conclusions justified
- Original[b]

[a]From question 30 of the "Peer Review Questionnaire" section in Appendix B.
[b]Perform a thorough PubMed search to assess whether your paper is original and document this in the Discussion of your paper.

FORMING A RESEARCH TEAM

PRINCIPLE 23 • Join or form a research team with the right chemistry.

The first step in performing a study is to build a research team. To produce high-quality science, experienced investigators have learned that a team must have the right blend of skills and personalities. They choose trustworthy people who have a reputation for doing their share of the work in a timely manner and avoiding academic politics.

When you participate in assembling a research team, select people who will work well together and show respect for one another (e.g., by coming to meetings on time). Check references and talk with candidates' previous research teams. Seek team members who have the free time and motivation to complete the project; an eminent scientist may not be the most suitable person for the job simply due to a lack of time.

The most productive medical research teams often are composed of highly skilled and experienced people with diverse backgrounds and academic degrees.

Choosing the right person to collect the data can be a challenge. Data collection often is more time-consuming than anticipated, and the ideal person for this task must have sufficient time funded for this work. For this reason, hiring a full-time research nurse may be more efficient than persuading a harried medical student, resident, or fellow to collect data. Also remember that many research projects require more than one person to collect data. This requires additional planning to ensure consistent, unbiased results.

The ideal data collection person for a clinical research project has the following characteristics:

+ Has years of experience in the medical field
+ Pays attention to detail
+ Follows instructions precisely
+ Asks questions when unsure
+ Is not overcommitted with other responsibilities
+ Remains objective
+ Has excellent data entry and database management skills

At least one team member must be skilled at creating professional medical research graphs that are publication quality. Ideally, this person is a skilled R programmer with years of experience at creating publication quality graphs with R packages such as ggplot2.

See https://www.r-project.org.

One team member should be proficient with data management tools, such as REDCap. The Coursera course "Data Management for Clinical Research" is an excellent way to develop these skills:

https://www.coursera.org/course/datamanagement

Recruit at least one team member who is a talented writer and editor. Discuss authorship early and candidly. Do not assume or promise that any member of a research team will, or will not, be a coauthor of your study. Authorship depends on, among other things, a "substantial contribution to the intellectual content of the study," so never list an author who has not met the full criteria for authorship.

One technique for ensuring that each coauthor does his or her fair share of the work is to list your name on the title page as "Smith et al." and then add the coauthors to the penultimate version—provided that they completed their sections in a timely manner. This avoids the awkward situation of having to delete names from the final version because they failed to do their work.

FOR MORE INFORMATION

See Appendix A and the following website for a full description of the updated authorship standards established by the International Committee of Medical Journal Editors:

http://www.icmje.org/recommendations/browse/roles-and-responsibilities
/defining-the-role-of-authors-and-contributors.html

Consider inviting the person who collects the data to coauthor the paper. Coauthorship motivates many people to do their best work. In addition, many studies hinge on the quality of the data collection, and some public accountability is only logical. Research nurses who made substantial contributions to the project should be invited to coauthor papers.

You do not have to be a chairperson with a large grant to form a research team. Medical students, residents, and junior faculty who have no budget or authority can form a research team by diplomatically asking the right people to collaborate. If you are polite and hardworking, many experienced researchers will work with you on worthwhile projects. Remember that today, you can form a virtual research team of experts from around the world by using modern technology. Be sure, however, that this team also has the right chemistry.

The Methodology

3

PRINCIPLE 24 • State the specific problem that your study will address.

The top priorities in the planning stage are:

+ Fully conceptualizing the problem
+ Formulating a robust approach to solving the problem

Conceptualizing a clinical research problem requires you to organize your thoughts and draw general conclusions from specific instances. Only when the problem and aim of the study are thought out and concisely defined can you begin to collect data. Ask your colleagues to critique your statement of the problem and make the recommended changes before you begin to collect data.

Adherence to traditional scientific methodology is essential. The steps in the scientific method are as follows:

Step	Section of the Manuscript to Describe in
1. State the problem.	Introduction
2. Formulate the (null) hypothesis.	Methods
3. Design the study.	Methods
4. Collect data.	Methods
5. Analyze the results.	Results/Discussion
6. Draw conclusions.	Discussion

Write one sentence for each step of the scientific method. Polish each sentence and be sure that it builds in a linear way on the previous steps.

STATING THE PROBLEM

Stating the problem is the first and most important step in the scientific method. The idea for a problem may come from anecdotal observations, the literature, ongoing or previous research, conferences, or conversations with colleagues. Whatever the source of the idea, quality research requires a polished problem statement. You must be able to provide a clear and concise answer to the question, "What is the main purpose of this study and how will it fill an important niche in the medical literature?" Write one sentence that completely describes the specific research problem that you are setting out to solve. Edit this sentence based on your literature review and feedback from colleagues.

One reviewer offered this advice: "Spend the majority of your time refining the clinical question. The time spent doing that will make the rest of the project much easier."

Example 3–1.
Approximately 30% of patients with spinal cord injury develop a pressure ulcer during the initial hospitalization; however, based on the current medical literature, there is currently no method

of quantifying this risk during the first hospitalization that is accurate for this unique patient population.

Note that the statement of the problem should not be as vague as "Spinal cord injury patients have a high rate of pressure ulcers." After this study is completed, that problem will still exist. The statement of the problem must define the specific niche in the published medical literature that, at the end of your study, will be filled and thus move science forward.

> *Example 3–2.*
> The following is an example of an appropriately specific statement of the problem: "The problem that this study will address is that it is unclear from the current medical literature whether a 1-year lifestyle coaching program to increase physical activity and decrease fat intake in participants with prediabetes will result in more weight loss than is seen in a parallel control group."

Unfortunately, many researchers will claim that their statement of the problem is something like this: "There is a diabetes epidemic in the US." Although that is true, that problem will not be solved by their study. This lack of precision creates unnecessary inefficiency. See Figures 22.1 and 22.2.

FORMULATING THE HYPOTHESIS

PRINCIPLE 25 • Formulate your (null) hypothesis.

After you state the problem, the next step in the scientific method is to formulate the hypothesis, which is defined as "a tentative explanation that accounts for a set of facts and can be tested by further investigation."[1]

Many experienced researchers prefer to start with the null hypothesis (H_0), which is a clear, testable statement about chance occurrence that assumes no difference between groups or association between two variables. Typically, the assumption involves an association between risk factors and outcome or a difference in outcome between patients who receive one treatment versus another. For example:

1. Preoperative serum albumin level is not associated with the occurrence of postoperative complications.
2. The infection rate will not be significantly different between patients given drug A and patients given drug B.
3. The prevalence of delirium will not be different between patients randomized to drug A and patients randomized to drug B.
4. On the index admission, the red cell distribution width is not significantly different between patients who are readmitted to the hospital within 30 days and those who are not.

The alternative hypothesis (H_a) is the opposite of the null hypothesis. Your research team should jointly develop a primary null hypothesis before you begin to collect data. Scrutinize this hypothesis and the major goals of the study and lay down the criteria to reject the null hypothesis.

Some researchers feel uncomfortable including a null hypothesis in their paper. Reviewers and editors, however, need this specific description of what you are actually testing to evaluate your manuscript. If you do not include a null hypothesis in the statistical section of your Methods, be sure to make it crystal clear to the reader what your main hypothesis is—in plain English.

FOR MORE INFORMATION

Hulley et al. (2013) provide additional details about methodology.

DESIGNING THE STUDY

PRINCIPLE 26 • Research the strongest appropriate study design.

The third step in the scientific method is to design the study. Obviously, different medical research problems require different types of study designs. For the typical clinical study of treatment, however, first attempt to use what commonly is considered the ideal design (Table 3.1).

This ideal design is not always possible; for example, clinical evaluation of the course of a disease cannot be "triple-blinded." Still, to achieve your objectives, use the strongest appropriate study design (Table 3.1).

The study design needs a rigorous methodology. You can strengthen your study during the planning phase by addressing problems that cannot be corrected after the data are collected.

VITAL POINT

A common flaw at this stage of a research project is lack of originality in study design. Successful scientists are creative at designing stronger study designs that maximize the signal to noise ratio and minimize bias.

A good study goes beyond testing whether Treatment A is better than Treatment B by including a conceptual framework or a theoretical model. Reviewers will be looking for a story about the mechanism of action and intermediate efficacy, which requires measuring the variables that will tell that story.

TABLE 3.1 Ideal Clinical Research Study Design

✔ **An unbiased sample that is**
- Large enough to answer the research question
- Homogeneous for the topic or research question (Many interventions are only effective if they are focused on high-risk patients and therefore require risk stratification or predictive modeling as a first step.)
- Representative of a broad population
- Drawn from several different hospitals (multicenter)

✔ **An intervention that is**
- Randomized
- Placebo-controlled (Patients in the control group receive an inactive substance.)
- Evaluated in a dose-response method
- "Double-blinded" (Patients and investigators are unaware of which group is subject to which intervention.)

✔ **An unbiased and rigorous measure of outcome that is**
- Well defined
- Specific
- Objective
- Widely accepted as a measure of success
- Directly observed by an independent observer
- Based on long-term, quality-of-life variables (ideally from questionnaires answered by patients)
- Measured prospectively
- Recorded as part of a comprehensive database, along with all potentially confounding factors, and quantified or coded properly

Avoid weak before–after designs without a randomized control group. These are often fatally flawed by regression to the mean, which is the statistical phenomenon of extreme values moving closer to the average on a second measurement. See Principle 30.

STUDY DESIGN TERMINOLOGY

PRINCIPLE 27 • Master study design terminology.

Figure 3.1 shows that study design flaws are the most important type of general flaw to avoid. Figures 3.2 and 3.3 provide more specific information to help you anticipate the most common and serious problems. The first step in improving your odds of publication is understanding the different types of study designs and the related terminology. The following terms are often misunderstood:

+ Incidence
+ Prevalence
+ Exposure

<u>Incidence</u> is the number of new cases of a disease in a defined population over a specific period.

> *Example 3–3.*
> In 2016, the number of new cases of HIV infection in residents of New York City was X per 100,000.

<u>Prevalence</u> is the total number of cases of a disease existing in a given population at a specific time.

> *Example 3–4.*
> The number of cases of HIV infection on January 1, 2016, was Y per 100,000 residents of New York City.

Prevalence depends on the incidence and duration of the disease. For highly lethal diseases, mortality rate also must be considered.

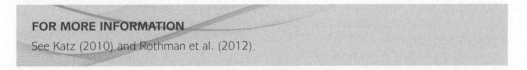

FOR MORE INFORMATION
See Katz (2010) and Rothman et al. (2012).

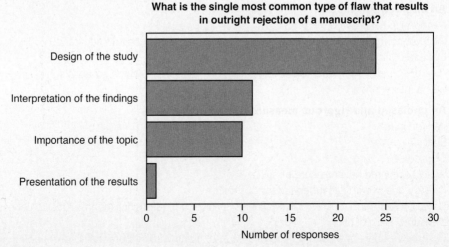

What is the single most common type of flaw that results in outright rejection of a manuscript?

FIGURE 3.1. The four major types of study flaws. From question 7 of the Peer Review Questionnaire (Appendix B). $P < .001$ based on a chi-square test.

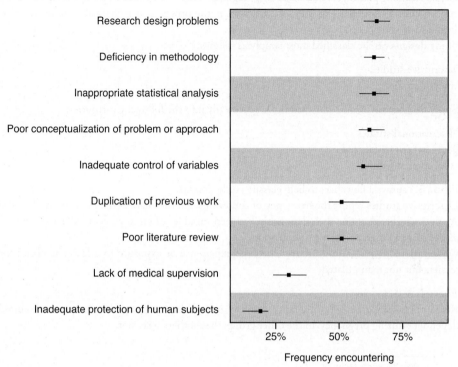

FIGURE 3.2. The frequency of specific study deficiencies. Answers are ranked by the median and bootstrap 95% confidence intervals using the sliding scale responses 0% (never) to 100% (always); from question 19 of the Peer Review Questionnaire (Appendix B). $P < .001$ based on the Friedman test.

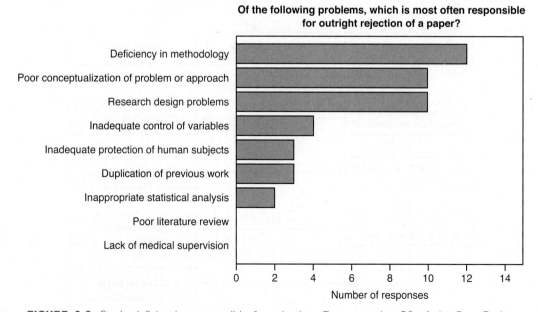

FIGURE 3.3. Study deficiencies responsible for rejection. From question 20 of the Peer Review Questionnaire (Appendix B). $P = .010$ based on a chi-square test.

<u>Exposure</u> describes whether a person was physically subjected to a suspected cause (an etiologic factor). For instance, among passengers of a cruise ship, exposure might be defined as those who used the ship's hot tub. In clinical research, exposure often describes the presence of a characteristic or preexisting condition, such as diabetes.

Study designs can be classified most simply as follows:

1. Descriptive studies
2. Analytic studies

Study designs can also be classified more specifically into the following categories:

1. Observational studies
2. Quasi-experimental studies
3. Experimental studies

Figure 3.4 shows a flowchart to help classify study designs.

Descriptive studies report the frequency of conditions and the characteristics of the study sample.

Analytic studies examine the relationship between variables often to detect risk factors and make inferences from a sample to a larger population.

<u>Observational studies</u> are those in which the experience or exposure to a factor is observed by researchers but not manipulated.

Example 3–5.
Researchers compare newborn infants from two groups. In one group, the mothers were opioid dependent during pregnancy. In the other group, the mothers were not.

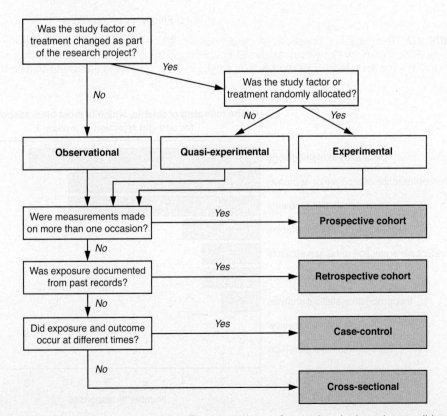

FIGURE 3.4. Flowchart of study designs. These questions refer to what the investigators did as part of this research project.

In <u>quasi-experimental studies</u>, a study factor or treatment is changed, but the change is not randomly allocated.

> *Example 3–6.*
> Researchers compare the outcome of infants born in two cities. In one city, a new law was enacted to test pregnant women for opioid use and enroll those who had positive test results in a treatment program. The other city had no such law or program.

In <u>experimental studies</u>, a study factor or treatment is actively changed by the investigators, and this change is randomly allocated. The investigators then measure the effect on an outcome. Experimental studies are stronger for proving causation.

> *Example 3–7.*
> Researchers compare newborn rats from two randomized groups. In one group, the researchers had given the pregnant rats opioids. The rats in the other group were not given opioids during pregnancy.

REPORTING GUIDELINES

An important part of improving your methodology is following the appropriate reporting guidelines for your study design. The guidelines are organized on the EQUATOR Network website.

EQUATOR - Enhancing the **QUA**lity and **T**ransparency **O**f health **R**esearch.

   http://www.equator-network.org

Randomized clinical trials (Table 3.2)	**CONSORT**	**CON**solidated Standards of Reporting Trials http://www.consort-statement.org/
Observational studies	**STROBE**	**ST**rengthening the Reporting of **OB**servational studies in Epidemiology http://www.strobe-statement.org
Systematic reviews	**PRISMA**	**P**referred **R**eporting **I**tems for **S**ystematic Reviews and **M**eta-**A**nalyses http://www.prisma-statement.org
Diagnostic accuracy studies	**STARD**	**STA**ndards for **R**eporting of **D**iagnostic accuracy http://www.stard-statement.org
Clinical trial protocols	**SPIRIT**	Standard Protocol Items: Recommendations for Interventional Trials http://www.spirit-statement.org/

PRINCIPLE 28 • Choose the optimal design for your study.

The major types of research studies (Fig. 3.5) are as follows:

   Treatment studies:
      Randomized controlled trial
      Nonrandomized trial (quasi-experimental)
   Observational studies:
      Case-control study
      Cohort study
      Prospective cohort study
      Retrospective cohort study, historical prospective study
      Cross-sectional study

TABLE 3.2		**CONSORT 2010 checklist of information to include when reporting a randomised trial***

Section/Topic	Item No	Checklist item	Reported on page No
Title and abstract			
	1a	Identification as a randomised trial in the title	_____
	1b	Structured summary of trial design, methods, results, and conclusions (for specific guidance see CONSORT for abstracts)	_____
Introduction			
Background and objectives	2a	Scientific background and explanation of rationale	_____
	2b	Specific objectives or hypotheses	_____
Methods			
Trial design	3a	Description of trial design (such as parallel, factorial) including allocation ratio	_____
	3b	Important changes to methods after trial commencement (such as eligibility criteria), with reasons	_____
Participants	4a	Eligibility criteria for participants	_____
	4b	Settings and locations where the data were collected	_____
Interventions	5	The interventions for each group with sufficient details to allow replication, including how and when they were actually administered	_____
Outcomes	6a	Completely defined pre-specified primary and secondary outcome measures, including how and when they were assessed	_____
	6b	Any changes to trial outcomes after the trial commenced, with reasons	_____
Sample size	7a	How sample size was determined	_____
	7b	When applicable, explanation of any interim analyses and stopping guidelines	_____
Randomisation:			
Sequence generation	8a	Method used to generate the random allocation sequence	_____
	8b	Type of randomisation; details of any restriction (such as blocking and block size)	_____
Allocation concealment mechanism	9	Mechanism used to implement the random allocation sequence (such as sequentially numbered containers), describing any steps taken to conceal the sequence until interventions were assigned	_____
Implementation	10	Who generated the random allocation sequence, who enrolled participants, and who assigned participants to interventions	_____

(continued)

TABLE 3.2		CONSORT 2010 checklist of information to include when reporting a randomised trial* *(continued)*

Section/Topic	Item No	Checklist item	Reported on page No
Blinding	11a	If done, who was blinded after assignment to interventions (for example, participants, care providers, those assessing outcomes) and how	_____
	11b	If relevant, description of the similarity of interventions	_____
Statistical methods	12a	Statistical methods used to compare groups for primary and secondary outcomes	_____
	12b	Methods for additional analyses, such as subgroup analyses and adjusted analyses	_____
Results			
Participant flow (a diagram is strongly recommended)	13a	For each group, the numbers of participants who were randomly assigned, received intended treatment, and were analysed for the primary outcome	_____
	13b	For each group, losses and exclusions after randomisation, together with reasons	_____
Recruitment	14a	Dates defining the periods of recruitment and follow-up	_____
	14b	Why the trial ended or was stopped	_____
Baseline data	15	A table showing baseline demographic and clinical characteristics for each group	_____
Numbers analysed	16	For each group, number of participants (denominator) included in each analysis and whether the analysis was by original assigned groups	_____
Outcomes and estimation	17a	For each primary and secondary outcome, results for each group, and the estimated effect size and its precision (such as 95% confidence interval)	_____
	17b	For binary outcomes, presentation of both absolute and relative effect sizes is recommended	_____
Ancillary analyses	18	Results of any other analyses performed, including subgroup analyses and adjusted analyses, distinguishing pre-specified from exploratory	_____
Harms	19	All important harms or unintended effects in each group (for specific guidance see CONSORT for harms)	_____

(continued)

Section/Topic	Item No	Checklist item	Reported on page No
Discussion			
Limitations	20	Trial limitations, addressing sources of potential bias, imprecision, and, if relevant, multiplicity of analyses	_____
Generalisability	21	Generalisability (external validity, applicability) of the trial findings	_____
Interpretation	22	Interpretation consistent with results, balancing benefits and harms, and considering other relevant evidence	_____
Other information			
Registration	23	Registration number and name of trial registry	_____
Protocol	24	Where the full trial protocol can be accessed, if available	_____
Funding	25	Sources of funding and other support (such as supply of drugs), role of funders	_____

TABLE 3.2 CONSORT 2010 checklist of information to include when reporting a randomised trial* *(continued)*

*We strongly recommend reading this statement in conjunction with the CONSORT 2010 Explanation and Elaboration for important clarifications on all the items. If relevant, we also recommend reading CONSORT extensions for cluster randomised trials, non-inferiority and equivalence trials, non-pharmacological treatments, herbal interventions, and pragmatic trials. Additional extensions are forthcoming: for those and for up to date references relevant to this checklist, see **www.consort-statement.org**.
From Schulz KF, Altman DG, Moher D. CONSORT 2010 Statement: updated guidelines for reporting parallel group randomised trials. *PLoS Med*. 2010;7(3):e1000251.

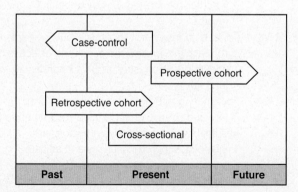

FIGURE 3.5. Study design and time. In case-control studies, outcome is determined in the present and subjects are asked to recall whether they were exposed in the past. In prospective cohort studies, exposure is measured in the present and outcome is recorded at some point in the future. Randomized controlled trials are a specific type of cohort study. For retrospective cohort (or historical prospective) studies, exposure is determined from past records and outcome is determined in the present. For cross-sectional studies, exposure and outcome are measured at the same time.

Case-control studies (also known as case-referent or retrospective studies) use two groups of subjects: those with and those without a disease. The history of these two groups is studied to determine whether differences between them could help explain why the disease developed in one group. The investigators then try to determine whether previous exposure or a particular attribute is responsible for the development of the disease.

In case-control studies, the study participants with the disease are obviously the cases, but choosing a control group is a challenging task. By definition, control subjects are members of the reference group: they do not have the disease but are drawn from a population similar to the group with the disease.

Example 3–8.
Food poisoning develops in one-third of the customers at a restaurant. Investigators question all of the customers about what they ate. The results are compared between the cases (with the food poisoning) and the controls (without the food poisoning).

Case-control studies can be completed in less time and for less money and ordinarily are more efficient than studies that follow patients over time. Case-control studies are useful for studying rare conditions and conditions with long intervals between exposure and outcome.

FOR MORE INFORMATION
See Chapter 7 of Hulley et al. (2013) and the books by Haynes et al. (2011) and Spilker (1991).

Cohort studies (also known as follow-up, prospective, or incidence studies) take measurements over time in a group of people, and they track new cases of a disease. Study subjects are classified by exposure status and are followed to determine whether the disease develops. Cohort studies are time-consuming, expensive, and often inadequate for rare conditions. They are effective for proving causation, measuring incidence, assessing the course of a condition, and studying conditions that cause sudden death.

Longitudinal studies are a type of cohort study in which subjects are followed over time to observe the natural course of a disease. These studies do not always use a control group. Although the term "prospective" is sometimes used to describe this type of study, this term can be confusing. "Prospective cohort study" is clear, but "prospective study" is too vague.

Randomized controlled trials (also called "intervention studies," "experimental studies," or "randomized clinical trials") are another form of cohort study and ordinarily are considered the strongest study design. They are considered the strongest because the prevalence of potential confounding factors, even those that the researchers are unaware of, should be similar in the control group and the treatment group. As a result of this randomization procedure, these two groups should, for example, have similar numbers of smokers. Therefore, randomization can often simplify the statistical analysis.

Randomized controlled trials are ideal for proving causation. Over the years, many ethical randomized controlled trials have been conducted that have contributed greatly to our understanding of medicine. Sometimes, however, the ideal randomized study is not ethical for research in humans. See Table 3.3 for a comparison of study designs.

Modern health care and the medical literature need more randomized controlled trials. There are too many weak, biased evaluations, with poor study designs that are polluting the medical literature and slowing the progress of improving health outcomes.

Retrospective cohort/historical prospective studies identify a group of people and then determine from past records whether they were exposed to a certain factor or had a particular attribute. Researchers determine whether, after that baseline point, the outcome of interest occurred.

TABLE 3.3	Comparison of Study Designs

Study Type	Advantages	Disadvantages
Experimental:		
Randomized controlled trial	Strong, unbiased cause–effect evidence	Can be expensive, not feasible for some questions
Randomized crossover	Efficient, eliminates between-patient variation issues, increases power	Not feasible for many questions, carryover effect issues
Pragmatic clinical trials	Determines benefit in routine clinical care and real-world settings	Can be challenging to overcome resistance of nonreseachers
Cluster randomized controlled trials	Solves problems of randomizing at patient level, real-world effectiveness	Increases needed sample size, increases complexity of analysis
Delayed-start designs/ stepped wedge design	Useful when a typical control group is unacceptable	Challenging to conduct and collect all of essential data, expensive
Nonexperimental/Observational:		
Prospective cohort	Exposure measured before outcome, good for assessing causation and incidence	Can be time-consuming, expensive
Retrospective cohort/ historical prospective/ historical cohort	Inexpensive, good for rare conditions	Potential for bias and confounding
Historical control trial/ before–after trial/ pre–post	Inexpensive, smaller sample size, useful when a permanent control group is unacceptable	New treatment often falsely appears to be superior due to bias and regression to the mean
Case-control study	Inexpensive, good for rare conditions	Potential for recall/selection bias
Cross-sectional study	Good for estimating prevalence quickly, inexpensive	Potential for bias, reverse causation, no temporality
Case series	Simple, inexpensive	Weak cause–effect evidence

Example 3–9.
A registry was created of trauma patients who were admitted to a hospital. After each patient was discharged or died, a research nurse reviewed the hospital chart. Baseline factors, recorded on admission to the hospital, were analyzed to determine whether they were predictive of complications that developed during the hospital stay. This investigation is a retrospective cohort study.

Cross-sectional studies provide a snapshot of the problem at a specific point in time. They also are called "prevalence studies" because only people with the specific disease or condition under study at the time of the snapshot are considered diseased. Cross-sectional studies make all measurements on a single occasion. A survey is an example of a cross-sectional study.

Example 3–10.
On a given day, researchers might measure the serum albumin and presence of pressure ulcers in 100 patients in a nursing home.

Obviously, a cross-sectional study is not a strong design for proving causation because they measure risk factors and disease concurrently; however, they are comparatively easy, fast, and economical.

Before you begin a cross-sectional study, plan how you will document whether exposure to the study factor preceded the effect or disease. Fixed characteristics, such as height, race, and sex, must be analyzed separately from variable characteristics, such as weight, marital status, and blood pressure, so be sure to word your questions appropriately.

Example 3–11.
People often stop exercising when a disease develops. In a cross-sectional study, this lack of exercise could be misinterpreted as a risk factor for the disease. This is reverse causation.

In summary, most studies can be classified by answering two questions:

1. Were the events under study (exposure or treatment) changed as a part of the study?
   If they were, the study was experimental. If they were not, the study was observational.
2. Were the measurements in this study made on more than one occasion?
   If not, the study was cross-sectional.
   If they were, the study was longitudinal.

After you answer these two questions and understand this basic terminology, you can move on to planning the finer points of the study design.

REFERENCES

1. *The American Heritage Dictionary of the English Language.* 5th ed. Boston, MA: Houghton Mifflin Harcourt; 2012.

Minimizing Bias

PRINCIPLE 29 • Plan to minimize but carefully measure bias.

Bias is a "systematic error introduced into sampling or testing by selecting or encouraging one outcome or answer over others."[1] All studies contain random errors that are determined by chance. When errors are not determined by chance alone and produce results that depart systematically from true values, bias exists. In science, bias cannot be ignored.

Bias reduces the representativeness of the sample studied. A biased sample is a common problem in study designs and often is responsible for the rejection of manuscripts. During the planning phase, be careful to develop a sophisticated protocol that minimizes bias.

> **VITAL POINT**
>
> An increase in the sample size will increase your precision but does not guarantee a decrease in bias. Selection bias and measurement bias, in particular, will not be solved with larger samples sizes. Increasing the sample size will only give you a more precise estimate of your biased measurement.

The three main types of bias are:

1. Selection bias
2. Response bias
3. Information/measurement bias

Selection bias is a systematic difference between people who are selected for a study and those who are not selected. This type of bias is both common and lethal to your chances of publication. Selection bias can be caused by patient referral patterns, survival differences, or loss to follow-up, which refers to participants who are unreachable resulting in incomplete ascertainment of outcomes.

To minimize selection bias in cohort studies, devise a strategy that will allow you to choose a random sample from a stable population and obtain an appropriate follow-up. A stable population is one in which you are able to obtain complete and accurate follow-up information on all or most members. To minimize selection bias, you should strive to identify a group of people who plan to live in the same area for a long period and who are willing and able to cooperate with follow-up investigators.

What is an adequate follow-up period? The answer depends on the topic, but if you can show a longer follow-up period than the landmark papers, you will certainly improve the odds of publication. Develop a plan to obtain follow-up information for the entire sample, or at least a large percentage.

To some extent, you can control for the effect of selection bias statistically if you have variables to measure the direction and effect. For example, you can record why patients were lost to follow-up and the exact cause of death. In other situations, you can document why people did not participate in the study. In general, however, it is better to invest in planning ways to minimize bias rather than trying to adjust for it statistically.

In clinical research studies, selection bias, particularly attrition bias, is a common problem. Attrition is a reduction in the number of patients who remain in a study. Attrition bias occurs when the patients who drop out of a study are systematically different from those who complete the study. Reviewers will study your CONSORT flowchart to look for signs of attrition bias.

Berkson's bias is a clinical selection bias that occurs when the rate of hospitalization differs between the cases and the controls. Patients with two overlapping conditions often are more likely to be admitted to the hospital. Researchers then may make the mistake of assuming an association between the two conditions if they analyze only the patients who are admitted to the hospital. Also, when one creates a control group from hospitalized patients, Berkson's bias can create problems with interpretation; for example, the control group will most likely have a higher percentage smoking than the population.

Prevalence-incidence (Neyman's) bias is caused by risk factors that prolong the disease rather than cause it. For example, suppose that marathon runners are more likely to survive an acute myocardial infarction (AMI). Analysis of AMI survivors might appear to show that marathon training is higher than in a control group, and researchers might conclude that it causes AMI—but this is simply a bias.

Response bias is a specific type of selection bias in which respondents (e.g., people who answer your survey) differ systematically from nonrespondents.

Example 4–1.
People with a certain disease may be more likely to respond to a questionnaire about the disease than people who are unaffected by the disease. One solution to this problem is to offer incentives for those who respond. Consult with an experienced survey methodologist to learn techniques for increasing the response rate and minimizing bias.

Example 4–2.
Participants in a weight loss program who are losing weight are more likely to return for follow-up visits. Those who gain weight or fail to lose weight are much more likely to drop out. The study design needs to anticipate and minimize the impact of this; for example, a strong financial incentive for a final private assessment.

Information/measurement bias is a systematic difference between the measurements recorded in different study groups. In cohort studies, patients with a risk factor may be tested for the outcome more frequently and carefully than those without the risk factor. This situation is a special type of information bias called "surveillance" bias or "diagnostic suspicion" bias.

Recall bias, another type of information bias, occurs when people with a certain condition are more likely to "remember" exposure to the variable under study than people without the condition.

Example 4–3.
Parents of children with cancer may "remember" more information and provide greater detail about exposure to potentially carcinogenic factors than parents of children without cancer, even if both groups had identical exposure levels.

This situation can easily occur in case-control or cross-sectional studies, but not in cohort studies. In cohort studies, it is very unlikely that anyone involved knows in which people the disease will develop in the future. Therefore, it is highly unlikely that these people can report a different level of exposure.

Example 4–4.
A group of patients hospitalized for a heart attack are asked, "Did you eat bacon for breakfast on the morning of your heart attack?" The control group is asked, "Did you eat bacon for breakfast last Tuesday?"

Other forms of bias include the following:

Confounding bias is the effect of extraneous variables that must be adjusted for before the research question can be answered. Confounding variables are the variables that may account for the association between exposure and disease. Sometimes they mask the true association.

Example 4–5.
A hospital that serves a disadvantaged population may have a higher neonatal mortality rate than the national average. Although the difference between these crude (unadjusted) mortality rates may be statistically significant, interpreting this difference as an indication of poor obstetrical care probably would be incorrect. The confounding variables associated with the population probably create a bias. These factors must be adjusted for before valid conclusions can be drawn.

Table 4.1 shows additional forms of bias reported by reviewers and editors. Table 4.2 provides a summary of the most common forms of bias.

Failure to recognize and control for these and other forms of bias is a classic mistake that researchers make when analyzing medical research data.

Bias is a complex subject, but the main points to remember are as follows: Plan to reduce bias to a minimum. Measure the effect of bias so you can adjust for it statistically in your analysis. During the planning phase, you can strengthen your study design by researching the specific types of bias and epidemiologic methods important for your particular study design and topic. Learn from previous researchers, and customize your study design to reduce bias. In your paper, document your efforts to minimize and understand the effect of bias (Table 4.3).

VITAL POINT

Minimizing bias and improving study design are much more important than using complex statistical methods to fix problems.

Sensitivity analyses can be used to cope with bias by showing the effect of varying assumptions (Greenland, 1996).

TABLE 4.1	Bias Reported by Reviewers and Editors

Sampling bias
Ascertainment bias (a measurement problem that can often be avoided by "blinding" the outcome measurement)
Data collection bias
Publication bias toward 'positive' results (Studies with 'positive' results are more likely to be published, leading to problems with meta-analysis interpretation; many researchers are reluctant to pursue and publish 'negative' results.)
Reviewer bias (against an unknown author from a "minor" institution)
Self-promotion or agency promotion bias
Uncontrolled variables bias

TABLE 4.2	Forms of Bias in the Medical Literature

Type of bias	Systematic error caused by:
Selection bias	Selection of nonrepresentative research participants with respect to exposure or outcome
Response bias	Response data that differ from the truth in the entire study population due to some failing to provide data
Publication bias	Editorial preference for publishing particular academic findings, for example, positive results
Recall bias	Recollections retrieved inaccurately or incompletely
Observer bias	Researchers influenced responses of or recording of data
Nonresponse bias	Nonresponders, for example in a survey, differing from responders
Cognitive bias	Holding onto one's beliefs, which obstructs recording the truth
Attentional bias	Recurring thoughts, which block accurate data recording
Information/measurement bias	Misreporting or misclassifying of exposure or outcomes
Time lag bias	Publication speed that depends on findings (positive vs. negative)
Detection bias	Diagnostic or outcome differences creating artifacts
Attrition bias	Differences in loss to follow-up and missing outcome data
Interviewer bias	Social nature of the interviews distorting responses
Lead time bias	Earlier detection of disease distorts outcomes findings
Length bias	Identifying cases before onset of symptoms
Learning bias	Changes associated with gained experience
Temporal bias	Outcomes occur before exposure—reverse causality
Surveillance bias	Increased attention for those with known exposure
Immortal time bias	Inclusion criteria require surviving a specified period
Channeling bias	Therapies prescribed to patients based on prognosis
Berkson's bias/admission rate bias/Hospital admission bias	Hospitalized patients differing in some exposure
Screening bias	Healthier people volunteering for screening and therefore screening appears to have greater benefit
Diagnostic suspicion bias	Knowledge of exposure increases search/detection of disease
Exposure suspicion bias	Knowledge of outcome increases search/detection of exposure (in case-control studies)
Acquisition bias	Differences in publications not obtained in a meta-analysis
Affirmation bias	Seeking data to support preconceived notions
Confirmation bias	Searching/interpreting information in a way that confirms one's preconceptions, tilting the analysis toward preconceived ideas
Loss to follow-up bias	Differences in health responses between lost and retained research subjects; assumption of noninformative censoring is violated
Incidence-prevalence bias	Differences in survivors (e.g., with mild forms of a disease); also called Neyman's bias
Sampling frame bias	Differences in the sample compared with population
Bias toward the null/attenuation	Nondifferential error in exposure measurement that reduces the effect of exposure on outcomes; odds ratios move closer to 1.0
Ascertainment bias	Type of patient included
Accidental bias	A randomization that did not produce balanced groups; nuisance factors affect experimental units

TABLE 4.3	Editors and Reviewers Report Lessons Learned about Writing and Publishing[a]

- Keep it simple! Reduce the text in the Introduction, Results, and Discussion but do not scrimp on details in the Materials and Methods section.
- (a) Don't try to solve world hunger in one study. (b) Be focused and clear about a single, specific, answerable question with a simple methodologic approach. (c) Work hard to keep the writing simple, short, and clear. (d) Don't make more out of the results than they deserve. (e) Be a ruthless editor or find one. (f) Learn how to take apart clinical studies and manuscripts so you know how to write yours.
- It is important to write clearly, concisely, and avoid excessive jargon. It is critical to acknowledge and cite the work of others and to frame the discussion in a way that moves the field forward and shows why the current work is important.
- Structure. Write an outline before writing the paper. So-called originality is highly overrated and often impedes a field's progress.
- Summarize the methods succinctly but with sufficient detail so that the reader understands clearly how the research question is being answered. Summarize data with a balance of narrative and figures/tables—with more emphasis on figures than tabular data. Make the discussion lucid, brief, but inclusive of the pertinent literature and limitations of the study.
- It is critical for researchers to carefully share their methodology in order for others to understand their approach and be able to replicate the work if indicated.
- Framing the question at hand; understanding the population being studied; proper methodology; managing intellectual bias
- Be consistent with the methods used, results obtained. Be consistent in the different part of your manuscript.
- The clear presentation of the data as expected by the social group/audience for whom you write is critical. Clear, careful writing demonstrates clear, careful thought and is key.
- A rigorous, almost formulaic approach to write the paper
- The writer has to answer the question of why would anyone want to read his or her article. In other words, the writer has to answer the "So what?" question satisfactorily. The next most important thing that I learned independently is if you want to become a good writer, read a lot of high quality articles. I have learned the most by following the example of more senior researchers whose work I respect.
- The importance of well thought out rationale for the study
- If you do not have a lot of methodologic and statistical training, make sure you are working with someone who does.
- Construct a rational, meaningful narrative that guides the reader through the research questions in the context of past findings and current pressing unanswered questions. Describe methods in as much detail as possible. As complicated as the findings may be, present them in as straightforward a manner as possible. Stay focused! Write as if your father (or mother) is the primary reader.
- How to write clearly
- First say what you want to do, then do what you said.
- Be clear, comprehensive, do not try to hide your design's flaws/limitations and explain how you have accommodated them. Acknowledge the main findings in the field (internationally) and explain how your study is different/moves the field forward. Try to explain your results with reference to existing research but do not overreach—acknowledge when you don't know why you have found what you have found.

(continued)

TABLE 4.3	Editors and Reviewers Report Lessons Learned about Writing and Publishing[a] *(continued)*

- Need to articulate the objective/hypothesis to be tested with the data available clearly and succinctly, need to get critiques from colleagues, need to rewrite multiple times, need to read the literature, need to include collaborators who are subject matter experts
- Clarity with brevity. Don't extend data findings or overgeneralize. Follow the data.
- A good paper starts with a well-conceived research design and solid execution. A poor experimental design cannot lead to a good manuscript.
- Writing a paper is akin to telling a story: It has a beginning, a middle, and an end. Lead the reader through the story in a logical manner giving enough detail that readers who are not experts in the topic can understand. And most important, let the data speak for themselves: If the data are strong and convincing, there is no need to overinterpret; the reader will see the implications of the work without the author overselling the message.
- Taking consideration of reviewer comments is critical—don't be defensive in response. If reviewer didn't understand something or misread it, it was probably not well written. Share your drafts with colleagues early—the more feedback you get, the better. Almost all research is publishable these days—finish those papers that are 95% completed and resubmit those papers which have been rejected.
- Almost any reasonable manuscript can find a journal. A careful and measured presentation of one's own data garners respect from reviewers and editors. Be sure to appropriately frame your question/problem for the readership of the journal you are submitting to. Looking at what journals you're citing is a good guide for selecting a journal to submit to. From the reader's perspective, the quality of the writing is a sign of the quality of research being presented. Anything less than an outright rejection is a positive result from peer review.
- How to demonstrate the importance of a topic
- Proper grammar, what information to put in each section of the manuscript
- Get the stats and methods people to provide help before doing the study rather than afterwards. Develop a team of collaborators.
- How to design a clinical trial to give meaningful results
- The importance of detailed methodology and statistical consideration. To stick with the important results and avoid excessive information that takes away from the important results that are to be highlighted.
- Start with a power analysis. Make sure your statistical analyses are determined ahead of time. Always replicate before publishing.
- Brevity, clear writing, avoidance of jargon, appealing tables and figures, compelling research question, careful interpretation, collaboration with a statistician
- Parsimony and multiple rewrites before submission
- (a) Proper background review of literature; (b) appropriate experimental design including the n, the length of follow-up, and appropriate controls; (c) reasonable appreciation of the importance of the results
- Use a few important primary sources as opposed to multiple ho-hum sources. Write in clear, specific language and use active voice. Have a biostatistician involved at the outset.
- How to be more effective in writing a persuasive paper
- Focused, clear, simple, meaningful for the field
  - (a) How to recognize the nature of chance and recognize and accept the consequences of chance; (b) how to recognize and accept the limits of one's certainty—conversely,

(continued)

TABLE 4.3	Editors and Reviewers Report Lessons Learned about Writing and Publishing[a] (continued)

the magnitude of the uncertainty; (c) emphasis on implications of causality from study designs that cannot prove causality; (d) importance of a priori declaration of primary endpoint(s) and analytical design and whether the data support or don't support conclusions about the endpoint(s). In this context, the importance of registering every study, including observational ones.
- How to write a good abstract that reflects the key content of the research paper
- Be clear, be concise, and be incisive.

[a]Based on question 14 in the Peer Review Questionnaire (Appendix B).

FOR MORE INFORMATION

The *Encyclopedia of Biostatistics* is an excellent source for more information about bias. Also, see Fleiss (1980); Fletcher et al. (2012); Friedman (2003); Friedman et al. (2015); Haynes et al. (2011); Hulley et al. (2013); Last (2000); Mausner and Kramer (1985); Morton et al. (2001); Rothman et al. (2012); Sackett (1979).

MINIMIZE THE AMOUNT OF MISSING DATA

One of the most important ways to minimize bias is to limit the amount of missing data. Careful planning, attention to detail, and early data audits are all useful techniques. For more information, see the articles by Little et al. (2012) and Ware et al. (2012) and Chapter 13.

PRINCIPLE 30 • Avoid being fooled by regression to the mean.

Regression to the mean is a statistical phenomenon in which extremely large or small values are followed by a second measurement that is closer to the average. To be successful at publishing medical research papers, you must truly understand regression to the mean (or regression toward the mean) and design studies that separate this effect from the intervention's effect. Whenever one selects extreme values in a variable that fluctuates (or has error), there is a strong tendency for the next measurement of that variable to be closer to the average. For example, if we take a group of patients and select the 10% subset with the highest systolic blood pressure ($\geq$180 mmHg) and then measure their blood pressure 1 hour later, with no intervention in between, we will find a significant drop in pressure. In a study in which 77 patients met this criterion, the pressure dropped from 193.8 to 173.3 mmHg, $P < .001$. This change of 20.5 mmHg is both clinically and statistically significant. Likewise, if we select the 10% of patients with the lowest initial pressures ($\leq$110 mmHg), we find that the blood pressure increases from 105.4 to 127.7 mmHg, $P < .001$ (Fig. 4.1). Researchers often confuse regression to the mean with the effect of their intervention. Without a randomized parallel control group, these are almost impossible to distinguish. Science needs more reliability research, for example, studies of changes that happen with a placebo, to show the strong impact of regression to the mean.

Regression to the mean is a natural and predictable change that was discovered by Galton in 1877 and yet many people in our modern health care system are unaware of this phenomenon and take

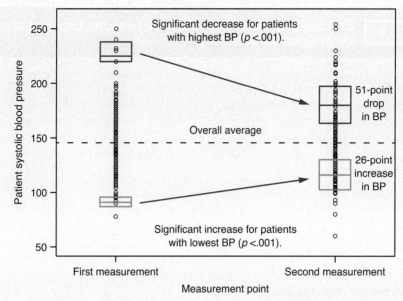

FIGURE 4.1. Regression to the mean. This graph illustrates the statistical phenomenon of regression to the mean in which extremely high or low values will move closer to the average on a second reading. This effect will happen without any intervention. Note that these changes are both statistically and clinically significant. P values based on the Wilcoxon signed-rank test. BP, blood pressure.

personal credit for it. Hospital administrators must also be aware of this and not reward those who have not actually improved patient outcomes but are simply advancing their career via regression to the mean.

FOR MORE INFORMATION

See Barnett et al. (2005); Friedman et al. (2015); James (1973); and Kahneman (2013).

REFERENCES

1. *Merriam-Webster's Collegiate Dictionary.* 11th ed. Springfield, MA: Merriam-Webster; 2008.

5

The Data Collection/Case Report Form

DESIGNING THE FORM

PRINCIPLE 31 • Design a comprehensive data collection form.

A common mistake that many researchers make is not investing enough time in creating a quality data collection form or case report form (CRF). Whether this form is a questionnaire for patients or a chart abstracting form for a research nurse, devoting ample resources to its creation enables one to avoid common mistakes and costly problems. The following principles related to questionnaires also can be used to improve most data collection forms.

Start with your most important questions and focus on solving your principal research problem. Then decide how many variables you can include. Short questionnaires may have higher response rates than long ones, but a questionnaire that is too short may not solve the research problem at all. Always number each question. Use questions with defined choices rather than open-ended questions except in the rare cases where you need this unstructured free text input. For example, in quality improvement projects, it is often useful to have a question of this form: "Please suggest three ways that the quality of this service could have been improved from your perspective." Also, use branching logic to collect additional free text detail when items are rated poorly or problems are identified. The additional text box will only open if a question is answered in a particular way.

As you design the data collection form, write a coding guide (data dictionary) to explain how to use the form. For example, explain how many decimal places to use, what units to use, and whether measurements should be recorded in metric units or the US equivalent.

Ensure that the choices for each question cover all possibilities. Include questions to verify inclusion and exclusion criteria. Line up the choices vertically and include the code with each choice on the data collection form to simplify data entry (0 = No, 1 = Yes). When you convert the CRF into a database, use variable names that are in the form of questions, for example, "died" rather than "outcomes" and "male_gender" rather than simply "gender." In this way, there will not be any confusion that 1 = died and 0 = survived and 1 = male and 0 = female. The 0–1 coding with 1 representing the higher risk group (e.g., smokers, males) makes it easier to interpret the statistical output associated with odds ratios. Note: Coding females as zero is not sexist; in fact, it is caused by the fact that women have better outcome in almost all medical research studies. Therefore, to have logical odds ratios, males need to be coded as 1.

Ask an experienced methodologist to critique your questionnaire before you administer it. A methodologist can identify and solve problems you may not notice, such as questions that will result in unanalyzable data.

FOR MORE INFORMATION

Spilker and Schoenfelder (1991) provide several hundred examples in their book *Data Collection Forms in Clinical Trials*.

PRINCIPLE 32 • Understand how your sample differs from the larger population.

Decide how you will compare respondents with nonrespondents, especially for surveys and mailed questionnaires. You may have basic information from a mailing list about the population, such as age and sex. Or, you may be able to compare your respondents with a published report.

A different approach is to compare early respondents with late respondents. Nonrespondents tend to be similar to late respondents (Babbie, 2015). To make this comparison, you must record the date sent and date received for each survey. The information that you obtain from this comparison will allow you to assess the direction and strength of response bias.

PRINCIPLE 33 • Conduct a thorough pilot test of your questionnaire to assess clarity and ease of use.

Use a pilot test on an available small group similar to your sample to determine whether the wording of the directions or specific questions is confusing. Use a system of logical choices that makes sense to your sample.

Including too many questions or too many of a certain type, such as open-ended questions, is an obvious problem. For the most part, omit repetitive questions, although to assess the consistency of a respondent's answers, some researchers repeat one or more questions, usually strategically separated from each other.

Delete or revise questions that most respondents in your pilot test misunderstood. Make abstract questions concrete by including straightforward, neutral examples respondents can evaluate. During the pilot test, determine whether the respondents thought that some questions were asked merely for effect, with no answer expected. Delete these rhetorical questions; respondents will be annoyed that you wasted their time with these. Do not ask questions that lead the respondent toward a particular choice. If, in the pilot test, most people circled one choice, such as "occasionally," convert to more specific choices in the final version (e.g., "once a day," "once a week," "once a month").

From a statistical point of view, you ordinarily would want to collect data on a continuous scale. An outcome expressed as a continuous variable is often superior to outcome expressed categorically and requires a smaller sample size.

Including "dummy" questions can reduce various forms of bias but only if respondents are unaware of the main risk factor or outcome you are testing. For example, if you are conducting a survey about alcohol use, you also can include questions about smoking, exercising, and eating habits.

Before you administer your questionnaire, try to solve the potentially devastating problems of respondents selecting more than one answer or not answering a question at all. Develop clear guidelines for defining invalid questionnaires that will be excluded from the analysis. For example, you might prespecify that at least 80% of the questions must be answered for a questionnaire to be considered valid.

If you spend adequate time creating, testing, and revising your questionnaire, your paper will have a much better chance of being published. Many investigators do not allow enough time or resources to develop a quality questionnaire. Always consult a colleague who has successfully designed questionnaires or better yet, make this person part of your research team.

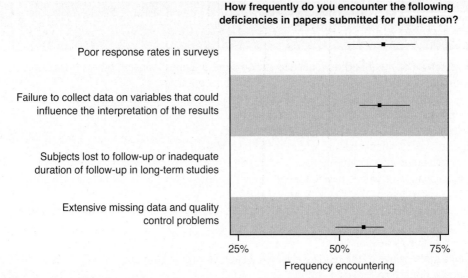

FIGURE 5.1. Frequency of problems with data quality. From question 25 of the Peer Review Questionnaire (Appendix B). $P = .026$ based on the Friedman test.

FOR MORE INFORMATION

See Appendices B and C for examples with solutions to many of these data collection form problems.

PRINCIPLE 34 • Improve your response rate.

The success of a study that is based on a mailed or e-mailed questionnaire often depends on obtaining a satisfactory response rate (Figs. 5.1 and 5.2). To improve your response rate for mailed questionnaires, consider the ideas shown in Tables 5.1 and 5.2.

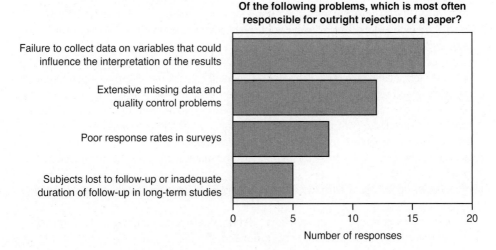

FIGURE 5.2. Data quality problems that result in rejection. From question 26 of the Peer Review Questionnaire (Appendix B). $P = .082$ based on a chi-square test.

TABLE 5.1	Elements to Include in the Invitation/Cover Letter of a Questionnaire

An estimate of the (brief) time needed to complete the questionnaire; time a few people completing the survey to make this as accurate as possible

The respondent's name in the salutation. Use the "Piping" feature in the survey invitation. For example, in REDCap use "Dear Dr. [last_name]"[a]

Relevance of the topic to the respondent

Answers to questions that arose during the pilot testing

An explanation of your intentions

An explanation of who is paying for the study (University sponsorship is better than corporate sponsorship; Fox, Crask, & Kim, 1988.)

An incentive for responding (A report of the findings may be a better incentive than a small sum.)

The deadline for responding

Language sensitive to the reading level and health literacy of your audience

A postscript asking for cooperation

[a]https://redcap.vanderbilt.edu/redcap_v6.11.1/DataEntry/piping_explanation.php

TABLE 5.2	Suggestions for Improving the Response Rate

Design your survey in a way so the rewards to the participant outweigh the cost of completing. There is an immediate tipping point at which people will decide to participate.

Make the participant feel important in an authentic way and explain that you need their expert input.

Explain that something important will be done with the results.

Pilot test your questionnaire to identify deal-breakers for participating and areas of misunderstanding.

For lengthy questionnaires or those on a sensitive topic, send a prenotification e-mail (or postcard/letter) explaining that a questionnaire will arrive soon (Fox et al., 1988). People are much more likely to respond if they know you, even if it is just from this prenotification.

Find a special third party contact, ideally someone respected by the respondents (e.g., a union leader, society president). This contact person can ask the group for cooperation in completing and returning the surveys. A manager or supervisor may not be the ideal contact person and may have a negative effect by creating a bias; you do not want subjects to feel pressured into completing the questionnaire. An article in a newsletter from an organization to which the respondents belong also may be helpful.

Allow the respondents to express their concerns and make suggestions with large open text fields.

Send a follow-up survey in 1 to 2 weeks; you can often double your response rate with a second invitation.

Three to four weeks after your initial mailing, send a thank you to those who have replied and a reminder to those who have not responded.

(continued)

TABLE 5.2	Suggestions for Improving the Response Rate *(continued)*

For those who say that they do not wish to respond, be sure to delete their names from the future reminders otherwise this can be viewed as harassment.

For printed questionnaires, print on green paper. Research suggests that questionnaires printed on green paper have a higher response rate (Fox et al., 1988). Any color that stands out from the white paper on most desks probably will improve the response rate. Avoid colors that make the survey difficult to read or appear unprofessional.

Consult early with an experienced survey methodologist.

Master the various skills required for creating a REDCap survey and sending invitations for participants long before your deadline. One option is the Coursera course "Data Management for Clinical Research."[a]

[a]https://www.coursera.org/course/datamanagement

FOR MORE INFORMATION

See the American Marketing Association's book, *Handbook for Customer Satisfaction* (NTC Business Books), or Chapter 5 of Hulley et al. (2013) for more details about questionnaire design. If you are planning to use an existing questionnaire, consult with an experienced survey methodologist and someone who has published papers using that questionnaire.

Mailing and e-mailing your questionnaires are not the only options. For example, you can administer them during mandatory training sessions. If you use this approach, ensure confidentiality and recruit someone whom the respondents trust to ask for their cooperation. Consultation with a community advisory committee can also provide valuable insights to increase the response rate.

PRINCIPLE 35 • Test for reliability and validity.

While reliability and validity of your measurements are always important in clinical research, they are essential in questionnaire research.

Reliability assesses consistency of measurement. Reliability is the degree to which an investigator can depend on a measurement instrument. When reliability is high, a test that is repeated on the same patient and under the same conditions will yield the same result. For reproducible research, medical researchers need to be performing much more research on reliability. Often, you can add a reliability component to your research project and describe it in your paper—or in a separate paper. This can raise the level of science and help future researchers.

Example 5–1.
A low-reliability variable is self-reported duration of exposure to passive smoke among women who are breastfeeding their infants. A high-reliability variable is a biomarker for exposure to tobacco smoke, such as the cotinine (a metabolite of nicotine) concentration in the mothers' breast milk.

Interrater reliability measures how well different data collectors obtain the same information. In studies that have more than one person abstracting information from hospital charts, reporting your interrater reliability is important to the credibility of your conclusions.

Intrarater reliability measures how well a person records the same information a second time. This factor is evaluated with the kappa (for nominal variables), weighted kappa (for ordinal variables), and the Bland–Altman method (for continuous variables). Consult an experienced biostatistician if you are not familiar with these methods.

When you evaluate studies performed by others, do not simply accept a statement that reliability testing was done. Look carefully to determine whether the fundamental variables were tested for reliability. A good study provides sufficient information to permit evaluation of its reliability. Inexperienced researchers sometimes have trouble assessing the reliability of their own research and critically evaluating reliability in published reports.

Validity is an index of how well a test or procedure measured what it is intended to measure.

Example 5–2.
Malnutrition could be assessed by asking patients to score their nutritional intake on a scale of 1 to 10, but measuring each patient's serum albumin level would have more validity.

During the planning phase, consider whether your questionnaire or data collection form is valid in comparison with other measures previously tested and published. When you write your paper, you may have to include the questions, or at least a sample of your wording, in your manuscript. Consider including your entire questionnaire or data collection form as an appendix in your paper. You may also have to explain why you chose to use a new instrument rather than an existing instrument.

Internal validity refers to how accurately your conclusions described what actually occurred in the study. Self-reported cholesterol levels may have internal validity problems because many people confuse the high density lipoprotein cholesterol (HDL-C), low density lipoprotein cholesterol (LDL-C), and total cholesterol values.

External validity is the generalizability of your study or the appropriateness of your conclusions to larger populations represented by your sample. A generalization is a broadly applicable statement, law, or principle derived from specifics.

Example 5–3.
A database of trauma patients pooled from major trauma centers around the country may be weighted toward disadvantaged inner city patients. In a study that uses this database, conclusions about priorities for injury prevention may not be valid for suburban or rural populations. This study has a problem with external validity.

AGREEMENT

When assessing agreement for a continuous measure between a gold standard and a new device, researchers often use a Pearson correlation. This is the incorrect approach. Suppose investigators develop a watch that can report serum glucose levels, and they wish to show agreement with a hospital lab. If the watch reported glucose levels that were exactly half of the lab's values, the Pearson correlation would show perfect correlation ($r = 1.0$, $P < .001$). Obviously, this is poor agreement. The correct method is a Bland–Altman plot of the average of the two devices on the x-axis and the difference between the two devices on the y-axis. See Bland and Altman (1986).

6

Reproducible Eligibility Criteria

PRINCIPLE 36 • Define your inclusion and exclusion criteria meticulously.

In some studies, the goal is to learn about a treatment or condition in a broad and representative population. In other studies, you must select a group of patients that is as homogeneous as possible to answer your research question. In these studies, your research conclusions will be stronger if you study a group of patients with one diagnosis or with unilateral, simple, or isolated injuries. Do not make the common mistake of including a mixture of diseases or procedures. Do not add dissimilar types of subjects simply to increase the sample size. Do not increase the sample size if it will increase the variability or noise. Adding noise decreases the statistical power of a study. Your goal is to increase the signal to noise ratio, that is, increase the size of the difference in the primary end point between the intervention and control group compared with the background variability (often the standard deviation).

Improper selection of patients reduces validity. To avoid this problem, define your inclusion criteria early in the planning phase. With the help of your colleagues, refine your definition until it is impossible to misunderstand. Ask yourself: "Could my colleagues obtain a similar sample by following my written instructions?" When the answer is "yes," you have completed an important part of the methods for reproducible research. Formalizing this definition of inclusion will prevent many problems during the study.

Many interventions are only effective when they are focused on patients at highest risk. For example, Hansen et al. (2011) showed that none of the interventions tested to reduce hospital readmissions were effective unless they were focused on the patients at highest risk of readmission. When the inclusion criteria are limited to just patients at highest risk of hospital readmission, then it is possible to apply interventions that are effective. When hospitals try to apply these interventions to all patients, even those at low risk for readmission, the interventions are inconsistently applied and the readmission rates are not decreased. The challenge to identifying the high-risk patients is solved by building a predictive model of hospital readmission into the electronic health record that computes the probability of readmission based on existing data. This probability is then updated each day based on the most recent data.

Much of the medical literature is confusing with flip-flopping messages about which interventions improve outcomes. Failing to use real-time predictive models to compute probability of the outcome and then focus interventions on those with the highest risk contributes to this confusion. Using a high-risk homogeneous group for a study enriches the sample and reduces the required sample size.

PRINCIPLE 37 • Be careful if you use a "mixed" sample.

Inclusion and exclusion decisions should be made by the entire research team and only after careful consideration of the statistical and clinical implications. Careless exclusion decisions can quickly destroy a study. For studies with many criteria, consider creating a table of inclusion and exclusion criteria. For a good example, see Ewigman et al. (1993). If you included conditions that may raise eyebrows, plan to describe them in the Methods and Results sections.

VITAL POINT

Including different conditions and disease states in the same study requires careful consideration regarding what conclusions can be drawn.

Some studies must include patients with different severities of a disease or complexities of a procedure. For this type of study, be prepared to explain your rationale. Specifically, clarify why patients with less severe conditions should be included in the study. Describe the distribution of the disease severity and explain why you are studying patients across this distribution. Plan a method to show that you have statistically adjusted for differences among these patients. In small clinical studies, a dilemma occurs when the number of subjects with a specific poor outcome is too small to permit reasonable statistical analysis. Trying to solve this problem by combining different types of poor outcome leads to the following types of reviewer criticism:

"Lumping many adverse outcomes under one end point obscures the true relation between the tests and the individual end points. Apparently, the authors found this necessary because of the relatively small number of cases."

"Creating a single group ('adverse outcome') from multiple types of adverse outcomes is concerning. These outcomes are unlikely to have a single common source."

Remember, be careful when your dependent (outcome) variable includes several diverse conditions. If combining many adverse outcomes into one category is necessary, anticipate criticism. Include only those that are potentially predictable by the independent variables in the study. Provide data, justification, and references for each type of outcome. Explain your rationale for including each different outcome in the dependent variable. Provide results for both the individual types of adverse outcomes and the combined group. In your final draft, describe, discuss, and compare with the literature both ways of looking at this problem (combined and separated). For more information, see Friedman et al. (2015).

When there are several ways to analyze your results, you can run these and show reviewers that your conclusions are valid in these various ways as a form of sensitivity analyses. For example, you might show the results with various components excluded from the composite end point.

Finally, composite end points require caution with screening studies. When you evaluate screening tests, your analysis will be more convincing if it is limited to one specific outcome, especially one that is biologically plausible to predict from such a screening test (Haynes et al., 2011).

PRINCIPLE 38 • Use a reproducible method to define your study subjects.

After you define your sample, the next step is to verify that your criteria are not subjective. When you define the inclusion and exclusion criteria for the final analysis, use a method that is clearly objective. Verify that this definition is consistent throughout the manuscript.

For the definition of a disease, the International Classification of Diseases (ICD) codes are a good place to start. Verify that the codes include and exclude precisely what you intended. For the definition of a procedure, Current Procedural Terminology (CPT) codes provide more detail.

All diagnoses and procedures must be encoded for optimal analyses. In question 45 of the data collection form in Appendix C, notice how multiple diagnoses are recorded with ICD codes. In the analysis phase, an unlimited number of variables can be created by defining ranges of codes.

Example 6–1.
By recording diagnoses with ICD codes, you can create a new variable called "hip_fx" for hip fractures by instructing the computer to search for the ICD-9 codes from 820.00 through 820.99 in the diagnosis fields (diagnosis_1_code, diagnosis_2_code, etc.). A broader variable for all

fractures can then be computed with the ICD-9 codes from 800.00 to 829.99. In the ICD-10 system, hip fractures are coded as S72.0 to S72.2. In the Methods, you would write this as "the inclusion criteria were patients with a hip fracture as a primary diagnosis according to ICD-10 codes S72.0, S72.1, and S72.2." You also can create a checklist for major groups of diagnoses. Checklists are useful when the ICD coding system does not provide enough detail for your project.

The following website provides an online converter from ICD-9 to ICD-10:

http://www.icd10data.com/Convert

7

Randomization, Blinding, and Confidentiality

> *"Randomize the first patient."*
> —Tom Chalmers

RANDOMIZATION AND BLINDING

PRINCIPLE 39 • Use randomization and blinding to strengthen the study design and minimize bias.

Whenever it is ethical and practical, consider using a randomized design. With random allocation, chance determines the assignment of subjects to study groups. To randomize subjects, most researchers use random number tables, which can be customized for your study with software such as R (https://www.r-project.org). If you use a randomized design, follow all of the principles of rigorous randomization and document your work (see the CONSORT checklist—Table 3.2, items 8 to 10; also see Friedman et al., 2015).

The study design in which patients are randomly assigned to either receive or not receive the intervention under study is called a "randomized controlled trial." This type of study design is particularly strong because it permits researchers to assess whether the intervention is related to the outcome of interest by reducing the effect of other factors.

Equipoise is a state of uncertainty on the part of investigators regarding the comparative therapeutic merits (advantages and disadvantages) of each arm in a trial. Clinical equipoise is an essential first step in randomized controlled trials. An effective modern learning health care system needs to use randomization much more often and early in the assessment of new interventions. If one waits too long, it can be too late to randomize. Most new interventions are rolled out on a subset of patients or units in a hospital, but if this is haphazard, there is no learning. By randomizing which patients receive new interventions at this early stage, one can learn whether the intervention improves outcomes.

Some clinicians are uncomfortable with randomization. It can be useful to realize that there is often variability in what patients receive in a clinical or hospital setting. If this variability is haphazard, we cannot learn about whether a treatment improves outcomes. If, however, we control the variability with randomization, we can learn what improves outcomes. It is not a question of whether there is variability but whether we control it and can learn from it.

> *"If a man will begin with certainties, he shall end in doubts; but if he will be content to begin with doubts he shall end in certainties."*
> —Sir Francis Bacon

A randomized controlled trial is the ideal way to avoid problems associated with regression to the mean. Remember, whenever patients who have an extreme value are selected, there is a tendency for their next measurement to be closer to the average. In Chapter 4, we saw that if patients are selected who have very high systolic blood pressure values, when these values are measured at any future point, the group will be closer to the mean (see Fig. 4.1). Without a control group, it is easy for investigators to attribute this change to their intervention. This happens often in hospitals and the flawed conclusions are often published. For example, if several units in a hospital are selected because they had high complication rates, regression to the mean will almost guarantee that the complication rates in these units will be lower in the future. Without a randomized control group, it is easy to believe that a new intervention solved the problem. In fact, the same intervention applied to the units in the hospital with the lowest complication rates would "prove" that the intervention made the problem worse. One solution to this problem is rather than selecting the three units with the highest complication rates, select the six units with the highest complication rates and randomize half to the intervention and half to a control group. Then after 6 months, switch the units to other arm in a crossover design. Hospital administrators often try to rush and fix problems without including a rigorous evaluation plan.

During the planning phase of your study, decide how you will use randomization (Table 7.1). Some researchers believe that the methods of randomization are standardized, but this is not true (Friedman et al., 2015). Many clinical research projects can be significantly improved with new and creative randomization strategies, for example, random permuted blocks, minimization randomization, biased coin, and other adaptive designs.

TABLE 7.1   Types of Randomization

Fixed Allocation Randomization

- **Simple**—single sequence of random assignments, as if flipping a coin
  - Might not result in 50/50 split, especially in small trials or if stopped early
- **Blocked**—randomize participants into groups (ABAB, ABBA, etc.)
  - Useful if the sample size is large ($n > 200$)
- **Stratified**—randomization within groups based on baseline characteristics (e.g., hospital, gender, and smoking history)
  - Important for multicenter studies and if $n < 100$

Adaptive Randomization

Covariates and previous assignment of participants used to change the allocation probability to assign treatment during the study.
Useful if large number of prognostic factors exists and outcome is known quickly

- **Baseline covariate adaptive**—to correct imbalances based on baseline variables
  - Biased coin—begin with simple randomization, if randomization is more than a preset limit from 50%, change probability to 60%, for example—increases complexity.
  - Urn design—change the probability of assignment based on the size of the imbalance by adding different colored balls to an urn. After selecting a white ball, replace white ball and add a black ball to the urn.
  - Minimization—allocate to minimize differences in covariates in treatment groups
- **Response adaptive**—adjust allocation probabilities based on response to intervention
  - Play the winner—if previous participant had a successful response, assign to same arm; if not successful, assign to the other arm.
  - Two-armed bandit—assign participants based on proportion successful among previous participants.

Blocks refer to units for which the treatment groups (e.g., A vs. B) are balanced; for example, for two treatments, with a block size of four, there are six possible sequences: ABAB, ABBA, BABA, AABB, BAAB, and BBAA. If the trial is stopped early but after a block is completed, the trial will be balanced. In this example, because the blocks consist of four participants, if the investigators were able to crack the code, they would be able to know what the fourth participant was to be randomized to. To avoid this problem, we can vary the size of the blocks, for example, between four and six and the order of these blocks can be randomized, for example: ABAB, AABABB, and BAABBA. This is referred to as random permuted blocks.

A Latin square design is one in which interventions/treatments are arranged so that they appear once, and only once, in each row and column. Latin refers to the use of Latin letters A, B, C. This is a balanced block design used to eliminate the variability from the rows (e.g., different patients) and the columns (e.g., order of the drugs given).

Patient	Phase_1	Phase_2	Phase_3
1	A	B	C
2	C	A	B
3	B	C	A

Stratified randomization refers to a study design in which the randomization occurs within important subgroups, for example, stage of cancer or hospital. Strata are created for important prognostic variable and then permuted blocks are used to achieve balance. Stratified randomization is particularly important for small studies with stratification factors known to greatly influence outcomes. Avoid the ABABAB design. This is not random and will cause problems.

With the R software, you can create a simple randomization table of 100 cases for a control versus intervention experiment with simple commands such as this:

```
>   random_table <- data.frame(seq(1,100), sample(c(0,1),100, replace=TRUE))
>   colnames(random_table) <- c("Case", "Random.Number")
>   random_table
```

In Excel, you can create a randomization table of numbers between 0 and 1 with a function such as this:

```
=rand()
```

Excel is not recommended for statistical analysis but can be useful for simple tasks such as this. In IBM SPSS, you can use the following menu commands:

```
Transform
Compute Variable . . .
random_number (in Target Variable box),
select Random Numbers in the Function group
select Rv.Uniform from the Function and Special Variables list
Rv.UNIFORM(1,100)
OK
```

Online randomization calculators are also available, such as http://www.randomization.com. Example wording:

"The randomization scheme was generated by using the website Randomization.com (http://www
    .randomization.com)."
"Randomization was stratified according to study hospital with the use of variable-sized blocks."

Then add more detail such as the type of randomization and how it was implemented to make it reproducible.

For clinical trials, document the elements of treatment in detail and describe your motivation for comparing these factors. You should have a theoretical model driving your project. So record in your research notes the rationale for each element of treatment. For all randomized controlled trials, be prepared to report all of the items shown in Table 3.2. Remember, randomization can also strengthen many other research designs, such as mailed questionnaires, processing lab samples, and even chart reviews.

> *Example 7–1.*
> A study is being planned in which five research nurses will review the hospital charts of patients who were admitted to 15 hospitals. Investigators who are planning the study design are concerned about problems with interrater reliability. They know from a pilot study that two of the research nurses are much more aggressive in searching the charts for complications. To minimize this potential bias, they use a random number table to assign monthly blocks of charts to be reviewed at the 15 hospitals by the five research nurses. Although this study is not a randomized clinical trial, the use of randomization strengthens the study design and reduces bias.

> *Example 7–2.*
> A study is conducted comparing biomarkers from patients with cancer to a control group. The order of processing the lab samples is randomized to minimize bias. If there is no randomization and the cancer patients' samples are processed on one day and then the controls the next day, the instrument measurement drift in the machine can result in a serious measurement bias.

Blinding, which refers to keeping participants unaware of the treatment being given, also requires careful planning. With a double-blind design, investigators are unaware of which patients receive the active treatment and which receive the placebo. With a triple-blinded design, which is used for the interim analysis, the data and safety monitoring board is unaware of which group received active treatment. Ophthalmologists prefer to use the term "masked" rather than "blinded."

To assess the effectiveness of the blinding, consider asking every patient at the end of their study period to guess which group they were randomized to. Participants should be forced to guess one group or the other and not allowed an "I don't know" option. You can then report the kappa statistic with the 95% confidence interval for the agreement between the guesses and actual assignment. Also ask participants to rate their certainly of the guess and give a reason for their guess. Report all of this in great detail. See Friedman et al. (2015).

Example wording:

"The treatment was not effectively blinded. Study participants correctly judged the intervention vs. placebo greater than would have been expected by chance (kappa level of agreement of 0.85, 95% confidence interval 0.80 to 0.90, $P < .001$) indicating inadequate blinding."

Note: Effective blinding would result in a kappa of approximately 0 and a P value $> .05$.
Example wording for triple blinding to use in the "Statistical Analysis" section of the Methods:

"Data were analyzed without knowledge of treatment assignments."

CONFIDENTIALITY

PRINCIPLE 40 • Protect the confidentiality of all participants.

Institutional review board (IRB) approval and informed consent are important parts of the modern research design. Even if IRB approval is not likely to be required, budget sufficient time for this review early in your project. A major element of IRB approval is confidentiality. Protecting patient, hospital, and physician confidentiality not only is ethical but also protects everyone from legal problems.

In your research database, use sequential "case numbers" (i.e., 1, 2, 3 . . .) for patients, hospitals, and physicians. Using case numbers instead of names protects patient confidentiality, which is especially important in studies that involve sensitive subjects. The principal investigator should keep a key matching names and case numbers in a password-protected file along with the research files and backup files.

Be sure to review the 18 identifiers related to protected health information and remove these before sharing your data with your biostatistician (https://en.wikipedia.org/wiki/Protected_health_information).

Be prepared to explain in the Methods section of your manuscript what steps you took to protect confidentiality and when IRB approval was obtained. Documentation of IRB approval is typically a requirement of publication.

Example wording:

"Patients who met the entry criteria were enrolled after providing written informed consent."
"This study was approved by the institutional review board at each participating center, and all participants provided written informed consent."
"The study was approved by the research ethics board at each participating center, and written informed consent was obtained from all participants."
"The study was approved by the independent ethics committee at each participating site and was conducted in accordance with the International Conference on Harmonization Good Clinical Practice guidelines."

Note: Avoid the terminology "patients were consented." Instead, stress that patients were informed about the risks and benefits of the research and then chose to give their consent to participate.

FOR MORE INFORMATION

See Hulley et al. (2013) and Friedman et al. (2015) or the U.S. Food and Drug Administration (FDA) website. The FDA provides information sheets, such as "A Guide to Informed Consent." Also refer to the Declaration of Helsinki (World Medical Association, 2013) and the International Conference on Harmonisation. See Leibson and Koren (2015) for informed consent in pediatric research.

CHAPTER 8

End Points and Outcome

UNIT OF ANALYSIS

PRINCIPLE 41 • Choose the optimal unit of analysis before you begin to collect data.

The unit of analysis usually is an individual patient, but not always. For some studies, it is a hospital, a population of residents of a particular country, or a knee replacement. Note: One patient might have both knees replaced and therefore the unit of analysis might not be the patient but the knee replacement.

> *Example 8–1.*
> A group of investigators is planning a study of pregnant women to evaluate the accuracy of screening for fetal problems. The group must answer several questions: How should twins be analyzed? How should a woman who has two deliveries during the study period be analyzed? Should abortions and stillbirths be excluded? Should the unit of analysis be (a) a pregnant woman, (b) an infant, (c) a pregnancy, or (d) a singleton (one fetus) pregnancy that continues beyond 28 weeks of gestation?

To choose an appropriate unit of analysis, you must think through the research question and intended data analysis. You can save time and money by collaborating with a biostatistician, particularly one who is willing to invest the time to learn your research subject thoroughly.

VITAL POINT

You must decide on the unit of analysis before you collect any data. Think of the rows in your spreadsheet as your unit of analysis and the columns as your variables.

CONFOUNDING FACTORS

PRINCIPLE 42 • Anticipate confounding factors.

Confounding factors, or confounders, are all of the "other things" that could explain your results. They are predictor variables that must be controlled before you can truly analyze your data. Confounding factors are correlated with both the predictor (independent variable) and the outcome (dependent variable).

Confounding factors are extraneous variables that distort the apparent association between exposure and disease or distort the size of the effect of a study factor. When investigators do not adjust for important confounding factors, their results must be interpreted carefully.

Crude rates are statistics not adjusted for confounding factors. Crude rates are calculated as the number of events in a population over time. They are tabulated without being broken down into classes.

"Adjusted rates are summary statistics that have undergone statistical transformation to permit fair comparison between groups differing in some characteristic that may affect risk of disease" (Mausner & Kramer, 1985).

Case mix or patient mix refers to baseline differences (in severity of illness or injury, preexisting conditions, or the characteristics of patients) among a group of patients.

Example 8–2.
If an investigator plans to compare survival rates among hospitals for patients who underwent a specific surgical procedure, crude survival rates are almost meaningless. The investigator must adjust for confounding factors, such as differences in the patients (e.g., age), preexisting conditions (e.g., diabetes), and whether the procedure was performed on an emergency or an elective basis. Collectively, these factors are referred to as "case mix" or "patient mix."

VITAL POINT

Before you collect any data, develop a strategy to control for as many confounding factors as possible, especially those that could affect the outcome of interest.

Perform a literature search to identify other variables that may be correlated with your outcome. Record these variables so that you can confirm or refute these reports through your analysis. You may decide to reproduce the tables and figures from landmark papers with your data.

Recording potential confounding factors, such as smoking history, during data collection saves time and money. If you overlook an important confounding factor, you may need to search for the information later. This retrospective search not only wastes time but also may produce poor quality data.

Identify several strategies to control for confounding factors and anticipate the problems associated with each strategy. Choose the strongest design that fits your budget and schedule. Document your strategy and cite a reference to support it. Ignoring this step may lead to the following comments from reviewers:

"This study is interesting in concept, but flawed in execution."

CLASSIFICATION OF VARIABLES

PRINCIPLE 43 • Distinguish between independent and dependent variables.

Independent or input variables ordinarily have values that are autonomous of the dependent or outcome variables (Fig. 8.1). Usually, independent variables are graphed on the x-axis (horizontal axis). Because independent variables precede dependent variables, they often are called "predictors." In epidemiology, independent variables are called "risk factors" or "exposure variables." Remember, independent variables are antecedents (smoking); dependent variables are consequents (lung cancer).

Dependent or output variables have responses that are contingent on independent variables. They usually are graphed on the y-axis (vertical axis) and often are called "outcome variables."

Example 8–3.
In a study to identify patients at high risk for pneumonia, pneumonia is the outcome or dependent variable. To predict this outcome, the investigator can analyze age, sex, and smoking history.

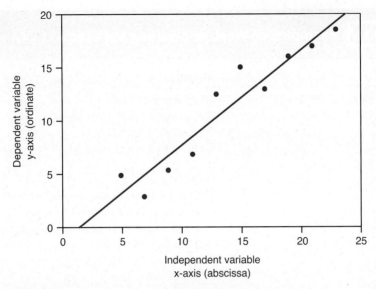

FIGURE 8.1. Independent and dependent variables.

These are the independent variables. During the analysis, the investigator might decide to control for age and determine whether sex is a significant predictor of pneumonia—independent of age. In this case, age is treated as a covariate that is adjusted for statistically.

A covariate is a patient factor (e.g., age, sex, smoking history) that may or may not be related to the outcome (pneumonia). If a covariate is related to both the risk factor and the outcome, then it is a confounder. For example, to assess the impact of the risk factor drinking history on the outcome pneumonia, smoking history would be a confounder because it is related to both drinking and pneumonia.

FOR MORE INFORMATION

About confounders, mediators, moderators, and covariates, see:

https://significantlystatistical.wordpress.com/2014/12/12/confounders-mediators-moderators-and-covariates/

PRINCIPLE 44 • Record outcome with several secondary end point variables but do not try to game the system.

Always prespecify one primary end point and document this in your analysis plan. In addition, identify several secondary end point variables that you can use to measure short-term and long-term outcome in your study. If you have technical problems with one dependent variable, you may be able to use another variable to answer the research question. When your success rests on one dependent variable, choose the strongest possible variable (Table 8.1). The ideal dependent variable is reproducible, objective, standardized, and patient-centric. Ideally, it is also measured as a continuous variable.

Continuous variables are measurements (e.g., hematocrit). Categorical variables are labels for groups (e.g., anemia). Dichotomous variables are categorical variables with only two groups, such as alive versus dead. For dichotomous dependent variables, the statistically ideal situation is to have 50% of patients with each outcome.

| TABLE 8.1 | Examples of Weak and Strong Variables |

Weak	Strong
Complications [text field]	Complication 1 [text]
	Complication 1 ICD-10 code
	Complication 2 [text]
	Complication 2 ICD-10 code
	etc.
Anemic	Hematocrit and hemoglobin level
Obese	Body mass index, height, and weight
Hypertensive	Systolic and diastolic blood pressure
Do you exercise? yes/no	How many days each week do you get at least 30 minutes of moderate to vigorous physical activity? (e.g., brisk walking, cycling, aerobics, hard physical labor) ☐0 ☐1 ☐2 ☐3 ☐4 ☐5 ☐6 ☐7
Was the patient readmitted to the hospital? yes/no	Was the patient readmitted to the hospital? yes/no
	Date of readmission
	Days from discharge to readmission?
	Was this a planned readmission?
	Reason for readmission [text]
	Reason for readmission ICD-10 code
Percentage change in weight from baseline	Baseline weight
	Baseline height
	Follow-up weight
	If missing, reason for missing data

ICD-10, International Classification of Diseases, Tenth revision.

Ask yourself: "How could reviewers see my dependent variable as inadequate or problematic?" Include additional dependent variables as secondary end points to control for these problems. Also consider the patient's perspective. For example, does your dependent variable measure success in the same way that patients define success?

Use caution when you define your end point as a change in a variable. Change variables have numerous statistical weaknesses. Use an end point that is clinically meaningful and then compare the postintervention measurements, adjusted for baseline using a method such as analysis of covariance (ANCOVA).

FOR MORE INFORMATION

Before you begin to collect data, research the current methods of assessing quality-of-life outcomes. See Fayers and Machin (2016), Testa and Simonson (1996), and the six articles on the quality of care that were published in *The New England Journal of Medicine* in 1996 (Berwick, 1996; Blumenthal, 1996, part 1 and part 4; Blumenthal & Epstein, 1996; Brook et al., 1996; Chassin, 1996; Kassirer & Angell, 1996). For randomized clinical trials, see Chapter 15 of the book by Bulpitt (2013).

PREPARING FOR DATA ENTRY

PRINCIPLE 45 • Quantify, quantify, quantify!

You can simplify data analysis by addressing these important points during the planning phase. First, choose variables that can be quantified and will thereby provide the strongest statistical analysis. Then strive for ways to measure these variables more precisely.

Example 8–4.
If smoking is a central factor in your study, do not classify patients simply as smokers or non-smokers. Quantify their smoking by including questions such as the following:

1. Have you smoked at least 100 cigarettes in your entire life?*

   0 ☐ No
   1 ☐ Yes

2. Do you now smoke cigarettes?

   0 ☐ Not at all
   1 ☐ Some days
   2 ☐ Every day

3. How many cigarettes do you smoke each day? ☐ ☐

4. How many years have you been smoking? ☐ ☐

5. If you are a former smoker, how many years ago did you quit smoking? ☐ ☐

6. At what age did you begin smoking daily? ☐ ☐

*Question 1 may appear peculiar, but it is a reproducible method of distinguishing people who "tried smoking" from those who were actual smokers.

Example 8–5.
Many people are reluctant to disclose their exact annual income, but on a questionnaire, many respondents will check off an income range such as <\$20,000, \$20,000–\$39,999, \$40,000–\$64,999, \$65,000–\$99,999, and >\$100,000. If you use this approach, make the categories meaningful by doing some homework. For example, What is the median income? What ranges will produce income groups with even numbers of respondents (such as quintiles)? This investment in planning will pay off during data analysis.

Always use a pilot test to determine how to convert text answers into numeric categories. Remember, for statistical analysis that will draw out the truth from your numbers, you must quantify the exposure of the key variables.

Use a logical coding system and avoid awkward conversions, such as the following:

   1 = none, 2 = one, 3 = two
   0 = first degree, 1 = second degree, 2 = third degree

For statistical analysis, the most effective coding is as follows:

   0 = no, 1 = yes

Most variables should be coded as 0 and 1. Variable names should be in the form of questions: diabetes (Does this person have diabetes?) 0 = no diabetes, 1 = diabetes.

Avoid mixing text and codes: Provide a code for "other" and create a separate field for a text description of the "other" option. Create numeric codes for variables such as county, town, and race. Do not record data that cannot easily be analyzed with statistical software.

If you must use text, keep it short and uniform, such as the two-letter uppercase abbreviations for states used by the US Postal Service. Avoid using embedded blanks in text. When an age is missing, use a code (e.g., −1) or leave the space blank. Do not enter text, such as "NA" or "Not Doc." Example 8–6 shows coding for computerized statistical analysis.

Example 8–6.

Problematic format	**Preferred format**
Restraint device used	Was the occupant wearing a seat belt?
_____	0 = No 1 = Yes 9 = Unknown

Possible text answers	**Possible numeric answers**
SEAT BELT	0
SEATBELT	1
Seatbelt	9
Unknown	
None	
NONE	
NA	
Not Doc	
(Blank)	

Avoid dichotomania—the habit of turning all continuous variables into binary variables. Use an interval/continuous scale when possible. For certain variables, however, a checklist of ordinal choices (see Table 10.1) can provide more accurate and complete data.

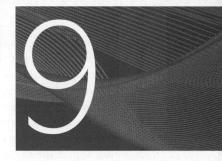

CHAPTER

9

Sample Size and Power

> *"We need less research, better research, and research done for the right reasons."*
> —Douglas G. Altman (1994)

> *"Only about a third of highly cited animal research translated at the level of human randomized trials . . . major opportunities for improving study design and methodological quality are available for preclinical research."*
> —Daniel G. Hackam (2006)

ESTIMATING SAMPLE SIZE

PRINCIPLE 46 • Calculate the sample size required to definitively address your research question.

Too many papers are published with inadequately small sample sizes. Science needs more studies with much larger sample sizes and studies that have sufficient statistical power. The good news is that it is becoming much easier and less expensive to access big data. For example, Noto et al. (2015) showed that it is possible to obtain a large sample size by using a pragmatic cluster randomized crossover study design using the electronic health record for the entire data set. This is an example of a modern learning health care system that can answer important questions at low cost with a large sample size.

Before you collect any data, determine whether your sample size will be adequate. You can use free software such as PS or a commercial software package such as nQuery Advisor to calculate sample sizes.

PS:

biostat.mc.vanderbilt.edu/PowerSampleSize

nQuery Advisor:

http://www.statsols.com

In addition to the formal power calculations, an experienced researcher (such as your mentor) can also help you weigh the necessary information (e.g., cost, time required) to estimate the sample size. This nonstatistical perspective is often equally as valuable. In some cases, a small sample of high-quality information is preferable to a large sample of questionable data.

Calculating a sample size often requires statistical judgments based on experience. Always consult an experienced biostatistician for this input. A biostatistician can help you estimate the size of your sample, design your data collection form, design the study, and write a detailed analysis plan. An experienced biostatistician will tailor this plan for statistical analysis based on your specific data set. Avoid biostatisticians who use a template approach and do not consider the specific needs of your study. When you consult a biostatistician about the sample size needed, be prepared to provide specific information about your study, such as the primary end point, the expected event rate (or mean and standard deviation [SD]), the expected dropout rate, and how certain you must be in detecting a difference.

Avoid using Cohen's standardized effect size in your sample size justification. This is an outdated method that is not rigorous enough for modern medical research (Lenth, 2001, 2007; http://homepage.stat.uiowa.edu/~rlenth/Power/). Instead use a clinically meaningful end point with a clinically meaningful change. If your end point is a continuous variable, use the standard deviation from your pilot study or from the published literature to estimate the sample size. Do not use the difference between groups from previous studies in estimating your sample size. The difference must be what you determine is a clinically important difference. Pilot studies can provide you with feasibility and variability but not this difference or effect size. For categorical variables, the pilot study or the literature can provide you with the percentage, with the outcome (event rate) in the control group.

Consult with your research team and review sample sizes from similar published studies to determine whether your sample is too small to allow worthwhile conclusions to be drawn. If your sample is too small, enlarge it by collecting data on more patients, or refocus your study.

If you cannot collect your own data, consider using existing databases, such as disease registries, hospital electronic health records, databases from the health department, and the Centers for Medicare & Medicaid Services (CMS). Academic medical centers are leading the way in this area by building the capacity to learn from the medical data collected. For example, Vanderbilt has created BioVU and the Synthetic Derivative as resources for investigators. BioVU is a biorepository of DNA extracted from discarded blood collected during routine clinical testing and linked to deidentified medical records in the Synthetic Derivative.

https://victr.vanderbilt.edu/pub/biovu/

Secondary data analysis has limitations, however, and you may not have the precise variables or quality of data you need.

PRINCIPLE 47 • Consider the various sample size requirements of your research early in the planning phase.

An important part of planning your study is choosing not only the size of the overall sample but also for important subgroups. Many investigators have problems with analysis because they end up with small subgroups. Your overall sample may appear large, but when the findings are broken down into different types of patients and different types of treatment, your subgroups may be too small to provide meaningful information. Having the power to analyze subgroups, such as ethnic minorities, individuals with low socioeconomic status, etc., is becoming more important for some funding agencies. If a treatment is effective, will you have enough patients younger and older than 60 to be able to assess this? Prespecify an analysis plan for assessing heterogeneity of the treatment effect, for example:

> "We prespecified two variables to examine heterogeneity of treatment effects, following the approach proposed by Kent et al. (2010)—baseline age and stage of disease."

VITAL POINT

Plan to study a large sample, with an adequate number in the control group and in important subgroups.

Prespecify the subgroup analysis and follow the advice of Wang et al. (2007). Reckless analysis of subgroups can be used to show that almost anything is related to poor outcome, even astrologic birth signs (see ISIS-2 [Second International Study of Infarct Survival] Collaborative Group, 1988).

STATISTICAL POWER

To plan your study effectively, you must understand the concept of statistical power. The formal definition is "the probability of rejecting the null hypothesis where it is false." In other words, the power of your study is the probability that if the treatment is effective, you will be able to show a statistically significant effect. Power is equal to 1-Beta. Beta is the probability of a type II error (see Principle 128). Larger studies usually have greater power. Remember that the P value is the probability that a difference (or association) as large as the one you observed (or larger) could have occurred by chance alone, given the null hypothesis is true.

Table 9.1 shows sample size requirements.

Example 9–1.
Suppose that drug A has a 25% success rate and the investigators are interested in whether drug B will increase the success rate to 50% or more. If a study randomizes 66 patients into the drug A group and 66 patients into the drug B group, the investigator will have an 80% chance of detecting this difference and showing a statistically significant difference ($P < .05$). The investigator also has a 20% chance of not detecting this difference and might incorrectly conclude that the success rates of these two drugs are similar. The power of this study is 80%. Note: in Table 9.1 the required sample size is 65 rather than 66 computed in the PS program. Different methods will provide similar but often slightly different estimates.

Use the following steps to reproduce Figure 9.1, Figure 9.2, and Example 9–1.

1. Download the PS software:

   biostat.mc.vanderbilt.edu/PowerSampleSize

2. Continue.
3. Select the "Dichotomous" tab for the end point.
4. Select "Sample size" for "What do you want to know?"
5. Select "Independent" for "Matched or Independent?"
6. Select "Prospective" for "Case control."
7. Select "Two proportions" for "How is the alternative hypothesis expressed?"
8. Select "Fisher's exact test" for type of test.
9. Enter .05 for a, .80 for *power*, .25 for p_0, .50 for p_1, 1 for m (ratio of patients in two arms). Click on the blue links for help.
10. Calculate, read the sample size displayed.
11. Change "Sample size" to "Detectable" alternative in "What do you want to know?"
12. Calculate.
13. Graph.
14. Select "Power" for "What should be on the Y axis?"
15. Enter 0 and 0.60 for the "X axis range."
16. Plot.

Example 9–2 shows how to use Table 9.1.

Example 9–2.
Suppose that you wish to estimate the sample size that is necessary to determine whether a new treatment can improve the cure rate from 75% to 85% (assuming a power of 80% and an alpha level [P value threshold] of .05). Find 75% along the top row of Table 9.1. Then find 85% along the left column. These numbers intersect at the number 270, which means that you must include 270 patients in each of these two groups. If the difference actually is this large, you would have an 80% chance of detecting the difference and showing a P value of less than .05.

TABLE 9.1 Sample Size Requirements for Each of Two Groups[a,b]

Group I	Group II (The Smaller of the Two Groups)																	
	5%	10%	15%	20%	25%	30%	35%	40%	45%	50%	55%	60%	65%	70%	75%	80%	85%	90%
10%	474																	
15%	160	725																
20%	88	219	945															
25%	58	113	270	1,134														
30%	43	71	134	313	1,291													
35%	33	50	82	151	348	1,416												
40%	27	38	57	91	165	376	1,511											
45%	22	30	42	62	98	175	395	1,573										
50%	18	24	32	45	65	103	182	407	1,605									
55%	16	20	26	34	47	68	106	186	411	1,573								
60%	14	17	21	27	36	48	69	107	186	407	1,573							
65%	12	14	18	22	28	36	49	69	106	182	395	1,511						
70%	10	12	15	18	22	28	36	48	68	103	175	376	1,416					
75%	9	11	13	15	18	22	28	36	47	65	98	165	348	1,291				
80%	8	9	11	13	15	18	22	27	34	45	62	91	151	313	1,134			
85%	7	8	9	11	13	15	18	21	26	32	42	57	82	134	270	945		
90%	6	7	8	9	11	12	14	17	20	24	30	38	50	71	113	219	725	
95%	5	6	7	8	9	10	12	14	16	18	22	27	33	43	58	88	160	474

These estimates use an alpha = 0.05 and a power = 0.80.

[a]How to use this table: To find the sample size required to compare the proportions in two groups of equal size:

1. Find the percentage in group I in the left column.
2. Find the percentage in group II along the top row.
3. If the percentage in group II is greater than the percentage in group I, reverse row and column in steps 1 and 2.
4. The number at the intersection is the sample size required for each of the two groups.

[b]For details of the calculations and formulas used to compute the values in this table, see the original source. Data from Fleiss JL. *Statistical Methods for Rates and Proportions.* 2nd ed. New York, NY: Wiley; 2003, 260–280 and Fleiss JL, Tytun A, Ury HK. A simple approximation for calculating sample sizes for comparing independent proportions. *Biometrics.* 1980;36(2):343–346.

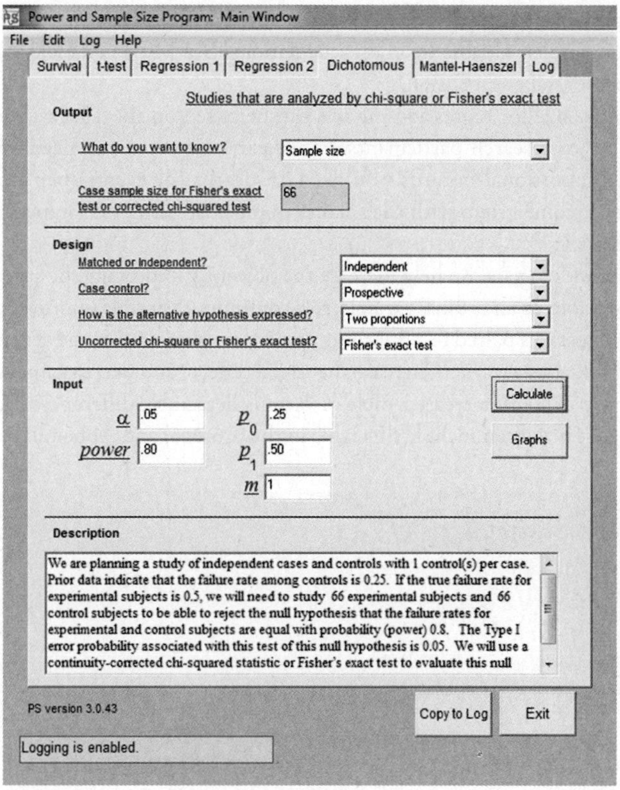

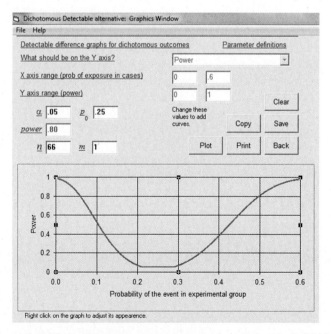

FIGURE 9.1. Screenshot of the PS sample size software. See Example 9–1, steps 1–10. (Courtesy of Bill Dupont and Dale Plummer.)

FIGURE 9.2. Screenshot of the detectable alternative graphics window from PS. See Example 9–1, steps 11–16. (Courtesy of Bill Dupont and Dale Plummer.)

Sample size can also be based on precision, for example, the width of the 95% confidence interval; the nQuery Advisor software is valuable for these calculations. See Mitjà et al. (2015) for an example of how to power a study based on precision.

Finally, the sample size for regression models can be based on the 15:1 rule of predictors in the model to the number of research participants. For linear regression, you need 15 patients for every predictor. For Cox proportional-hazards, you need 15 deaths (or events) per predictor. For logistic regression, find the outcome group with the smaller number of patients. You need 15 patients in that group for every predictor.

Experienced methodologists can help increase the power by improving the study design. Changing from a categorical variable, to an ordinal variable, to a continuous variable improves power. Also, changing from an unpaired test to a paired test improves power, for example, a crossover trial. Methodologists can also help you think about ways to increase the signal (effect) and decrease the noise (variability).

Successful scientist will often create a table of various detectable differences that are possible with the given sample size. They often include this table in the protocol and Appendix.

FOR MORE INFORMATION

See Hulley et al. (2013).

Preparing for Modern Statistical Analysis

PLANNING THE ANALYSIS

PRINCIPLE 48 • Consider the level of measurement for each of your variables.

To apply the appropriate statistical tests, you must understand the three basic levels of measurement (Table 10.1):

1. Nominal/categorical
2. Ordinal
3. Interval/continuous/scale

A simple analogy may help. In a horse race, a nominal variable would be "Did the horse come in first place? Yes or no?"; an ordinal variable would be "What was the horse's place? First, second, or third?"; and an interval variable would be "How many seconds did it take the horse to cross the finish line?" Note that there might be a small difference between the first and second horse but a large difference between the second and the third horse. The ordinal variable would not measure this gap but the continuous variable would because it has a meaningful <u>interval</u> between numbers.

PRINCIPLE 49 • Organize your variables into clinically logical buckets.

Your prespecified analysis plan should clearly distinguish between inclusion criteria variables, risk factors, outcome variables, and confounding factors. Be careful if using the same variable for more than one of these groups. The success of your statistical analysis may depend on how well you plan the collection and grouping of risk factors. Other useful groupings are:

+ Variables routinely known within the first 24 hours of a hospital admission
+ Variables known after the first 24 hours of a hospital admission
+ Variables that are inexpensive and readily available
+ Those that are expensive and infrequently ordered

Risk factors can be further subdivided into those that:

+ Can be modified on a daily basis (exercise)
+ Can be modified long term (body mass index)
+ Cannot be modified (age)

TABLE 10.1	Levels of Measurement

Level	Explanation
1. Nominal (categorical variables)	Numbers are only labels for categories.
Examples:	0 = no, 1 = yes
	0 = nonsmoker, 1 = smoker
	1 = White, 2 = Black, 3 = Hispanic, 4 = Asian, 9 = Other
	0 = female, 1 = male (Note: Males are generally at increased risk.)
Note:	The categories can be numbered in any order without affecting the results:
	1 = Black, 2 = Hispanic, 3 = Asian, 4 = Other, 9 = White
2. Ordinal	Numbers are used to provide rank ordering (as in a horse race); these variables may be subjective.
Examples:	1 = first, 2 = second, 3 = third
	0–10 Apgar score
	0 = nonsmoker, 1 = light smoker, 2 = moderate smoker, 3 = heavy smoker
3. Interval (scale) (continuous variables)	Numbers have equal intervals between successive points; this type of measurement typically is more objective than the other types.
Examples:	Age
	Hematocrit
	Serum albumin level
	Cigarettes smoked per day

PRINCIPLE 50 • Demonstrate that the study groups are comparable.

Use the same selection criteria for all treatment and control groups. Uniformity of treatment groups is a major concern of reviewers, as shown by the following comment:

"Are patients in one group weighted in one direction? Do they have more severe or chronic problems? Is the average age different between the groups?"

PRINCIPLE 51 • Establish a valid and robust control group.

A control group is a set of subjects who are treated in the same way as a treatment group—absent the intervention being tested. The control group is the standard of comparison in judging experimental effects.

An absent or inappropriate control group is a major problem in many clinical studies. The entire research team should help define the ideal control group and then critique it. Reviewers will reject a well-written paper if they perceive that the control group is weak. When you search the literature, study how various types of control groups are used for your particular topic. A control group can be improved by using randomization and avoiding an easy-to-access group—a convenience sample. If it is impossible to use a randomized control group, you can often find large population studies that can be used as a benchmark; for example, the Behavioral Risk Factor Surveillance System (see Byrne et al., 2011). Avoid the weak before–after designs with historical controls. Without a randomized control group, it can be very difficult to prove that your intervention caused the changes that occurred from a before to after period.

FOR MORE INFORMATION

See Baker (1986); Bulpitt (2013); Friedman (2003); Hulley et al. (2013); Last et al. (2000); Mausner and Kramer (1985); and Morton et al. (2001).

PLANNING THE FOLLOW-UP

PRINCIPLE 52 • Include an impressive length of follow-up with quality of life outcome measures that are important to patients.

When you plan a study, strive for a longer than average follow-up period. For some orthopedic journals, the required follow-up period is 2 years. Consult clinical specialists from several disciplines to establish the optimal "window of follow-up" for each outcome.

For studies of long-term outcome, record each patient's first name, last name, middle initial, date of birth, gender, Social Security number, Medicare number, father's surname, country of birth, age at death (if known), race, marital status, state of residence, and state of birth. You can use the National Death Index (http://www.cdc.gov/nchs/ndi.htm) to determine whether patients, who were lost to follow-up by conventional methods, have died. Since 1979, the National Center for Health Statistics has maintained a database of all deaths in the United States. You should also record the name, address, e-mail, and telephone number of the patient's physician and the name, address, e-mail, and telephone number of a friend or relative of the patient. Note there are very specific rules for formatting the data that you submit to the National Death Index. To be efficient, record the data in this format to avoid having to recode the values. See

http://www.cdc.gov/nchs/data/ndi/ndi_users_guide_chapter2.pdf

PRINCIPLE 53 • Consider the implications of differences in follow-up time.

Establish a plan to analyze your data that addresses the possibility that the average follow-up time may differ between the treatment and control groups. Measure the range of time "at risk" for both groups—time from start of the study to the end point or lost to follow-up. Control for time at risk in the analysis since this is likely to be an important confounding variable. Cox proportional-hazards analysis will allow you to analyze the factors associated with time to death or the first occurrence of an event. Poisson regression will allow you to analyze factors associated with the number of events. Each method has several assumptions that must be met. Therefore, to assess these assumptions, collaborating with a biostatistician for these complex analyses is wise.

Example 10–1.
Before an investigator can analyze the results of a study of occupational stress, the investigator must consider each participant's length of time at the job and the various types of bias that could affect the follow-up data.

Include in your study the number and percentage of patients who are lost to follow-up at the close of the study and explain (in the Discussion section) how this number affects your results. If you plan to use survival analysis to adjust for follow-up differences, recognize the assumptions that must be met. One assumption is that the "censored" patients are similar to the uncensored patients. Resolve these problems during the planning phase of your study. Work with your biostatistician to address this issue of independence of censoring.

"Censored" is a term that is used to refer to a patient who was alive at the last contact with the researchers. For life-table analysis, this term is used to identify patients who have follow-up data to enter the particular time interval but whose most current follow-up data do not extend to the end of the interval. The number of patients withdrawn (who died) during this interval is used for survival analysis calculations.

Intention-to-treat (ITT) analysis includes data from all patients who were randomized into treatment or control groups, regardless of their compliance or the treatment they actually received. Analyzing only the patients who completed the study (actual on-therapy analysis, on-randomized treatment [ORT], or per protocol analysis) can create bias problems and seriously hinder your chance of publication in a high-quality journal. Often, the analysis is performed using both methods and the ORT is included in the appendix.

FOR MORE INFORMATION
See Bulpitt (2013).

Avoiding Common Criticisms

PEER REVIEWERS' RESPONSES

PRINCIPLE 54 • Anticipate and avoid common criticisms.

Table 11.1 shows the answers that peer reviewers gave when they were asked to identify their most common criticisms of manuscripts.

Four major categories of criticism were identified by Kassirer and Campion (1994). Problems with study design are the most common problems (see Fig. 3.1); be sure, during the planning stage, to identify and address these problems.

EDITORS' RESPONSES

Table 11.2 shows the responses of editors who were asked to report their most common criticisms of manuscripts.

As with reviewers, editors were most concerned with study design. Editors also were concerned with the importance of the topic, whereas reviewers focused on the interpretation of the findings.

TABLE 11.1a   Reviewers' Most Common Criticisms of Manuscripts[a]

- (a) Inadequate control experiments; (b) selected images that show only one cell in a frame; (c) incremental advance
- Poor quality and/or overinterpretation of data. Data do not support conclusions. Results are minimal and/or do not advance the field sufficiently.
- (a) Does not clearly differentiate their work from past work; (b) contains no historical perspective; (c) authors are clearly biased and cherry-pick data to support their views.
- Incorrect study design; inadequate power; discussion/conclusions that go unreasonably beyond the data presented
- The manuscripts do not have a clear objective. The manuscripts have grammatical errors which were not carefully fixed prior to submission. Often discussions do not address the results provided.
- Poor reporting of methods and results; inadequate methods; overoptimistic conclusion
- Not a full consideration of explanations of the results; a topic/result not important enough for the level of journal; unclear presentation of a critical argument
- Lack of rigor in writing; overstate the findings; overemphasis of statistical differences without clinical importance
- (a) A poorly written article with numerous typos, formatting issues, and grammatical errors is hard to overcome, regardless of the science; (b) inappropriate or poorly explained methodology including statistical analysis; (c) discussion has to tell the story of where the current study lies within what we know from the literature including an explanation for discrepant findings. The results also need to be put into context regarding the larger public health, medical practice, health care, and/or policy ramifications.
- (a) Overinterpretation of the results; (b) too much information in the Background section—get right to the crux of the research; (c) unclear methods
- Lack of novelty/innovation; inappropriate analyses; poor methodology
- Methods insufficiently described so that replication (or even understanding) is not possible; needless complexity in presenting results, particularly in statistical models. There is a needless focus on relative effects and P values without understandable results that allow the reader to easily understand the effect size; unfocused introductions and discussions.
- Inconsistency between study hypothesis and methodology; lack of clear clinical plausibility; too much enthusiasm in support of study hypothesis
- Writing not clear; poor understanding of study design and analytical methods; poor understanding of the elements of a scientific hypothesis
- (a) Poor design; (b) unappreciated bias; (c) conclusions unsupported by the data
- Being sent manuscripts that are not in compliance with journal guidelines—usually manuscripts that greatly exceed limits; being sent manuscripts that are clearly not suitable for consideration in the journal due to poor content, offensive tone, or not in line with journal priorities; conducting a second review of a manuscript only to see that author has not responded to suggestions
- (a) Quality of statistical analysis; (b) external validity of findings; (c) measurement of variables in secondary data analyses
- (a) Insufficient data analysis/adjustment for confounders; (b) incomplete review of prior literature (especially older papers); (c) inappropriate sampling of subjects (usually convenience) without consideration of generalizability or influence on conclusions

(continued)

TABLE 11.1a   Reviewers' Most Common Criticisms of Manuscripts[a]
(continued)

- Inadequate statistical analyses; poor editing; lack of translation
- Statistical rigor; conclusions not supported by discussion; methodology issues—control group not properly set up, others
- (a) Methodology not sound; (b) statistical issues; (c) conclusions not supported by results
- (a) Poor description in the Methods section of the actual scientific methodology used; (b) criticism of the actual methodology used; (c) points made either in the Introduction or the Discussion that appear unclear or undocumented
- Lack of clarity regarding methods; overinterpretation of the importance of the results; incremental value of research question
- (a) Inadequate data—no or improper controls, insufficient number of patients or inadequate follow-up, or inappropriate statistical analysis; (b) overextension of the authors' conclusions—basically saying they have proven something that they have not proven; (c) poor use of the English language to the extent that the manuscript is unreadable
- Poorly written; not useful information; poor methodology
- Poor study design; no clear hypothesis; too small numbers
- (a) Sloppy writing; (b) poor description of methods and what was actually done in the study, such that it would actually be impossible to replicate the study based on the paper; (c) overly enthusiastic conclusions and making too much out of modest findings
- The reporting of the data is not consistent with established guidelines (e.g., PRISMA, CONSORT); poorly formed hypothesis. Statements in the manuscripts are not supported by the data or addressed by the design of the study.

TABLE 11.1b	**Reviewers' Most Common Criticisms of Manuscripts**[a]

Design of the Study
- Poor experimental/study design
- Vague or inadequate description of methodology
- Biased data collection or inadequate sample
- No control or improper control
- Methodologic flaw, methodology not sound
- Poor description in the Methods section of the actual scientific methodology used
- Poor description of methods and what was actually done in the study, such that it would actually be impossible to replicate the study based on the paper
- No clear hypothesis or poorly formed hypothesis
- Small sample size
- Nonrandom samples
- Statistically inadequate
- Univariate statistics when multivariate statistics were needed

Interpretation of the Findings
- Erroneous and unsupported conclusions
- Conclusions not supported by results
- Overextension of the authors' conclusions—basically saying they have proven something that they have not proven.
- Overly enthusiastic conclusions and making too much out of modest findings
- Conclusions based on noncontrolled data
- Study design that does not support inferences
- Over interpretation of data
- Inadequate link of findings to practice or policy
- Failure to consider alternative explanations of results
- Inadequate discussion

Importance of the Topic
- Overinterpretation of the importance of the results
- Incremental value of research question
- Rehash of established facts
- Insignificant research question
- Irrelevant or unimportant topic; not useful information
- Low reader interest
- Little clinical relevance

Presentation of the Results
- The reporting of the data is not consistent with established guidelines (e.g., PRISMA, CONSORT).
- Poorly focused
- Poorly organized
- Poorly written, sloppy writing
- Points made either in the Introduction or the Discussion that appear unclear or undocumented
- Poor use of the English language to the extent that the manuscript is unreadable
- Statements in the manuscripts are not supported by the data or addressed by the design of the study.

[a]From question 1 of the Peer Review Questionnaire (Appendix B). Table 11.1a is from the survey conducted for the second edition of this book. Table 11.1b is from the survey conducted for the first edition of this book.

TABLE 11.2a	Editors' Most Common Criticisms of Manuscripts[a]

- Unclear writing; incomplete information; conclusions that are not supported by the results presented
- Poor organization; inadequate literature review; statistical fishing expeditions
- (a) Language and grammar; (b) short view of the hypothesis; history of the issue goes back only a couple of decades despite a long trail of data; (c) overreach (and at times under reach) of the conclusion
- (a) Overinterpretation of findings; (b) confusing presentation of findings; (c) failure to acknowledge methodologic limitations
- Incomplete reporting of items; loss of data during follow-up; lack of clarity about limitations of the study
- Not explaining the rationale for a study, analysis, or article; selective reviewing of the literature, that is, US researchers tend to only include other US research (even if there is international research that is relevant); failing to (try to) explain why results have been found
- (a) Inadequate adjustment in MV models; (b) overstating, reaching with conclusions; (c) data splitting
- Incomplete submissions and noncompliance with the guidance in our Information for Authors; lack of detail in the manuscript to make an informed decision on what was actually done or how the data were analyzed; overinterpretation of data
- Overstating the importance of the research findings being presented; not fairly presenting the strengths and weaknesses of the research; lack of clarity describing either the study population or the data collection methods
- Poor methodology, weak positioning in the literature, unclear research question
- (a) Lack of prespecification of the statistical methodology used; (b) overestimation of the effect size of an intervention; (c) failure to differentiate between an association and a true causal relationship
- Do not answer the question they claim to have answered; not of broad interest; data are not novel.
- (a) Nothing new; (b) inadequate powered study; (c) employing inappropriate databases
- Poor sourcing—format is incorrect; source is not a primary source or does not support the statement for which it is cited; use of ambiguous language; lack of detail
- (a) Overstatement of novelty; (b) poor writing; (c) issues with modified image data
- (a) Inappropriate statistical prediction model validation; (b) irrelevant or missing comparison of statistical model with alternative; (c) unclear handling if missing data/values
- (a) Trial question; (b) faulty experimental design; (c) post hoc manipulation of data to ensure results that are "positive" with respect to the investigator's allegiance biases
- (a) Data mining; (b) salami slicing; (c) missed biases and confounders
- As a journal editor-in-chief, my most common criticisms are lacks breadth of impact or significance, lacks sufficient support for conclusions, and has weaknesses in design or interpretation.

TABLE 11.2b | **Editors' Most Common Criticisms of Manuscripts**[a]

Design of the Study
- Lack of prespecification of the statistical methodology used, data mining
- Inadequate or faulty experimental study design
- Poor methodology, yielding potentially faulty results
- Failure to account for confounding factors
- Methods lacking sufficient rigor
- Biased protocol
- Lack of validity and reliability
- Inappropriate use of statistics
- Inappropriate comparisons
- Statistical methods not applied or used improperly
- Too few patients to permit meaningful conclusions, inadequate powered study
- Employing inappropriate databases

Interpretation of the Findings
- Do not answer the question they claim to have answered
- Overestimation of the effect size of an intervention
- Failure to differentiate between an association and a true causal relationship
- Unfounded conclusions
- Conclusions disproportionate to the results
- Uncritical acceptance of statistical results
- Improper inferences
- Unexplained inconsistencies
- Failure to acknowledge methodologic flaws
- Inflation of the importance of the findings
- Interpretation of the results not concordant with the data
- Weak positioning in the literature; inadequate literature review
- Missed biases and confounders

Importance of the Topic
- Lacks breadth of impact or significance
- Trivial question
- Incremental advance
- Not of broad interest
- Data are not novel; overstatement of novelty
- Lack of originality
- Nothing new; insufficient new information
- Not generalizable
- Repetitious data (already in the literature or adding little)
- Unclear research question

Presentation of the Results
- Statistical fishing expeditions
- Too long; verbose
- Excessively self-promotional
- Poor grammar, syntax, or spelling
- Somewhat anecdotal
- Poor organization

(continued)

TABLE 11.2b	Editors' Most Common Criticisms of Manuscripts[b] *(continued)*

- Inappropriate statistical prediction model validation
- Irrelevant or missing comparison of statistical model with alternative
- Unclear handling if missing data/values
- Poor writing; poorly written Abstract
- Failure to communicate clearly
- Poor organization
- Selected images that show only one cell in a frame
- Issues with modified image data
- Post hoc manipulation of data to ensure results that are "positive" with respect to the investigator's allegiance biases
- Poor sourcing—format is incorrect; source is not a primary source or does not support the statement for which it is cited.
- Use of ambiguous language—lack of detail
- Salami slicing

[a]From question 1 of the Peer Review Questionnaire (Appendix B). Table 11.2a is from the survey conducted for the second edition of this book. Table 11.2b is from the survey conducted for the first edition of this book.

12

Preparing to Write a Publishable Paper

ORGANIZING YOUR MATERIAL INTO A MANUSCRIPT

PRINCIPLE 55 • Organize your information into the sections of a manuscript as soon as possible.

Before you collect any data, develop a clear plan for organizing your paper. Having such a plan will allow you to enter information into your manuscript file efficiently. Medical manuscripts typically are arranged as shown in Table 12.1.

Always create an outline to build a framework for your paper before you write any text. A good mentor will insist on an outline before writing and will help you create this structure. A good mentor will also give you specific weekly assignments such as "By next Monday, please complete Table 1" rather than, "Go write the paper."

CHOOSING A JOURNAL

PRINCIPLE 56 • Select a target journal before you begin to write your paper.

Plan to submit your paper to the journal most appropriate to the strength of your study and reader interest in your topic. The most prestigious journal in your field may not be the most appropriate for your paper. Although some researchers always send their manuscripts to a leading journal first, these journals usually have a low acceptance rate, and it can harm your reputation to submit papers that are obviously inappropriate.

In selecting a journal, consider the following factors:

+ Reader interest
+ Impact factor
+ Circulation
+ Acceptance rate
+ Publication lag

Tables 12.2 through 12.5 provide information on circulation, impact factor, and acceptance rate for a selection of journals.

Publication lag is the interval between acceptance and publication; 15 years ago, the average lag was 7 months. This has decreased substantially in recent years, for example, *The New England Journal of Medicine* reports a 3-month lag.

The impact factor is a useful citation metric to compare journals. It gives you a sense of how often papers from that journal are cited by other researchers. For example, for a given journal, take the number of citations in 2016 from articles that were published in 2014 and 2015. Divide this by the total number of articles published by this journal during 2014 and 2015. For example, if a journal published 400 articles in 2014–2015 and had 20,000 citations in 2016 related to these 400 articles, the impact factor would be 50.00 (20,000/400).

TABLE 12.1	Order of Manuscript Sections with an Example of Page Limits for a Typical Journal	

Manuscript Section	Pages[a]
Cover letter	1–2
Title page	1
Abstract and keywords	1–2
Text	
Introduction	1
Methods	4–6
Results	3–4
Discussion, with conclusions	3–5
Acknowledgments and support information	1
References	3
Tables, with titles and footnotes	3
Figure legend page	1
Figures	4
Total	26–33

[a]Pages refer to double-spaced formatting with the exception of the cover letter, which should be single-spaced.

TABLE 12.2	Medical Journals Commonly Accessed Electronically

1. *The New England Journal of Medicine*
2. *Nature*
3. *Proceedings of the National Academy of Sciences of the United States of America (PNAS)*
4. *Journal of Biological Chemistry*
5. *Cell*
6. *The Journal of Neuroscience*
7. *Circulation*
8. *Blood*
9. *Pediatrics*
10. *The Lancet*
11. *Nature Neuroscience*
12. *Nature Genetics*
13. *Neuron*
14. *Cancer Research*
15. *Nature Medicine*
16. *The Journal of Immunology*
17. *Nature Methods*
18. *Clinical Infectious Diseases*
19. *Nature Biotechnology*
20. *NeuroImage*

NOTE: Based on 2015 journal usage statistics from the Vanderbilt University Eskind Biomedical Library.

TABLE 12.3	Impact Factor for a Selection of Medical Journals

Journal	Impact Factor
CA: A Cancer Journal for Clinicians	144.80
The New England Journal of Medicine	55.87
Chemical Reviews	46.57
The Lancet	45.22
Nature Reviews Drug Discovery	41.91
Nature Biotechnology	41.51
Nature	41.46
Annual Review of Immunology	39.33
Nature Reviews Molecular Cell Biology	37.81
Nature Reviews Cancer	37.40
JAMA (Journal of the American Medical Association)	35.29
Science	33.61
Cell	32.24
Nature Genetics	29.35
Nature Medicine	28.22
Journal of Clinical Oncology	18.44
Annals of Internal Medicine	17.81
BMJ (British Medical Journal)	17.45
Circulation	15.07
JAMA Internal Medicine	13.12
Proceedings of the National Academy of Sciences of the United States of America (PNAS)	9.67

NOTE: The first 10 journals are those with the highest impact factor; the others are a selection of notable journals.
Sources: ISI Web of Knowledge, Journal Citation Reports, 2014 JCR Science Edition, Thomson Reuters; or reported directly by the journal.

To find a journal's impact factor, see the Science Citation Index/Journal Citation Reports or ask the reference librarian at your medical library. The website for Web of Science, Journal Citation Reports ranks journals by impact factor within different medical specialties.

For example:

+ View a group of journals by (Subject Category)
+ Submit
+ Select a category (for example Endocrinology & metabolism)
+ View Journal data - Sort by: (Impact Factor)
+ Submit

To determine whether a journal is included in PubMed and currently indexed for MEDLINE, see http://www.ncbi.nlm.nih.gov/nlmcatalog/journals. Although many medical researchers ignore these lists, if you want your message to reach a large audience, these sources can be helpful.

| TABLE 12.4 | Approximate Acceptance Rate for Unsolicited Manuscripts for a Selection of Medical Journals | |

Journal	Approximate Percentage of Unsolicited Manuscripts Accepted (%)	Impact Factor[a]
The New England Journal of Medicine	<5[b]	55.87
Nature Genetics	5[c]	29.35
The Lancet	5[d]	45.22
Science	<7[e]	33.61
Annals of Internal Medicine	7[f]	17.81
BMJ (British Medical Journal)	7[g]	17.45
Nature	8[h]	41.46
The Journal of Clinical Investigation	8.7[i]	13.26
JAMA (Journal of the American Medical Association)	9.5[j]	35.29
Circulation	11[k]	15.07
Gastroenterology	10–12[l]	16.72
Journal of Bone and Joint Surgery British Volume	12.5[m]	3.31
Circulation Research	13[n]	11.02
JAMA Internal Medicine	13[o]	13.12
Diabetologia	<15[p]	6.67
Cell	10–20[q]	32.24
Mayo Clinic Proceedings	15–20[r]	6.27
Proceedings of the National Academy of Sciences of the United States of America (PNAS)	18[s]	9.67
JAMA Surgery	19[t]	3.94
Academic Medicine	20[u]	3.06
Emergency Medicine Journal	20[v]	1.84
The Journal of Pediatrics	22.8[w]	3.79
Journal of Ultrasound Medicine	26[x]	1.54
Diabetes	34[y]	8.10

NOTE: Acceptance rates are based on those reported on the journal's website or from personal communication with the journal's editors and staff.
[a]ISI Web of Knowledge, Journal Citation Reports, 2014 JCR Science Edition, Thomson Reuters; or reported directly by the journal.
[b]The New England Journal of Medicine office staff.
[c]http://schpubreviews.blogspot.com/2015/01/nature-genetics-with-abbreviation.html.
[d]http://www.thelancet.com/lancet/information-for-authors.
[e]http://www.sciencemag.org/site/feature/contribinfo/faq/#pct_faq.
[f]http://annals.org/public/press.aspx.
[g]http://www.bmj.com/about-bmj/resources-authors.
[h]http://www.nature.com/nature/authors/get_published/.
[i]https://acr.confex.com/acr/2011/recordingredirect.cgi/id/404.
[j]http://jama.jamanetwork.com/article.aspx?articleid=2110953&resultClick=3.
[k]http://circ.ahajournals.org/site/misc/stats.xhtml.
[l]http://www.gastrojournal.org/content/authorinfo.

(continued)

| TABLE 12.4 | Approximate Acceptance Rate for Unsolicited Manuscripts for a Selection of Medical Journals *(continued)* |

[m] http://www.bjj.boneandjoint.org.uk/site/menubar/info_authors.xhtml.
[n] http://circres.ahajournals.org/site/misc/stats.xhtml.
[o] http://archinte.jamanetwork.com/public/About.aspx.
[p] http://www.diabetologia-journal.org/aboutthejournal.html#supplements.
[q] Based on an e-mail from the Editorial Operations Supervisor from January 2016.
[r] http://www.mayoclinicproceedings.org/content/aims.
[s] http://www.pnas.org/site/authors/authorfaq.xhtml.
[t] http://archsurg.jamanetwork.com/public/About.aspx.
[u] http://journals.lww.com/academicmedicine/Documents/Academic%20Medicine%20Frequently%20Asked%20Questions%20for%20Authors.pdf.
[v] http://emj.bmj.com/site/about/.
[w] http://journalinsights.elsevier.com/journals/0022-3476/acceptance_rate.
[x] http://www.jultrasoundmed.org/site/misc/about.xhtml.
[y] http://diabetes.diabetesjournals.org/site/misc/stats.pdf.

| TABLE 12.5 | A Selection of High-Profile Medical and Biomedical Research Journals |

Journal Title	Impact Factor[a]	Acceptance Rate (%)
1. *The New England Journal of Medicine*	55.87	<5[b]
2. *Science*	33.61	<7[c]
3. *Nature*	41.46	7.8[d]
4. *JAMA (Journal of the American Medical Association)*	35.29	9.5[e]
5. *The Lancet*	45.22	5[f]
6. *Cell*	32.24	10–20[g]
7. *Annals of Internal Medicine*	17.81	7[h]
8. *Proceedings of the National Academy of Sciences of the United States of the America (PNAS)*	9.67	18.0[i]
9. *The Journal of Clinical Investigation*	13.26	8.7[j]
10. *Nature Genetics*	29.35	5[k]

NOTE: Approximate percentage of unsolicited manuscripts accepted.
[a] 2014 Impact Factor, Thomson Reuters Journal Citation Reports or reported directly by the journal's editor or staff.
[b] *The New England Journal of Medicine* Associate Editors.
[c] http://www.sciencemag.org/site/feature/contribinfo/faq/#pct_faq.
[d] http://www.nature.com/nature/authors/get_published/.
[e] http://jama.jamanetwork.com/article.aspx?articleid=2110953&resultClick=3.
[f] http://www.thelancet.com/lancet-information-for-authors/how-the-lancet-handles-your-paper.
[g] E-mail communication from the Editorial Operations Supervisor, January 2016.
[h] http://annals.org/public/about.aspx.
[i] http://www.pnas.org/site/authors/authorfaq.xhtml.
[j] https://acr.confex.com/acr/2011/recordingredirect.cgi/id/404.
[k] http://schpubreviews.blogspot.com/2015/01/nature-genetics-with-abbreviation.html.

Many manuscripts are rejected because the editors consider the material inappropriate for their journal. However, submitting the same paper to more than one journal simultaneously is highly unethical. See *The New England Journal of Medicine* for a clear set of guidelines on redundant publications (Kassirer & Angell, 1995) if you are in doubt about what is redundant. You are, however, allowed to submit a presubmission inquiry simultaneously to multiple journals.

GUIDELINES FOR AUTHORS

PRINCIPLE 57 • Read and follow your target journal's instructions for authors.

Follow the Uniform Requirements for Manuscripts Submitted to Biomedical Journals (see Appendix A) for general concepts, but more important, read and follow your target journal's instructions for authors.

Editors and reviewers report that most authors do not adhere to the journal's format and policy. As one reviewer commented, "*You must follow a rigid and unimaginative style of presentation and thinking if you wish to publish in respected journals.*"

PLANNING THE LENGTH OF YOUR MANUSCRIPT

PRINCIPLE 58 • Plan to submit an article that is slightly shorter than the average article published in the target journal.

See Figure 12.1, which is probably the most important graph in this book, and read several articles in the target journal, especially original research papers. As was mentioned in the key principles (see Chapter 1), the length of your manuscript should be close to the target journal's average and, ideally, slightly shorter. The number of tables and figures can be slightly more than average for your initial submission. Although it is very important to follow the guidelines for authors, the one exception is that you can submit a few extra graphs and tables.

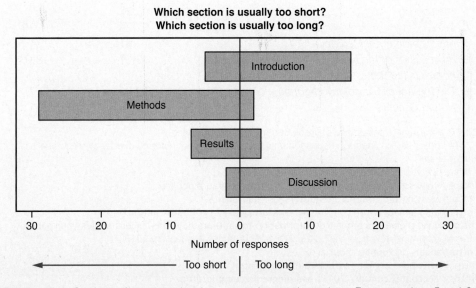

FIGURE 12.1. Sections of a manuscript that are too long and too short. From questions 5 and 6 of the Peer Review Questionnaire (Appendix B). *P* < .001 based on a chi-square test.

VITAL POINT

When in doubt, shorten.

Use short sentences and paragraphs. The best papers are concise. When asked which section of a manuscript usually is too short, one editor answered, "None!"

Journals measure article length by word count. *The New England Journal of Medicine* requires manuscripts to be less than 2,700 words. The *BMJ* no longer has a word limit but suggests about 4,000 words.

Authors address length limitations in two ways. Some authors write their findings, submit them for each coauthor to edit, and incorporate all of the changes into the final version, cutting material as necessary. Others set page limits for each section before they begin to write (see Table 12.1). This page limit method is generally much more efficient.

Plan the scope of your paper in detail. A detailed plan with an outline of section headings will help you to avoid writing a manuscript that is too long, too complex, has too many references, or is rambling.

Your paper should read like a published research report, not a dissertation, so do not include too many variables, hypotheses, or references. Remember, your goal is to convince the editor, reviewer, and eventually the journal's reader as simply as possible of the accuracy of your data and the utility of your results. As the distinguished pathologist Rudolf Virchow observed: "Brevity in writing is the best insurance for its perusal" (*Familiar Medical Quotations*, 1968).

Many researchers base the first paper that they submit for publication on their thesis or dissertation. Shortening this work to an acceptable length for publication is challenging and often never completed. Ask your advisor for permission to write your thesis or dissertation in two parts: an original research paper and a literature review, with all additional material placed in appendixes. This format makes it much easier to submit your thesis or dissertation for publication as two separate manuscripts. A change in medical and graduate school requirements for theses and dissertations to accommodate this two-part format (two manuscripts of publication length and quality) would have two benefits:

1. Students would learn how to write a publishable paper.
2. Students' findings would reach a broader audience.

If this is not an option, the good news is that your long thesis/dissertation should have all the information needed to write several publishable manuscripts. It is helpful to have a plan for how you will make this happen.

FOR MORE INFORMATION

The *Publication Manual of the American Psychological Association* (American Psychological Association, 2010) offers advice for converting a dissertation into a journal article.

WORKING WITH REVIEWERS AND EDITORS

PRINCIPLE 59 • Keep reviewers happy.

Table 12.6 offers suggestions for keeping reviewers happy.

Figure 12.2 ranks the reasons for outright rejection of manuscripts. The respondents reported that poor methods and inappropriate statistical analysis were most often responsible for rejection. In contrast, more than 20 years ago, Abby et al. (1994) reported that the most common reason for rejection was weak conclusions and discussion.

TABLE 12.6	How to Avoid Annoying a Reviewer[a]

What Reviewers Find Most Annoying

- When the abstract isn't crisp and the methods aren't clear, that creates confusion for me as a reviewer. Confusion is bad.
- It is challenging to read poorly written manuscripts. It is critically important for the senior author to really take the job of editing seriously. Many people do not know how to write. I know in my earlier manuscripts, my senior authors really challenged me to make my manuscripts better. It was harsh, but from their input, my papers were always accepted.
- Numbers don't add up; sloppy thinking and presentation
- Poor grammar and poor flow of ideas
- Poor syntax and punctuation; poorly written Methods section that defeats any fair evaluation of the study. At the very least, this means a reject and resubmit—and another review. Then only with that version can the manuscript be fairly evaluated, with the risk of further problems being identified.
- Poor writing and/or conceptualization; wordiness; excessive use of adverbs
- Excessive citation of authors' previous publications
- Manuscripts that far exceed word limits; failure to adequately discuss policy implications
- Poor grammar/need for proofreading; lack of inventiveness—seen the same type of study many times (but they don't realize it); poor/inappropriate data tables; discussion that ends with "More research is needed. . ."
- When the senior authors have clearly not read a junior's paper and allow it to be submitted with multiple English usage errors
- Poor methodology
- Poor style and sloppy presentation of data with obvious mistakes
- Self-promoting language with reference to own work only

Solutions to Avoid Annoying Reviewers

Methods
- Show a solid methodology and experimental design.
- Define the research question.

Results
- Identify the key elements in the text and consider placing them in tables.
- Use simple, easy-to-read tables and figures.
- Simplify busy tables.

Presentation
- Present the data in an unbiased manner and let the reader come to his own conclusions before interpreting the data in the Discussion.
- Organize the paper logically.
- Follow the rules of standard English usage.
- Be concise.
- Be sure the manuscript flows.
- Prepare the manuscript carefully.
- Correct all typographical errors.
- Avoid unnecessary complexity.
- Select and display good summary information.

(continued)

TABLE 12.6	**How to Avoid Annoying a Reviewer**[a] *(continued)*

Statistical analysis
- Use modern, robust analyses.
- Avoid, or control for, clear-cut bias.
- Explain all statistical methods clearly.
- Eliminate all statistical "snow jobs."

Discussion
- Explain the clinical relevance of the findings.

Originality
- Submit only work that has never been published.

Conclusions
- Explain how the evidence will be used.

Adherence to the journal's instructions
- Follow the journal's instructions for authors.
- Avoid having authors outnumber subjects.

[a]Paraphrased from answers provided to question 29 of the Peer Review Questionnaire (Appendix B).

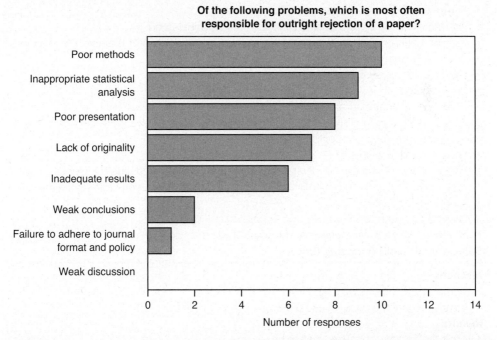

Of the following problems, which is most often responsible for outright rejection of a paper?

FIGURE 12.2. General problems responsible for rejection of manuscripts submitted for publication. From question 16 of the Peer Review Questionnaire (Appendix B). $P = .073$ based on a chi-square test.

PRINCIPLE 60 • Keep editors tickled pink.

Editors were bothered by many of the problems that reviewers mentioned, but editors were more concerned than reviewers about inappropriate statistical analysis. Table 12.7 gives specific suggestions for working with editors.

One editor wrote, "I get a lot of foreign manuscripts. I have learned to be patient with these authors, but I have absolutely no patience with English-speaking authors who send in poorly written manuscripts."

As you can see from Figure 12.3, the most common problems were poor presentation, lack of originality, and weak discussion.

Editors like to see that you have written a prespecified analysis plan and registered it with Clinical-Trials.gov (or the appropriate registry for your country). They are also interested in whether you have a clinically important study with quality data that will result in a high-impact paper.

When you have planned your study thoroughly, you are ready to move on to the second phase of the POWER principles: Observing.

TABLE 12.7	**How to Avoid Annoying an Editor[a]**

What Editors Find Most Annoying

- If the authors do not follow our requirements; format not in our journal style
- When author overinflates importance of work or writes to impress
- Failure to define knowledge gap
- Abstract is poorly composed and cannot be readily understood.
- Lack of manuscript transparency about the primary end point(s) of the registered study
- Jargon and poor grammar
- No page numbers, not double-spaced; horrible grammar
- Poor concept
- Poor writing; grammatical and typographic errors; sloppiness
- If submitted to an English-speaking journal, it is the failure to have the paper written by someone with adequate English writing skills
- Failure to follow guidance
- Lack of clarity: If you can't understand what the authors intended, and the manuscript is littered with typos, spelling mistakes, and grammatical errors, you can't send a manuscript out for review.
- Lack of pertinent detail to make an informed decision
- Having to work to figure out what the point of the manuscript is

Solutions to Avoid Annoying Editors

Methods
- Demonstrate a flawless study design.
- Clearly identify the problem and develop it logically with the research process.

Results
- Limit the number of figures and tables.
- Describe the tables and figures adequately.
- Verify that the tables and figures agree with the text.

(continued)

TABLE 12.7	How to Avoid Annoying an Editor[a] *(continued)*

Presentation
- Include an accurate summary of the results, correct inferences, and an appropriate discussion of both random and systematic error.
- Be clear, brief, and interesting.
- Ensure that the study is logical, with no obvious leaps.
- Organize the paper logically.
- Check spelling and grammar.
- Present the manuscript neatly and carefully.
- Eliminate redundancy.
- Use clear, precise language.
- Proofread the manuscript before submission.

Statistical analysis
- Include appropriate statistical analysis.
- Avoid technologic "pyrotechnics."
- Show that you understand your statistical analysis.

Discussion
- Do not repeat information in the Introduction, Discussion, and Conclusions.
- Explain the importance of the findings in a balanced way.
- Demonstrate an ability to understand the point.

Originality
- Explain the clinical relevance of the data.
- Show clinical correlation and follow-up.

Conclusions
- Be sure that the conclusions are completely supported by the Results and Methods.
- Include a well-written narrative and careful conclusions based on a good study design.

Adherence to the journal's instructions
- Prepare the manuscript according to the journal's instructions for authors.
- Follow the journal's format for the reference section.
- Follow the correct style for the target journal.

[a]Paraphrased from answers provided to question 29 of the Peer Review Questionnaire (Appendix B).

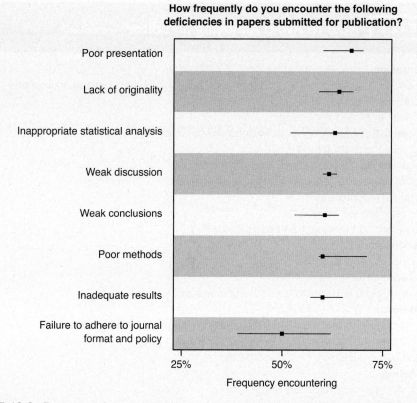

How frequently do you encounter the following deficiencies in papers submitted for publication?

FIGURE 12.3. Frequency of general problems with manuscripts submitted for publication. Answers are ranked by the median and bootstrap 95% confidence intervals using the sliding scale responses 0% (*never*) to 100% (*always*); from question 15 of the Peer Review Questionnaire (Appendix B). $P = .037$ based on the Friedman test.

OBSERVING

Key Questions to Answer in the Observing Phase:

- What if the study does not go as planned?
- How do I analyze these numbers?
- Has the trial been registered?
- Has the prespecified analysis plan and interim monitoring plan been documented?

Collecting Data and Handling Missing Data

MAKING OBSERVATIONS

PRINCIPLE 61 • Collect data in a scientifically rigorous and reproducible way.

After you have stated the problem, formulated the hypothesis, and designed the study, the next step in the scientific method is to collect your data or, in other words, make your observations. In this observing phase of your project, you obtain and record your findings. For experimental studies and randomized trials, in addition to observing, you manipulate exposure or treatment. Whichever study design you choose, recognizing the common pitfalls that occur during the observing phase will prepare you for the process of writing a publishable paper.

Successful research requires periodic monitoring of the study's progress. To ensure that the study is on track, the research team should meet regularly during the observing phase, either monthly or weekly, to ensure that the protocol is being followed, the data are complete and accurate, and the members of the team agree on all major points.

For studies that rely on recruiting research participants, consider using ResearchMatch.org (Fig. 13.1). This is a web-based recruitment registry that matches individuals who wish to participate in clinical research with investigators searching for volunteers (Harris et al., 2012).

http://www.researchmatch.org

KEEPING CAREFUL RECORDS

PRINCIPLE 62 • Record your research decisions as you conduct the study.

Writing within a well-organized framework will help readers to understand and follow the logic of your decisions. To build this framework, keep notes as you conduct the study and perform the data analysis to construct a chronological record of the project. This can be an appendix to your protocol.

Create an electronic folder of the following information:

1. The notes detailing your research decisions
2. The protocol along with any data coding conventions and abstracting guides
3. A blank data collection form/case report form
4. A full copy of the key papers that you plan to use as references in your paper
5. The instructions for authors from the target journal
6. A recent article from the target journal

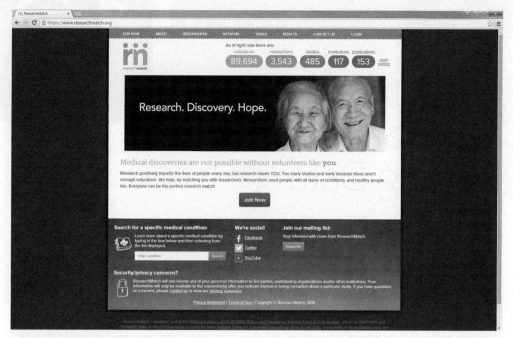

FIGURE 13.1. ResearchMatch.org. An online tool to help clinical researchers find research participants and to help those who are interested in participating in research find an appropriate project. See Harris et al. (2012). (Courtesy of Paul Harris.)

Keeping this information together and easily accessible will save you time. The biostatistician also will need this information during the analysis. Check with other members of your research team periodically at lab meetings to verify that you are all trying to answer the same exact research question. Record when and why your research team made major research decisions so that when you write the paper, you can describe these decisions clearly.

Be prepared to describe your decisions in sequential order, or reviewers may question your logic. For example, explain in detail why you excluded certain patients from the study. You had to solve the research problems in certain logical steps, so do not expect readers to understand the study in any other illogical sequence.

If your study involved unusual chemical substances, record their source, purity, potency, and lot number. For animal subjects, record details such as strain and supplier.

Record your notes and references in a document that is structured as a manuscript (i.e., Introduction, Methods, Results, Discussion, and References). Put additional detail in the appendix. With this approach, you will avoid redundant work and your paper will be partially finished before the analysis is completed. Remember, reviewers will be looking for a coherent framework in your study. This preparation will help them find it. Also document data sets, manuscripts, graphs, and protocols so that the next fellow in your lab could pick up your project and write another paper.

PRINCIPLE 63 • Follow the eligibility criteria precisely to be prepared for a scientific audit.

During the course of the study, the research team should ensure that the planned inclusion and exclusion criteria are being followed precisely as written in the protocol. Any changes should be made democratically, and the rationale for them should be well documented. Both the statistical and clinical implications of changes in eligibility must be considered carefully. Document the number of and reasons for missing eligible patients. Start to sketch out your CONSORT flowchart with this information.

PRINCIPLE 64 • Specify the randomization methods that you used.

To avoid ambiguity, explain in detail how randomization was conducted. For example, what was the temporal relation between randomization and treatment decisions? Describe the use of any "blocking" (randomization of subsets; e.g., randomizing within hospital or gender).

Example wording:

"Randomization was performed with the use of permuted blocks with stratification according to hospital center."

"A permuted, block-randomization plan was created with varying block sizes, with stratification according to hospital unit."

State which subjects were "blinded," during which phase, and to what information. During some blinded studies, participants discover which group they are assigned to and therefore become "unblinded." This situation must be described honestly.

Use blinding whenever it is ethical and improves your study, especially if the outcome variable is subjective. Use double-blinding when you can, evaluate how well it worked, and report your results carefully. Remember to assess blinding by asking participants at the end of their study to guess which group they were randomized to and report a kappa statistic for the agreement between their guess and actual assignment. Capturing this level of detail on all patients requires attention to detail.

DETECTING POTENTIAL PROBLEMS

PRINCIPLE 65 • Record the details of interventions and compliance in real time.

Compliance is the degree to which research participants followed the protocol. Poor compliance among research participants can create serious bias problems. Document and report compliance levels so that readers can draw sound conclusions. For randomized clinical trials, it is particularly important to explain how you monitored compliance with both arms of the study.

For studies of surgical procedures, describe the indications for the procedure and also the preoperative and postoperative conditions. Verify that you described the procedure accurately.

An experienced dedicated research nurse is essential to coordinate, manage, and document changes to the protocol and data collection forms.

PRINCIPLE 66 • Handle missing data using sophisticated modern methods.

Distinguish between missing data and the answer "no." A problem sometimes arises when researchers record the occurrence, but not the absence, of a factor (e.g., smoker). The data analyst does not know whether a blank means "no" or indicates a missing value. To avoid this problem, record the absence, not just the presence, of an outcome or risk factor. For surveys, provide options for "I don't know" or "undecided" so that these responses are not confused with missing data.

Although there are statistical methods of handling missing data, it is much more important and effective to work on minimizing missing data. A little effort in planning and oversight can greatly reduce the amount of missing data during a trial. You can set standards for maximal acceptable rates of missing data and monitor this. Educate your research staff regarding the importance of limiting missing data. Have them treat missing data as a continuous quality improvement project with graphs of percentage missing as a part of lab meetings. Work on continuously updating contact information to minimize loss to follow-up. Do record the reason that important information is missing. In your prespecified analysis plan, include a section on how you will minimize and handle missing data. Be transparent about how you handled missing data. Justify that the assumptions are valid if you use complete-case analysis or simple imputation methods such as last observation carried forward (LOCF) or baseline observation carried forward (BOCF). Consider using a more modern method such as multiple imputation or likelihood-based methods, which use your data to estimate the missing values. Other approaches to handling missing data include Bayesian methods and inverse probability weight methods. Collaborate with a biostatistician regarding these methods. Avoid case-wise deletion of missing data. With this approach, multivariate regression models exclude patients who have any missing data for any of the variables in the model, which can create a serious bias. For your key variables, analyze patterns of missing data. Include sensitivity analyses and tipping-point analyses in the appendix to show that the missing data does not change your conclusions and that your findings are robust.

FOR MORE INFORMATION
See Donders et al. (2006); Little et al. (2012); and Ware et al. (2012).

PRINCIPLE 67 • Use an adaptive design and monitor the sample size.

During a study, the research team may need to reevaluate the sample size. After some information is collected, investigators often have more realistic estimates of prevalence and effect size. Recalculating the sample size in accordance with these new estimates may help your research team to project a more realistic time frame. In addition, researchers often overestimate the number of recruitable patients, so monitor the sample size while there is still money in the budget to correct problems. Adaptive study designs that prespecify the rules for this can save time and should be used more often (Lorch et al., 2012). Also consider adaptive allocation methods, which use the accumulating outcomes data to determine treatment assignment.

Example wording:

"We used a group-sequential adaptive treatment-assignment design to minimize the number of participants exposed."

See the book by He et al. (2014), *Practical Considerations for Adaptive Trial Design and Implementation.*

14

Analyzing Data: Statistical Analysis for Reproducible Research

LAYING THE GROUNDWORK FOR STATISTICAL ANALYSIS

One editor provided the following three tips:

1. As John Tukey once said, "Far better an approximate answer to the right question, which is often vague, than an exact answer to the wrong question, which can always be made precise."
2. Get statistical help at the start of the study, during the study, when analyzing study data, and when writing the manuscript.
3. Recognize one's own biases and don't let these cloud objective interpretation of the data.

PRINCIPLE 68 • Build a database with reproducible statistical analysis in mind.

A common problem among medical researchers is finding an appropriate and efficient technique for data entry. Entering data in a spreadsheet is inefficient for most clinical research projects; using database management software or a web-based data entry tool, such as Research Electronic Data Capture (REDCap) (Harris et al., 2009), is usually more appropriate (Fig. 14.1). These methods make it easier to enter data and can prevent many forms of data entry errors. For very small projects with fewer than 25 patients and fewer than 10 variables, you can enter data in a spreadsheet or even directly into a statistical software package.

Whichever software package you use, when you enter data, use exact measurements. Avoid using subjective judgments that cannot be reproduced; if you cannot avoid subjective evaluations, at least give these variables numeric codes (e.g., 0 = no, 1 = yes). An example of subjective judgment would be "Was the patient at high risk of falling during the hospitalization?" Enter mutually exclusive data, such as "the most severe stage of the patient's disease," as one variable (stage 1 to 4), not as separate variables (e.g., stage 1: yes or no; stage 2: yes or no . . .). A good principle for data entry is MECE or "mutually exclusive and collectively exhaustive"—that is, a variable has options that do not overlap and cover all possibilities.

Sometimes, despite careful planning, you obtain text data (or string variables). When you build your database, look for ways to convert these data to numbers.

Make all necessary clinical research decisions before you begin to enter data. For example, did the patient have a stage 2 or a stage 3 pressure ulcer? Do not enter "2 to 3" and then wait until the analysis is performed to classify the patient.

Entering data as text, and without proper planning, limits the value of your database (Fig. 14.2). Remember that building a database is expensive. Because computer memory and speed are no longer rate-limiting factors, it is not necessary to record data in the least possible space. Recording data in a format that a statistical package can use for multivariate analysis is more important than conserving memory.

A common mistake is to ask a programmer or student with no data analysis experience to develop a custom database. These people often include informatics "bells and whistles" (unnecessary features that make the program look sophisticated) but produce a database that cannot be analyzed easily (Fig. 14.3).

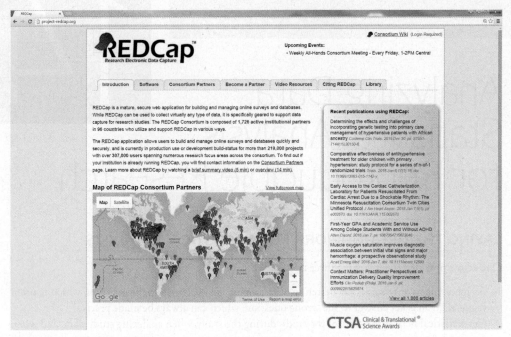

FIGURE 14.1. Research Electronic Data Capture (REDCap). This is a modern robust method of collecting data for a medical research project. See Harris et al. (2009). (Courtesy of Paul Harris.)

Ten Data Entry Commandments

1. Enter all, or most, of the data as numbers. Avoid entering letters, words, string variables (e.g., NA, 22%, <3.6), or anything that resembles a cartoon curse word grawlix (*&#%!@?!,). In Excel, all columns, with the exception of names and text comments, should be formatted as numbers or dates (not as general or text).

2. Give each column a unique, simple, one-word name, eight characters or less with no spaces, beginning with a letter, and place this name in the first row.

3. Put only one variable in a column. Do not combine variables in the same column.

4. Enter each patient (or unit of analysis) on a separate line, beginning on the second line/row.

5. Give each research participant or patient a unique case number (1, 2, 3, etc.) in the first column. Delete patient name, SS#, MR#, and any identifying information before sending it to a biostatistician. Always save the spreadsheet with a password.

6. Enter cases and controls in the same spreadsheet. Use one variable to define the control group (TREATED: 0 = no, 1 = yes).

7. Quantify. Enter continuous measurements when possible.

8. Create a simple guide (or key) using a word processor to explain variable abbreviations, value coding, and how missing values were entered. Be consistent.

9. Think through the analysis before collecting any data.

10. Have a biostatistician or other methodologist review the coding before data entry and again after the first 10 patients have been entered.

FIGURE 14.2. Ten data entry commandments. Guidelines for data entry.

	A	B	C	D	E	F	G	H	I	J	K
1	Comparison of Drug A and Drug B										
2	Drug A	Age of Patient	Patient Gender	Height (inches)	Weight (pound)	24hrhct	Blood pressure	Tumor stage	Race	Date enrolled	Complications
3											
4											
5	1	25	Male	61"	>350	38%	120/80	2-3	Hispanic	1/15/99	no
6	2	65+	female	5'8"	161	32	140/90	II	White	2/05/1999	yes
7	3	?	Male	120cm		12	>160/110	IV	Black	Jan 98	yes, pneumonia
8	4	31	m	5'6"	obese	40	140 sys 105 dias	?	African-American	?	
9	5	42	f	>6 ft	normal	39	missing	=>2	W	Feb 99	
10	6	45	f	5.7	160	29	80/120	NA	B	last fall	n
11	7	unknown	?	6	145	35	normal	1	W	2/30/99	n
12	8	55	m	72	161.45	12/39	120/95	4	African-American	6-15-00	y
13	9	6 months	f	66	174	38	160/110	3	Asian	14/12/00	y
14	10	21	f	5'							
15											
16	Drug B										
17	1	55	m	61	145	normal	120/80 120/90	IV	Native American	6/20/	3
18	2	45	f	4"11	166	?	135/95	2b	none	7/14/99	n
19	3	32	male	5'13"	171	38	140/80	not staged	NA	8/30/99	n
20	4	44	na	65	?	40	120/80	2	?	09/01/00	n
21	5	66	fem	71	0	41	140/90	4	w	Sep 14th	y, sepsis
22	6	71	unknown	172	199	38	>160/110	3	b	unknown	y, died
23	7	45	m	?	204	32	140 sys 105 dias	1	b	12/25/00	n
24	8	34	m	NA	145	36	130	3	w	July 97	n
25	9	13	m	66	161	39	166/115	2a	w	06/06/99	n
26	10	66	m	68	176	41	1120/80	3	w	01/21/58	n
27											
28	Average	45		65	155	38					

FIGURE 14.3. Spreadsheet from hell. An example of the improper way to enter data for a medical research project.

It is best to have someone with years of experience in analyzing data decide how the variables will be stored and oversee database design from the beginning (Fig. 14.4). For most clinical research projects, creating a database with database management software or a web-based tool (such as REDCap) is more efficient than hiring a programmer to customize a database with a low-level programming language.

Label each variable with a logical, easy-to-remember field name (variable name) that will be valid for most statistical software (i.e., eight characters or fewer, no spaces, and a letter at the beginning—age, male_gender, bmi1, diabetes, etc.). Using these field names simplifies the translation between the database and statistical software. Although many programs now allow for variable names longer than eight characters, it is wise to use short names where possible (Table 14.1). After your data are completely entered into the database program, transfer the information to a statistical software package for the data analysis. Run a report in the database program or use "File, Save As" to create a file that the statistical package can import (e.g., a CSV [comma-separated values] file or Excel; see Table 14.2).

If you have trouble translating files between software packages, you can use the Stat/Transfer software (Circle Systems). This software package allows you to translate your files into someone else's format or to translate someone else's files into a software package that you prefer. The most recent version of most statistical software packages can import and export computer files for a variety of software packages with simple commands of "File, Open, Data, and Files of type" or "File, Save As . . . , Save as type."

Whenever you transfer data, the following suggestions will simplify the process:

+ Whenever possible, store all data for a research project in one flat file/spreadsheet.
+ Make each row a case (i.e., each patient or unit of analysis is entered on a separate line).
+ Place each variable in a different column (i.e., avoid systolic/diastolic blood pressure [BP] in one column).
+ Avoid scientific notation (e.g., convert 3.2×10^{-4} to 0.00032).
+ Convert measurements that are extremely small or extremely large to a scale with absolute values between 1 and 1,000. For example, convert 0.0000023 g to 2.3 μg.
+ Assign patients to their correct groups before you enter any data. Moreover, because ambiguous values (e.g., 25% to 50%) cannot be analyzed, use actual values rather than ranges or inequalities. For example, the actual age is better than <65 versus ≥65. You can collapse into categories later, but you cannot "uncollapse" categories. Avoid this dichotomania.
+ Enter height and weight separately rather than entering a calculated body mass index or a category such as obese (yes/no).
+ Assign codes (e.g., −1, 999) for missing values or leave them blank.
+ Code results consistently. If "no" is coded as 0 for one question, be sure that "absent" is coded as 0 for the other questions. For example:

Perinatal mortality:	0[] No	1[] Yes
Diabetes:	0[] Absent	1[] Present

+ Always use a unique sequential case number to identify each patient.
+ Code variables as questions, such as "diabetes" (Does this patient have type 2 diabetes?).
+ Code most answers as 0 = No, 1 = Yes.

PREPARING THE DATA

PRINCIPLE 69 • "Clean" and then "freeze" the data well in advance of your deadline.

Before you perform any analysis, use a statistical software package to perform descriptive statistics, frequencies, and cross-checks to screen the data thoroughly and detect potential problems (e.g., pregnant males). Create new variables to check the entered data. For example, subtract the diastolic BP from the

	A CASE	B GROUP	C AGE	D SEX	E HT	F WT	G HCT	H BPSYS	I BPDIAS	J STAGE	K RACE	L DATE1	M COMPLIC
2	1	1	25	1	61	350	38	120	80	3	3	1/15/1999	0
3	2	1	65	2	68	161	32	140	90	2	1	2/5/1999	1
4	3	1	25	1	47	150	38	160	110	4	2	1/15/1998	1
5	4	1	31	1	66	161	40	140	105	2	2	4/1/1999	0
6	5	1	42	2	72	177	39	130	70	2	1	2/15/1999	0
7	6	1	45	2	67	160	29	120	80	1	2	3/6/1999	0
8	7	1	44	1	72	145	35	120	80	1	1	2/28/1999	0
9	8	1	55	1	72	161	39	120	95	4	2	6/15/2000	1
10	9	1	0.5	2	66	174	38	160	110	3	4	12/14/2000	1
11	10	1	21	2	60	155	40	190	120	2	2	11/14/2000	0
12	11	2	55	1	61	145	41	120	80	4	5	6/20/1999	1
13	12	2	45	2	59	166	39	135	95	2	1	7/14/1999	0
14	13	2	32	1	73	171	38	140	80	1	1	8/30/1999	0
15	14	2	44	2	65	155	40	120	80	2	2	9/1/2000	0
16	15	2	66	2	71	145	41	140	90	4	1	9/14/1999	1
17	16	2	71	1	68	199	38	160	110	3	2	1/14/1999	1
18	17	2	45	1	69	204	32	140	105	1	2	12/25/2000	0
19	18	2	34	1	66	145	36	130	75	3	1	7/15/1997	0
20	19	2	13	1	66	161	39	166	115	2	1	6/6/1999	0
21	20	2	66	1	68	176	41	120	80	3	1	1/21/1998	0

FIGURE 14.4. Spreadsheet from heaven. An example of the proper way to enter data for a medical research project.

TABLE 14.1 Example of a Fixed-Field or Fixed-Width Text Format File

Case	Group	BPs	Sex	Race	Age	LOS	ICU
1	3	120	1	1	24.6	22	9
2	2	80	2	3	0.5	15	1
3	3	130	1	5	−99.9	10	0

BPs = systolic blood pressure; LOS = length of stay; ICU = intensive care unit.

systolic to ensure that these values were not transposed. Most databases contain many types of human and technologic errors. Do not skip this important step. Although you may have deadlines and limited free time, if you hurry to analyze your data, you will be wastefully repeating the analysis as you uncover one error at a time. For this reason, invest enough time and effort to clean the data completely.

Budget your time backward from your deadline. Determine how much time you need for writing, creating graphs, performing analysis, cleaning, collecting data, and planning. After data for the first 10 patients are entered, check the accuracy and completeness of the data. Meet with your research team to discuss any problems and set minimum standards (e.g., all patients must have age and gender recorded). For long-term projects, clean the data periodically by checking all inconsistencies and correcting errors. Document all changes so that you are prepared for any type of scientific audit.

During the planning phase, you should have identified strategies to prevent many errors, such as upper and lower limits for age in the data entry screen. Some errors, however, always occur, despite the most careful planning, so expect them. Some errors cannot be spotted simply by looking at extreme values. With two highly correlated variables, such as hemoglobin and hematocrit, create a scatter plot to identify values that are improbable because they are off the diagonal trend line. Another way to screen your data for errors is to run a correlation between the sequential case identification (ID) number and all other variables. If you find a significant correlation for a variable, you can explore the reason and fix the errors. For example, the lab changed halfway through the study and the second lab reports the values with different units.

Cleaning is needed when data are stored using different units (e.g., age is recorded in years, months, and weeks). Recording age in years with one decimal place usually is adequate. For example, a 6-month-old infant's age would be recorded as 0.5 (years), and a 7-month-old infant's age would be recorded as 0.6 (7/12). Program your database to calculate the exact age from the date of birth and the date of admission.

You can simplify the cleaning process by recording the case number on each data collection form and all related laboratory slips or monitoring strips. Filing these forms in case number order will make it much easier to check suspicious values.

TABLE 14.2 Example of a Free-Field Format File or Comma-Separated Values File

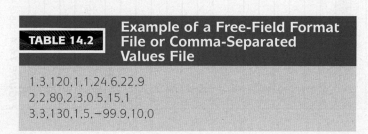

```
1,3,120,1,1,24.6,22,9
2,2,80,2,3,0.5,15,1
3,3,130,1,5,−99.9,10,0
```

Complete any missing data or code it as "unknown." Correct the original source of the data (the master home of the database or spreadsheet) and transfer the corrected data back to the statistical package. Check with the research team to determine whether any cases should be excluded from the analysis because essential data are missing. Document any changes made in the data and include this information in your research notes to create an audit trail. Build an audit trail to make your research reproducible. The appendix of your protocol or paper is a useful place to document any changes that might be needed for this audit.

After the database is completely cleaned, the research team should agree to freeze the data. Freezing the data means that no data will be added or changed during the next phase of the analysis. Freezing the data saves time and money, but freezing uncleaned data obviously is a waste of time.

FOR MORE INFORMATION

See Chapter 15 of Hulley et al. (2013).

AVOIDING COMMON PROBLEMS

PRINCIPLE 70 • Learn how to avoid common statistical problems.

Nature speaks but one language, and that language is mathematics. Unfortunately, many medical researchers become rusty with the language of mathematics, particularly the language of statistics. Because many health care professionals fail to learn how to use statistics as part of their formal education, mastering statistics often requires self-education. Fortunately, modern statistical software now makes statistical analysis much easier and more interesting to learn.

FOR MORE INFORMATION

The following books provide a good introduction to statistics: *Study Design and Statistical Analysis: A Practical Guide for Clinicians Public Health Researchers* (Katz, 2011), *Practical Statistics for Medical Research* (Altman, 1991), *Basic & Clinical Biostatistics* (Dawson & Trapp, 2005), *Basic Statistics for the Health Sciences* (Kuzma & Bohnenblust, 2004), *Essential Medical Statistics* (Kirkwood & Sterne, 2003), and *Basic Statistical Analysis* (Sprinthall, 2011).

Another excellent resource of statistical software instructions is the UCLA Statistical Consulting Group's Institute for Digital Research and Education (IDRE) (http://www.ats.ucla.edu/stat/). The "Data Analysis Examples" provide the recipes for common statistical tests for SAS, IBM SPSS, Stata, and R.

http://www.ats.ucla.edu/stat/dae/

If you are interested in learning the R software, Mike Marin has created an excellent series of YouTube videos.

https://www.youtube.com/user/marinstatlectures/playlists

Interpreting the Data

PREPARING FOR DATA ANALYSIS

PRINCIPLE 71 • Interpret the data.

After you collect and enter the data, and then correct errors and freeze the data, you are ready to analyze. Interpretation is the fifth step in the scientific method. Because this analysis is still part of the observing phase, remember to keep an open mind and let the numbers reveal the truth. Do not try to force the numbers to prove your point. Analyzing the results of a clinical research study can be complicated; therefore, collaborating with an experienced and resourceful biostatistician is always prudent. Even Einstein consulted mathematicians.

The key is to find a biostatistician who has adequate experience, a broad understanding of statistics, sufficient time, and the motivation to help you. To find such a person, ask a well-published colleague for a referral. Ideally, you will want to develop a long-term collaboration with a biostatistician. Avoid the mistake that many medical researchers make: They do not allot sufficient time, funding, or resources for data analysis. Although most modern statistical software packages now are fairly easy to use, it still takes considerable time and thought to analyze data. The lead author on the paper should reproduce all of the analysis that the biostatistician produces—ideally with different statistical software. This author should also be able to explain to colleagues in plain English how all of the statistical methods were performed and exactly what the results mean.

The following sections describe the more common statistical pitfalls (Table 15.1).

AVOIDING COMMON PROBLEMS

PRINCIPLE 72 • Avoid common problems with data analysis.

The Nobel laureate, Gertrude Elion, said that most data analysis errors occur when researchers make the following mistakes:

+ They do not apply common sense to the data.
+ They do not try to repeat experiments.
+ They have poorly matched control groups.

TABLE 15.1	Most Common Data Analysis Mistakes in Medical Research

The statistical tests are not appropriate or they do not provide necessary statistics to support their claim.

Use of P value without considering clinical implications

Distinguish the generalizability of the results

Understanding the "bias" or value placed on subgroup analysis

Searching and highlighting only statistically significant findings—data torturing

Conclusions not in line with their results

Focus on P value, failure to take into account the magnitude of the findings

Failure to look at the result in the context of other studies on the topic

Overbelief in positive findings

Sloppy interpretation of the findings

Overemphasis of statistical differences without clinical importance

Inferring no association based on P values of underpowered studies (clinical vs. statistical significance); giving too much credence to one study

Failing to know the limitations of meta-analysis

Incorrect interpretation of statistical measures (e.g., OR, RR)

Improper selection of statistical test

Invalid interpretation of statistical significance

Failure to use time-to-event analyses when there is censoring in the data

Inferring prediction and even causality from cross-sectional correlational data

Use of unvalidated measures

Failure to evaluate methodologic limitations

Failure to accurately assess clinical relevance

Complete dismissal or blind acceptance of author's conclusions

Failure to follow the intention-to-treat principle

Loss of data during follow-up

Lack of clarity about limitations of the study

They like the studies that support their hypothesis more than those which are contrary.

Analyses do not appear to have been justified or planned in advance, that is, it is a fishing expedition for a significant result.

Not controlling for confounding

Researchers often have access to variables that would control for sampling variation, for example, but do not use them to see if their primary outcome is real or not. Seeing nonsignificant results as unimportant—often, these are useful but overlooked.

Not being aware of how the selection biases inherent to participants in medical research projects

Not understanding how to handle missing data

Not accounting for possible confounders

Incomplete accounting for confounding and bias

Measurement error not accounted for

Missing data not handled appropriately

Mistaking associations for cause–effect

Results not generalizable

Ignorance of statistical methods

Failure to adequately conduct descriptive analysis prior to more advance analysis

(continued)

TABLE 15.1	Most Common Data Analysis Mistakes in Medical Research *(continued)*

Providing confusing tables and figures

Overstating the implications of their results

Inappropriate statistical modeling

Overfitting regression models

Lack of understanding of limitations on data measures

Basic statistical errors

Overinterpretation of data

Saving important data relevant to the current manuscript for a future publication ("salami slicing")

Reliance on P values to make conclusions

Use of multivariable models without appropriate considerations

Lack of attention to missing data

Lack of understanding of how the design of the study drives the kinds of conclusions that can be fairly drawn from a study leads to erroneous conclusions and overstatements.

The belief that a P value of $<.05$ means the finding is important and P value $>.05$ means the finding is meaningless

Making analytic decisions based on how it affects the P value rather than on what the correct approach is for the question being asked

Paying too much attention to P values and not enough to "The Full Monty"

Drawing incorrect conclusions

Not accounting for confounding variables

Using only basic tests like chi-square or t-test and make overly broad conclusions

They do not consider context.

They do not understand the limitations of the study.

They do not understand sample size.

Concluding that because the P value from a study is $<.05$, the observed effect must the "true"

Applying data beyond the limitations of the population that was studied

Conflating association with causality

Not accounting for confounding

Being very "P" centered

Unable to understand appropriate statistical tests and limitations

Frequently, they skip the methodology section and sometimes draw unwarranted conclusions about the results of the study that were either never the intent of the study or are not supported by the actual work done in the study.

Lack of understanding of statistical methods and presentation

A tendency to overexaggerate positive results particularly if they are presented as a relative benefit rather than an absolute benefit

Sample size too small

Methods not sufficiently rigorous to make the stated claims

Control group not analogous to experimental population

Inappropriate study design; inappropriate statistical analysis; overinterpretation of results

Not considering the study design

Not considering sources of bias

Acting on a small subset of research manuscripts on a particular clinical topic

Inadequate control group; inadequate follow-up; insufficient number of observations

Inadequate recognition of underpowered studies; inadequate knowledge of database limitations

(continued)

TABLE 15.1	Most Common Data Analysis Mistakes in Medical Research *(continued)*

Extrapolating results
Failure to put results in context
Poor reporting of data (Check the math!)
Incomplete data
Inadequate sample
Poorly controlled variables
Retrospective data given too much weight
Lacking deep knowledge regarding statistics/study design
Lack of mechanistic assessment around observed associations
Inappropriate statistical prediction model validation
Irrelevant or missing comparison of statistical model with alternative
Unclear handling of missing data/value
Confusing relative and absolute risk or benefit and not understanding the concept of NNT or NNH
Not understanding how the study population compares to their own patients, or doesn't
Confusing statistical significance with clinical importance
Choosing the wrong statistical approach
Failure to account for and correct for multiple observations (hypotheses tested)
Extending the conclusions beyond the limits of the data
Implying causality where they should not
Failure to do a power calculation to determine adequate sample size
Failure to control for key confounders and biases
Failure to account for or report on missing data
Failure to account for biases specific to the type of analysis
Failure to determine specific subgroup analyses a priori
Cohorts are too small to be meaningful.
Selection bias or insufficient controls
Incorrect method of statistical analysis of data
Incorrect use of statistical measures of association
Inadequate assessment of potential confounders and/or effect modifiers
Too little information about exposure and outcome variables

OR = odds ratio; RR = relative risk; NNT = number needed to treat; NNH = number needed to harm.
From question 2 on the Peer Review Questionnaire (Appendix B).

PRINCIPLE 73 • Avoid dichotomania.

Dividing a continuous variable, such as body mass index, into two categories, such as "not obese/obese" is generally problematic because there are few true discontinuities like this in nature. Researchers often dichotomize because they have learned a few statistical and graphical methods for categorical variables but lack the more advanced skills to use continuous and nonlinear variables. In addition, the "optimal" cut point rarely replicates, so it is better to use the continuous variable and report the odds ratio or slope. To avoid these dichotomania problems, learn how to use regression models with restricted cubic splines and how to create spline (nonlinear) graphs.

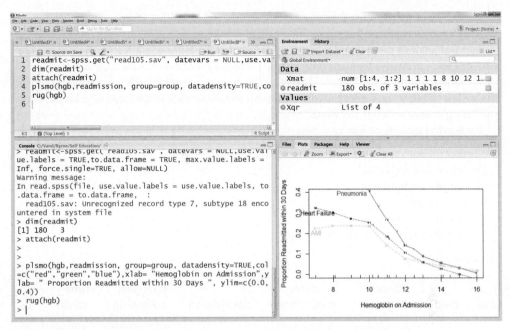

FIGURE 15.1. RStudio. An example of how to use the R software with the RStudio interface to create a spline graph. (Courtesy of Bill Carney, RStudio, Inc.)

Although the R software is difficult to learn, it is an excellent way of creating customized spline graphs. Follow these steps:

Download R.

https://www.r-project.org/

Download RStudio to provide an interface that makes the R software easier to use.

http://www.rstudio.com/products/rstudio/

Install and load the package Hmisc.

To create a spline graph of the risk of readmission by hemoglobin level for 3 diagnostic groups, you would use this command in R.

plsmo(hgb,readmission, group=group, datadensity=TRUE)

Note: plsmo = plot smoothed estimates.

Use the command "?plsmo" to see more advanced options (see Fig. 15.1).

PRINCIPLE 74 • Use epidemiologic methods to make the analysis and presentation of your data more sophisticated.

Epidemiology is the study of the spread and cause of diseases and injuries in a human population. Originally, epidemiologists studied epidemics, but now, most focus on clinical research, prevention, and population health. Many epidemiologic techniques can be used to strengthen clinical research papers. Here are just three examples:

1. Person-years
2. Survival analysis
3. The dose–response relationship

Person-years are the sum of the number of years that each member of a population has been afflicted by a certain condition (e.g., years of treatment with a certain drug).

Survival analysis can be used to compare groups that are followed up for varying periods. This technique also can be used for many other clinical problems in addition to survival. It allows you to adjust for varying lengths of follow-up and uses the maximum amount of information, even from patients who are lost to follow-up. Before you collect data that require survival analysis, consult a biostatistician who has experience with this technique.

For survival analysis, be sure to record:

+ Whether the outcome of interest occurred (died, 0 = no, 1 = yes)
+ The date of first diagnosis
+ The date of randomization
+ The date of death
+ The date of last follow-up
+ Whether the patient was lost to follow-up

For example:

case	died	date_diagnosis	date_randomized	date_death	date_last_follow-up	time_days	lost_fu
1	0	06/21/1995	07/15/1995	—	01/29/2006	3851	1
2	1	12/14/1996	01/15/1997	05/13/2007	—	3770	0
3	1	03/04/1997	05/14/1997	06/03/1998	—	415	0

Include several variables that measure the severity of disease and any potentially confounding factors. A thorough literature search is essential to identify all variables needed to answer the research question—convincingly. Record in detail why some respondents were lost to follow-up and analyze how the lost patients differ from the patients who remained in the study. This will be important when you are showing reviewers that you have an unbiased data set, or at least you understand the bias.

The dose–response relationship is a change in the amount, intensity, or duration of exposure associated with a change in the risk of a specified outcome. This gradient effect can improve a Results section that contains only borderline evidence of cause and effect by showing that outcome changes with each change in exposure.

Example 15–1.
The incidence of type 2 diabetes decreases with days of aerobic exercise per week.

Univariate Analysis

COMMONLY USED UNIVARIATE TESTS USED IN MEDICAL RESEARCH (TABLE 16.1)

PRINCIPLE 75 • Master the chi-square test and the Student's *t*-test.

Univariate is defined as "characterized by or depending on only one random variable."[1] Univariate analysis is a set of mathematical tools to assess the relationship between one independent predictor variable and one dependent outcome variable. A considerable proportion of medical research questions can be answered with two univariate tests: the chi-square test and the Student's *t*-test. Therefore, a good place to start your self-education in biostatistics is in mastering these two tools. Figure 16.1 can help you to decide which statistical test to use.

Because univariate analysis evaluates one predictor variable at a time, it cannot simultaneously adjust for other factors, such as age. And because univariate analysis is one-dimensional, it is too simplistic to definitively answer many clinical research problems. Still, it is an essential first step in data analysis.

> **VITAL POINT**
>
> Never bypass univariate analysis and proceed directly to multivariate analysis or regression models. Be sure that you understand the univariate results fully before you create complex multivariate regression models.

Bivariate is defined as "of, relating to, or involving two variables."[1] Because this term often is misused, I suggest that you avoid using it. Stick with univariate versus multivariate.

To master the chi-square and the *t*-test, you must learn the relationship between the statistic test value, degrees of freedom, and the *P* value. The following principles should make this clear. Most statistical tests are based on the concept of using a ratio of signal to noise to create a test statistic. This test statistic is combined with a conversion factor, called "degrees of freedom," that is based on the sample size or number of categories. This test statistic is then converted into a *P* value, or probability that results that you observed (or larger) could have occurred by chance alone—if we assume there was no difference.

> **VITAL POINT**
>
> Use two-sided tests and *P* values with the exception of rare cases where the study design requires a one-sided test, such as in noninferiority trials.

Signal/Noise = test statistic; test statistic + degrees of freedom → *P* value

Type of Test	Difference/Association	Pairing	Dependent Variable: Level of Measurement	Dependent Variable: Distribution	No. of Groups	N	Paired Links	Appropriate Statistical Method	Nonparametric Links
Question 1	Question 2	Question 3	Question 4	Question 5	Question 6	Question 7			
Univariate	Difference	Unmatched/independent	Interval	Normal	2			Student's t-test	
			Interval	Normal	≥2			One-way ANOVA	
			Ordinal	Nonnormal	2			Mann-Whitney U test/Wilcoxon rank-sum test	
			Ordinal	Nonnormal	>2			Kruskal-Wallis H test	
			Nominal		2	<20		Fisher's exact test/LRT	
			Nominal		≥2	≥20		Chi-square	
			Nominal	Time-to	≥2			Kaplan-Meier, log-rank	
		Matched/paired	Interval	Normal	2			Paired t-test	
			Interval	Normal	≥2			Mixed-effects, repeated measures ANOVA	
			Ordinal	Nonnormal	2			Wilcoxon signed-rank test	
			Ordinal	Nonnormal	>2			Friedman test	
			Nominal		2			McNemar's test/binomial/sign test	
	Association/correlation		Interval	Normal				Pearson's r	
			Ordinal	Nonnormal				Spearman's r_s	
			Nominal/ordinal					Chi-square for trend test	
			Nominal/nominal					Kappa	
Multivariate	Association	Unmatched/independent	Interval					Linear regression ANOVA/GLM ANCOVA	
			Ordinal					Ordinal regression	
			Nominal		≥2			Logistic regression	
	Difference		Nominal		≥2			Mantel-Haenszel test	
			Nominal	Time-to	≥2			Cox proportional-hazards	
		Paired			2			Conditional logistic regression	

ANOVA = analysis of variance; LRT = likelihood ratio test; GLM = generalized linear model; ANCOVA = analysis of covariance.

FIGURE 16.1. Flowchart of common inferential statistics. To use this chart, answer the following seven questions and follow the answers from the left to right on the flowchart.

1. Which type of test do you need: univariate or multivariate? (Start with a univariate test and then proceed to a multivariate test to adjust for confounding factors and regression modeling.)

2. Do you want to test for a difference between groups or for an association between variables? An example of an association between variables is the following: "Is length of stay in the hospital associated with age?"

3. Were the groups matched (paired) or were they unmatched (unpaired - independent)?

4. What is the level of measurement for the dependent (outcome) variable? Is it nominal (categorical), ordinal, or interval (continuous)?

5. Is the dependent (outcome) variable normally distributed? If your histogram forms a bell-shaped curve, assume that it is normal; otherwise, assume that it is not normal. Note: This is the classical method of selecting a statistical test. A more modern robust method is to assume nonnormal for all variables and use nonparametric methods. When analyzing time to death (or some event that has not occurred for all patients), select time-to methods.

6. How many groups are there for the independent (predictor) variable?

7. What is the total sample size?

TABLE 16.1	Most Commonly Used Inferential Statistical Techniques in Modern Medical Research

Rank	Test
1.	Kaplan-Meier method
2.	Logistic regression
3.	Cox proportional-hazards
4.	Log-rank test
5.	Chi-square (Pearson χ^2)
6.	Fisher's exact test
7.	Wilcoxon rank-sum test/Mann-Whitney U test
8.	Student's t-test or unpaired t-test
9.	Mantel-Haenszel method
10.	Linear regression analysis
11.	Poisson regression
12.	Mixed-effects models
13.	Analysis of covariance (ANCOVA)
14.	Generalized estimating equations (GEEs)
15.	Chi-square test for trend
16.	Kruskal-Wallis one-way analysis of variance (ANOVA) by ranks procedure
17.	Paired t-test
18.	One-way ANOVA
19.	Wilcoxon signed-rank test
20.	ANOVA (two-way)
21.	Kappa statistic/weighted kappa
22.	McNemar's chi-square test
23.	Likelihood-ratio chi-square test
24.	Ordinal logistic regression
25.	Conditional logistic regression
26.	Pearson's product-moment correlation
27.	General linear model/generalized linear model
28.	Repeated measures ANOVA
29.	Pooled logistic regression
30.	Binomial test

Based on a review of original articles and their protocols in the online supplementary appendix published in *The New England Journal of Medicine* in 2015, Volume 372, Issues 1–26.

USING THE CHI-SQUARE TEST

PRINCIPLE 76 • Use the chi-square test for most categorical variables.

Categorical variables are the simplest to analyze because they classify (e.g., smokers vs. nonsmokers) rather than measure (e.g., cigarettes per day) as continuous variables do. Figures 16.2, 16.3, and 16.4 show the concepts and terms that commonly are used with a two-by-two (2×2) table. The chi-square test is used to determine whether the actual proportion, in two or more groups, differs significantly from the proportion expected by chance alone.

Results of a screening test

		Positive	Negative
Diseased	Yes	a	b
	No	c	d

FIGURE 16.2. Results of a screening test in a 2 × 2 table.

Sensitivity	$\dfrac{a}{a+b} \times 100$	Percentage of subjects with the disease who have a positive test result
Specificity	$\dfrac{d}{c+d} \times 100$	Percentage of subjects without the disease who have a negative test result
Positive predictive value	$\dfrac{a}{a+c} \times 100$	Likelihood that a positive test result indicates disease
Negative predictive value	$\dfrac{d}{b+d} \times 100$	Likelihood that a negative test result indicates absence of disease
Likelihood ratio for positive results	$\dfrac{a/(a+b)}{c/(c+d)}$	Odds of a positive test result in patients with disease versus odds of a positive test result in patients without disease
Likelihood ratio for negative results	$\dfrac{b/(a+b)}{d/(c+d)}$	Odds of a negative test result in patients with disease versus odds of a negative test result in patients without disease

FIGURE 16.3. Predictive value measurements.

Results of an HIV test

		Positive	Negative
HIV status	Positive	True-positive	False-negative
	Negative	False-positive	True-negative

FIGURE 16.4. Example of a screening test.

Death × Sex Crosstabulation

			Sex		Total
			Female	Male	
Death	Survived	Count	678	192	870
		Expected count	665.8	204.2	870.0
		% within death	77.9%	22.1%	100.0%
		% within sex	95.0%	87.7%	93.2%
		Residual	12.2	−12.2	
	Died	Count	36	27	63
		Expected count	48.2	14.8	63.0
		% within death	57.1%	42.9%	100.0%
		% within sex	5.0%	12.3%	6.8%
		Residual	−12.2	12.2	
Total		Count	714	219	933
		Expected count	714.0	219.0	933.0
		% within death	76.5%	23.5%	100.0%
		% within sex	100.0%	100.0%	100.0%

Chi-Square Tests

	Value	df	Asymptotic Significance (two-sided)	Exact Sig. (two-sided)	Exact Sig. (one-sided)
Pearson chi-square	14.133[a]	1	.000		
Continuity correction[b]	12.999	1	.000		
Likelihood ratio	12.447	1	.000		
Fisher's exact test				.001	.000
Linear-by-linear association	14.118	1	.000		
N of valid cases	933				

[a]0 cells (0.0%) have expected count less than 5. The minimum expected count is 14.79.
[b]Computed only for a 2×2 table.

FIGURE 16.5. Results of a chi-square test. This statistical output shows that the mortality rate is 2.5 times higher in men compared with women (12.3% vs. 5.0%). The traditional chi-square P value can be found on the line "Pearson chi-square" under "Asymptotic Significance (two-sided)." The P value is .000170 but displays as .000. This would be reported in a paper as $P < .001$. The overall mortality rate is 6.8%. The expected values are based on this rate. The residual is the difference between the observed and expected. Avoid using the P value from the Yates continuity correction. Always check that the following assumptions are met: The overall sample size is >20 (in this case yes, 933), at least 75% of the cells have an expected count of at least 5 (in this case yes, 100%), and all cells have an expected count of at least 1 (in this case yes, 100%). If these assumptions are violated use the P value from either Fisher's exact test ($P = .001$) or the likelihood ratio test ($P < .001$). Note the linear-by-linear association is the chi-square test for trend and could be used for nominal/ordinal comparisons, for example, mortality by age in quartiles. (Reprint courtesy of IBM Corp. Copyright IBM Corp.)

The chi-square test is appropriate for most categorical (nominal) variables in 2 × 2 tables when the following three assumptions are met:

+ The sample size is greater than 20.
+ The expected frequency for each cell is greater than 1.
+ The expected frequency is at least 5 for at least three of the four cells.

Some statistical packages automatically detect when these conditions (assumptions) are violated. Nevertheless, you must be alert for this problem and be careful to use Fisher's exact test or a likelihood ratio test rather than the chi-square test when these assumptions are violated.

The Yates continuity correction is a variation of the chi-square formula designed for small studies. This correction increases the P value and makes it more conservative (Sprinthall, 2011). The Yates correction is controversial and is probably not appropriate for most clinical research (Conover, 1974). For this reason, you should use the unadjusted (Pearson) chi-square statistic in most situations (Fig. 16.5). Note: In the R statistical software, for the "chisq.test" function, the default is a Yates continuity correction. You must add the argument "correct = FALSE" to obtain an uncorrected chi-square.

The standard chi-square test also is inappropriate for variables with more than two ordered categories (e.g., age in quartiles). For these variables, either the "chi-square test for trend" or the "Mann-Whitney U test" is more appropriate.

STATISTICAL SOFTWARE

PRINCIPLE 77 • Learn how to use a full-featured modern statistical software package.

In modern medical research, the most commonly used statistical software packages are SAS, R, Stata, and IBM SPSS* (Table 16.2). Professional biostatisticians often use R or SAS; R is popular in academia, and SAS is popular in the pharmaceutical industry. For those who do not use this software routinely, it can be very difficult to remember the programming commands for these two packages. Therefore, for those who are not professional biostatisticians, the statistical software packages that have intuitive graphical user interfaces (menus), such as IBM SPSS Statistics and Stata, provide a better balance of power, flexibility, and ease of use.

To produce high-quality reproducible research, it is a good idea to have at least two separate biostatisticians, using different statistical software, perform and check all analyses in your paper.

Then cite this in the Methods as "All analyses in this paper were independently verified by an independent biostatistician."

TABLE 16.2	Most Commonly Used Statistical Software Packages Used in Medical Research	
Rank	Software	Company
1	SAS	SAS Institute, Inc.
2	R	The R Foundation for Statistical Computing (http://www.r-project.org)
3	Stata	StataCorp LP
4	IBM SPSS Statistics	IBM Corp.
5	StatXact	Cytel

Based on a review of original articles and their protocols in the online supplementary appendix published in *The New England Journal of Medicine* in 2015, Volume 372, Issues 1–26. Only packages that were used in at least three papers were included in this list. To encourage reproducible research, journal editors should require authors to identify in the Methods all statistical software used in the project. *Note*: R was often used for the graphics in papers that used other software for the analysis.

*SPSS Inc. was acquired by IBM in October 2009.

IMPORTING DATA INTO A STATISTICAL SOFTWARE PACKAGE

Comma-separated values data files can be imported into statistical software in the following ways:

| In R use: "my.data<-read.csv(file.choose(),header=T, sep=",")" |
| In IBM SPSS use: File, Open, Data, Files of type, text (*.csv), Select the file, Open. |
| In Stata use: File, Import, ASCII data created by a spreadsheet, Browse to find the file, OK. |

HISTOGRAMS

PRINCIPLE 78 • Examine the histograms of your continuous (interval-level) variables.

A histogram is a simple bar graph that shows the number of cases at each level for a particular variable. It provides you with a picture of the frequency distribution. Use your statistical package to create these histograms.

Creating a histogram for each continuous variable is the first step in analyzing continuous (interval) data because it permits you to see whether your data are normally distributed, skewed, or bimodal. When you know the distribution, you can choose the correct statistical test. A normal curve has a symmetrical, bell-shaped histogram which makes it possible to use parametric tests. An asymmetrical histogram suggests that the data may be skewed and therefore require nonparametric tests. A histogram that has two peaks is called "bimodal" (see Fig. 24.4). Remember, the modern approach is to use nonparametric methods regardless of the distribution. Also, work with your biostatistician to assess and understand the distribution of the residuals.

In R, a histogram can be created with the command "hist(variable_name)."

In IBM SPSS, the menu steps are Analyze, Descriptive Statistics, Frequencies, Select the variable, Charts, Histograms, Show normal curve on histogram, Continue, OK.

The syntax for this would be as follows:
FREQUENCIES VARIABLES=variable_name /HISTOGRAM NORMAL /
ORDER=ANALYSIS

In Stata: Graphics, Histogram, Select variable, OK.

The command for this would be as follows:
histogram variable_name

USING THE STUDENT'S *T*-TEST

PRINCIPLE 79 • Learn how to use the Student's *t*-test.

Although nonparametric statistical methods are more modern and robust, it is important to understand the classical parametric statistical approach. With this approach, when the frequency histogram approximates a bell-shaped curve, investigators would use the Student's *t*-test to compare two averages or means (Figs. 16.6 and 16.7). The Student's *t*-test (also called the "independent" or "unpaired" *t*-test) can help to detect whether the means for two unmatched groups are significantly different. (If the groups are matched or the variables are measured "before" and "after" within the same patient, use the paired *t*-test.)

You can calculate the Student's *t*-test in two ways:

1. The first method assumes that the two groups have similar variances and thus pools a variance estimate for the two. (The variance is simply the standard deviation squared.)

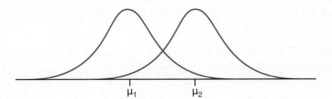

FIGURE 16.6. Two normal curves.

2. The second method compares means with variances that are not similar (i.e., one group has a much larger standard deviation than the other).

If *P* is less than .05 for the *F* ratio, then the variances are different enough to apply the unequal (separate) variance formula (the second method). See Figure 16.7 for an example.

With some statistical software, this *P* value is displayed as "Levene's Test for Equality of Variances" (Fig. 16.7). If the significance (Sig.) for this test is less than .05, use the results for "Equal variances not assumed."

Fortunately, you do not need to understand the intricacies of these statistical procedures; with most statistical software programs, running a *t*-test is straightforward. When two values are truly different, the difference usually is significant with both formulas.

Group Statistics

	Death	N	Mean	Std. Deviation	Std. Error Mean
Age at admission	Survived	870	75.0342	13.16537	.44635
	Died	63	82.1124	7.16893	.90320

Independent Samples Test

		Levene's Test for Equality of Variances		t-Test for Equality of Means							
		F	Sig.	t	df	Sig. (two-tailed)	Mean Difference	Std. Error Difference	95% Confidence Interval of the Difference	
									Lower	Upper
Age at admission	Equal variances assumed	13.502	.000	−4.221	931	.000	−7.07820	1.67697	−10.36928	−3.78713
	Equal variances not assumed			−7.026	95.574	.000	−7.07820	1.00747	−9.07813	−5.07828

FIGURE 16.7. Results of a Student's t-test for two unpaired (unmatched) groups. This test answers the following question: Is the age significantly different between patients who died and those who survived? For the 63 who died, the average was 82.1 years. For the 870 who survived, the average age was 75.0 years. There are two ways to perform a Student's *t*-test—equal variances assumed and equal variances not assumed. Because the standard deviations are quite different, 13.2 versus 7.2, the equal variances not assumed is the appropriate choice. If the *P* value for Levene's test (under Sig.) is <.05, use the unequal variance method—the bottom row. The *P* value for the Student's *t*-test would be reported as *P* < .001. It is found on the bottom row under "Sig. (two-tailed)." This is the classical statistical approach. A more modern and robust approach is to use nonparametric methods for all continuous variables, regardless of the distribution. The Mann-Whitney U test is the nonparametric equivalent to the Student's *t*-test. (Reprint courtesy of IBM Corp. Copyright IBM Corp.)

FOR MORE INFORMATION

See the following website for a video about how to use R for a *t*-test:
https://www.youtube.com/watch?v=RIhnNbPZC0A

PRINCIPLE 80 • Understand when to avoid using the Student's *t*-test.

When comparing more than two groups, using a Student's *t*-test repeatedly is not appropriate (e.g., comparing hospital length of stay among White, Black, and Hispanic patients). Instead, use a one-way analysis of variance (ANOVA). A one-way ANOVA is used to analyze continuous (interval) data and compare three or more groups. When one group has a mean that is significantly larger or smaller than that of the others, the *P* value is less than .05. However, to identify which groups are different, use a statistical test called a "multiple comparison procedure." Several multiple comparison procedures are available for different situations. Scheffé's procedure is a good robust choice for most problems.

See "The dead salmon study" for an entertaining account of what can go wrong if one fails to adjust for multiple comparisons:

http://blogs.scientificamerican.com/scicurious-brain/ignobel-prize-in-neuroscience-the-dead-salmon-study/

When your frequency histogram is skewed (does not resemble a bell-shaped curve), do not use a Student's *t*-test; instead, use a nonparametric test (see Chapter 17). A typical nonparametric test will sort your data and compare the ranks instead of the actual measured values, thereby avoiding problems associated with using parametric tests with skewed data. To compare only two groups with skewed data, use the Mann-Whitney U test (also known as the Wilcoxon rank-sum test). To evaluate three or more groups with skewed data, use the Kruskal-Wallis test.

VITAL POINT

The modern approach to analyzing medical research data is to use the nonparametric tests regardless of the distribution. This approach is more robust because no assumptions are made about the distribution.

REFERENCES

1. *Merriam-Webster's Collegiate Dictionary*. 11th ed. Springfield, MA: Merriam-Webster Inc; 2008.

Nonparametric Tests

PRINCIPLE 81 • Use nonparametric tests as your first option rather than as a backup plan.

Nonparametric is defined as "not involving the estimation of parameters of a statistical function"[1]; in other words, we do not have to make the assumption that the histogram has a symmetrical bell shape. When data are not normally distributed or when they are on an ordinal level of measurement, nonparametric tests are appropriate, but these methods also work perfectly fine for data that are normally distributed. Remember, ordinal data are rankings. For example, "level of psychological stress" may be reported as 0 = none, 1 = a little bit, 2 = moderate, 3 = quite a bit, or 4 = extreme.

A common mistake in medical research is using the wrong class of statistical test, such as a parametric test in place of a nonparametric test. The traditional approach was to use a parametric test for normally distributed (bell-shaped) data and a nonparametric test for skewed data. A more modern approach, however, is to use nonparametric tests routinely. Table 17.1 lists the nonparametric equivalents for several common parametric tests.

The Mann-Whitney U test, the nonparametric equivalent of the unpaired Student's t-test, is used to compare two groups, for example, length of hospital stay by gender. The rank-sum test for two independent samples ordinarily is called the "Mann-Whitney U test" (Mann & Whitney, 1947). Because Wilcoxon (1945) developed an almost identical test, however, sometimes it is called the "Wilcoxon rank-sum test" or "Wilcoxon-Mann-Whitney test."

The Kruskal-Wallis test, the nonparametric equivalent of the one-way analysis of variance (ANOVA), compares ordinal or skewed data with more than two independent groups, for example, length of hospital stay by type of insurance (A, B, C, D).

The Wilcoxon signed-rank test, the nonparametric equivalent of the paired t-test, is used only when the two groups were matched in some way (such as by age and sex) or when measurements were repeated within the same patient, for example, weight loss from baseline to completion of a diabetes prevention program. Do not confuse the Wilcoxon signed-rank test with the Wilcoxon rank-sum test.

The Friedman ANOVA by ranks is the nonparametric equivalent of repeated measures ANOVA. This test is appropriate for assessing differences for an ordinal or skewed variable measured several times for the same patient, for example, blood pressure at time 1, time 2, and time 3.

VITAL POINT

Nonparametric methods should be used routinely rather than only in situations in which the data are skewed.

Many investigators are concerned that nonparametric methods are not as powerful as parametric methods. There is approximately a 4% loss of efficiency. This, however, is outweighed by the robustness of nonparametric methods. In fact, when the data are not bell-shaped (non-Gaussian), the Mann-Whitney U test is generally more powerful than the Student's t-test. Because most medical research papers are

| **TABLE 17.1** | Corresponding Parametric–Nonparametric Tests |

Parametric	Nonparametric
Student's *t*-test	Mann-Whitney U test/Wilcoxon rank-sum test
One-way ANOVA	Kruskal-Wallis H test
Paired *t*-test	Wilcoxon signed-rank test
Repeated-measures ANOVA	Friedman ANOVA by ranks
Pearson correlation	Spearman correlation
Linear regression	Nonparametric regression

The classical approach was to use parametric test if the data were normally distributed; the modern approach is to use nonparametric regardless of the distribution.
ANOVA = analysis of variance.

focused on nonnormal patients, it is logical to assume that many of their variables will be nonnormal as well. Also, it is almost impossible to prove that your data are normally distributed unless you have a large sample. Therefore, reviewers can always question whether you have met the assumptions for parametric tests.

When reporting nonparametric methods, use the median and bootstrap 95% confidence interval (CI). If the variable has a large number of ties or zeros, the mean and bootstrap 95% CI may be more appropriate. The Hodges-Lehmann estimator, the median difference for all pairs, is technically more appropriate but may be too complex for some medical research papers. If the median and mean fail to appropriately summarize your findings, consult with a biostatistician regarding the Hodges-Lehmann estimator.

Example wording:

"We used the Hodges-Lehmann method to display the point estimates of absolute difference. These are the medians of all paired differences between observations in the two groups (Lehmann, 1963)."

VITAL POINT

In almost all cases, use two-sided tests with two-sided *P* values.

REFERENCES

1. *Merriam-Webster's Collegiate Dictionary*. 11th ed. Springfield, MA: Merriam-Webster Inc; 2008.

Matching and Propensity Score Analysis

PRINCIPLE 82 • Use matching but plan it carefully.

Matching is an important technique for creating a control group by pairing patients based on one or more confounding factors. Matching is often used when other methods of controlling for confounding variables are unsatisfactory.

Once you match patients on a variable, you cannot analyze the effect of that variable on the outcome. For this reason, be sure that you will not need to assess the effect of the matching variable. Sometimes, researchers decide to match patients on age and sex without giving adequate thought to whether they need to assess the outcome effect of age and sex.

Matching is most successful and efficient when it is planned before data are collected. You can match after data are collected but recognize the drawbacks. A major disadvantage is that, time and money can be wasted collecting data on unmatched cases.

When you report results for two comparison groups, always state whether and how you matched the groups. Matching completely changes which statistical analyses are appropriate. As you can see from Figure 16.1, matched cases require a different set of statistical tools, for example, a paired t-test rather than a Student's t-test. Also, in matched analyses, one would use conditional logistic regression rather than logistic regression.

PRINCIPLE 83 • Consider the hybrid method: matching and logistic regression.

Example 18–1.
Preventable deaths are a major issue in the field of trauma care. To analyze why preventable deaths occur, investigators must control for both the severity of injury and the mechanism of injury. The typical method of mathematically weighting the effect of the severity of injury and the mechanism of injury in regression modeling is inappropriate because it does not adjust for the severity of injury within each mechanism group. Alternatively, patients could be analyzed in groups according to the mechanism of injury (e.g., stabbings, motorcycle crashes, falls); however, stratifying patients into these groups may make the subgroup samples so small that they are often useless for statistical analysis.

One solution to this problem is the hybrid method, a statistical technique that combines matching and logistic regression to provide convincing evidence (Rothman et al., 2012). The hybrid method is useful for statistically controlling for the severity of injury within each specific mechanism of injury. Then with the hybrid method, researchers can simultaneously consider many types of trauma patients in their analysis.

Whenever you use matching, be prepared to describe the characteristics of the unmatched group. When a bias is present, describe it and explain how it could affect the results. Some patients cannot be matched; explain why this situation is not a drawback. The final matched sample may differ significantly from the initial study group. Explain why this situation is not a bias. For instance, suppose that among fatally injured victims of motor vehicle crashes in Example 18–1, you had a person who was decapitated. Obviously, you will not find a matching survivor, but this situation does not weaken your study because the decapitated person is so severely injured that nothing can be learned about trauma care from a comparison with a survivor.

Remember, matching is an effective but time-consuming statistical method for extracting truth from a set of numbers. In addition, it offers many advantages over using regression models to control for confounding variables. In practice, matching is often a useful way to strengthen the analysis of a paper by performing it in addition to regression analyses and propensity score analyses. Each of these three methods has weaknesses, but a paper that demonstrates the same conclusion based on all three methods will often convince reviewers and editors to accept it for publication. Because matching requires manual labor, it has been used less frequently in recent years, but it has advantages and should be used more often.

PRINCIPLE 84 • Use propensity score methods to adjust for differences in observational data.

For observational studies in which it is impossible to randomize the treatment, propensity score methods are increasingly used. Propensity score is the probability of choosing a treatment (or exposure) based on observed covariates and is used to adjust for nonrandom treatment assignments. For example, a researcher may be interested in whether a daily low-dose aspirin reduces the risk of some outcome. This researcher may be unable to randomize patients but may have access to a large observational data set. Suppose more educated patients are more likely to choose to take the aspirin and also have better outcomes. This creates a problem called confounding by indication. The investigator can create a logistic regression model of the patient characteristics, such as education level, and compute a probability (from 0 to 1) that a patient is likely to take a daily low-dose aspirin. Then the investigator can assess whether the aspirin is significantly associated with the outcome independent of this probability, the propensity score. In practice, the model for propensity score would include many more variables than education, such as age, gender, insurance type, comorbidities, etc. The propensity scores are used in four ways: propensity score matching, stratification of the propensity score, covariate adjustment, and inverse probability of treatment weighting using the propensity score.

FOR MORE INFORMATION

See Armitage and Colton (2005); Austin (2011); and Rosenbaum (2010).

Multivariate Analysis and Model Validation

> *"Essentially, all models are wrong, but some are useful."*
> —GEORGE E. P. BOX

PRINCIPLE 85 • Learn how to use modern multivariate analysis to create reproducible research.

Multivariate is defined as "having or involving a number of independent mathematical or statistical variables."[1] "Multivariable" is sometimes used interchangeably. Some argue that multivariable should be used to describe models with more than one predictor but only one outcome variable and multivariate should be used for models when there is more than one outcome measurement, such as repeated measurements. Because this distinction is rarely made in practice, I will continue to use multivariate for analyses in which more than one predictor is used with one outcome variable.

Unlike univariate analysis, multivariate analysis can evaluate the independent effect of several predictor variables simultaneously. Multivariate analysis assesses the independent contributions of multiple independent variables on a dependent variable and identifies those independent variables most significant in explaining the variation of the dependent variable. It also permits clinical researchers to statistically adjust for differences among patients.

Example 19–1.
Suppose that you wish to determine whether the cure rate of patients who received drug A differs from that of patients who received drug B. Even though you randomized patients into two groups (A and B), you find that the patients in one group are significantly older than those in the other group. You can use multivariate analysis to adjust for the age of the patients. Then you can determine whether the cure rate differs between the two groups independent of age. The univariate analysis will provide you with an odds ratio, and a multivariate analysis (such as logistic regression) will provide you with an adjusted odds ratio, by controlling for age. Multivariate models such as this one should be used more than simple univariate hypothesis testing (such as the chi-square and *t*-test), even in randomized controlled trials.

FOR MORE INFORMATION
See Kleinbaum and Klein (2010); Kleinbaum et al. (2013); and Steyerberg (2010).

PRINCIPLE 86 • Describe precisely how you used multivariate analysis to control for confounding factors.

A confounding factor is an extraneous variable that is related to both the risk factor and the outcome and can distort the interpretation of the causal effect of the risk factor on the outcome. An extreme example would be as follows: Researchers find that people who carry a lighter in their pocket are more likely to develop lung cancer. Obviously, the lighter does not cause cancer. Smoking causes cancer, and smokers often carry a lighter. In this example, smoking would be the confounding factor. It is related to the lighter and cancer.

Confounding factors that are not taken into account are a common and serious statistical problem. Multivariate analysis can solve this problem by adjusting for the effects of these variables. To allow the reader to judge the validity of your study, however, you must describe—in plain English—how you controlled for confounding variables. Reviewers expect you to search the literature and study the appropriate papers. Be aware of which variables cited in the current literature are potential confounding factors for your study. Even if you did not include these factors in your multivariate analysis, note in your paper that you are aware of them.

FOR MORE INFORMATION

https://significantlystatistical.wordpress.com/2014/12/12/confounders-mediators-moderators-and-covariates/

PRINCIPLE 87 • Master logistic regression analysis.

Logistic regression is a multivariate statistical technique that is commonly applied (and misapplied) in medical research. When outcome is recorded in two categories, such as diabetic versus nondiabetic, logistic regression is an effective way to examine the independent contributions of more than one predictor variable. Logistic regression will be even more important in the future. For this reason, it is wise to learn how to use it, or at least how to interpret the statistical output.

Hosmer and Lemeshow (2012) explained the fine points of logistic regression. Kleinbaum and Klein (2010) also wrote a self-learning text on logistic regression. Some logistic regression techniques are too complex and lengthy to include in a medical journal article; use the appendix of the manuscript to include this level of detail for the statistical reviewers. Do describe how you used modern data reduction techniques and avoided stepwise variable selection. Steyerberg (2010) is an excellent resource and reference for this.

Many researchers ignore the most valuable information provided by logistic regression: the outliers. After the predictor variables are mathematically weighted, logistic regression attempts to predict the outcome based on your model. Patients who clearly do not fit the model (outliers) are noted (e.g., patients who had a poor outcome but were predicted to have a good outcome). Review the outliers (sorted by the residuals), study the patients' records, and interview the patients or families to learn about other factors that are not included in your model. Remember, the experiment that came out wrong is trying to tell you something.

Example 19–2.
At Vanderbilt University, the Cornelius project was created to build logistic regression models to predict which hospitalized patients would be readmitted within 30 days, develop pressure ulcers, fall in the hospital, develop blood clots, develop hospital-acquired infections, etc. The equations for these models were then programmed into the hospital electronic health record for a random half of the patients to display real-time probabilities for complications. For patients at the highest risk of each complication, prevention specialists in the hospital ensure that all appropriate prevention efforts are implemented in a timely and reliable way. The control group continues to receive the current standard of care. By using a randomized controlled trial of all patients admitted to the hospital, we are able to know when this approach improves patient outcomes.

This is an example of a modern learning health care system. The old approach was to use science and randomization to learn what works and then operationalize it. The new approach is to learn what works as a natural part of hospital operations. There is always variability in how hospitals, units, physicians, and nurses care for patients over time. If this variability is haphazard, there is little learning. If, however, the variability is randomized, we can learn with rigor what works and what does not work. Changing the culture to accept this translational research in a hospital setting is a challenge, but hospitals that do not embrace the idea of a learning health care system are unlikely to survive in a future in which payments are tied to quality. Mastering logistic regression analyses will prepare you for the future.

Example 19–3.
In this hypothetical example, researchers develop a series of logistic regression predictive models for an employee wellness program to compute the probability that each employee will develop type 2 diabetes, hypertension, have a heart attack, etc. Those at highest risk are invited to participate in free prevention programs. Incentives are provided to those who attend an initial information session and a larger incentive to those who complete the prevention programs.

Such a system is likely to be an improvement over the current US health care system, in which the first time most patients learn that they have heart disease is when they have a heart attack. On that day, one-third die. For the survivors, the costs are huge. With this new approach, the investment in incentives is used to prevent chronic disease.

PRINCIPLE 88 • Get a second opinion before concluding that there were no differences between the study groups.

In clinical studies, the significant findings are usually found deep in the numbers, so deep that multivariate analysis often is required to control for differences among patients. Even randomized studies based entirely on univariate analysis should not be interpreted as showing that no significant differences existed.

These problems of concluding that no differences exist commonly occur when data are analyzed by people who do not have a solid understanding of both the research subject and the statistical methods. Incorrect conclusions also can be drawn when the analysis does not examine important subgroups or does not use the most powerful multivariate method.

An interaction is the combined influence that two or more variables can have on an outcome. Never overlook the importance of clinically important interactions but avoid post hoc fishing for significant interactions.

Example 19–4.
A group of investigators found that among people with spinal cord injury, both diabetes and smoking were moderate risk factors for pressure ulcers. However, all of the patients who had diabetes and also smoked had a history of pressure ulcers. This effect from a combination of factors is an interaction, which can be tested statistically.

Example 19–5.
Age was a significant predictor of pressure ulcer development for women but not for men. The age–gender interaction significantly improved the prediction model.

PRINCIPLE 89 • Clearly describe the methods you used to perform multivariate analysis.

Although you may use complex multivariate analysis to control for confounding factors, always simplify the presentation of the findings to make them useful for readers. Explain these results clearly and graph the main points. This task is not easy and may be time-consuming. If, however, you skip this step, reviewers may misinterpret the independent contributions of your key variables.

VITAL POINT

Always translate multivariate analysis into plain English and illustrate the findings with a professional graph, such as a forest plot or a spline.

"Everything should be made as simple as possible, but not simpler. Any intelligent fool can make things bigger, more complex, and more violent. It takes a touch of genius—and a lot of courage— to move in the opposite direction."

—ALBERT EINSTEIN

Most reviewers and editors are not statistical experts, and what they do not understand may hurt you. Their misunderstanding can lead to a rejection of your paper. To ensure that reviewers and editors understand your statistical analysis:

+ Explain how you used multivariate analysis to adjust for the overlap in variables and solved the problem of confounding factors.
+ Describe how you chose the variables that you used in the multivariate analysis and explain why you did not include other variables previously associated with your measure of outcome.
+ Indicate how and why you chose certain interactions and whether you examined other interactions.
+ Avoid assuming linearity for all predictors; instead, test restricted cubic splines to model the non-linear terms.
+ Show that you used modern data reduction methods and avoided stepwise variable selection.
+ Include a detailed appendix to transparently show the statistical reviewer an additional level of detail.

The strongest way to present a logistic regression model is to show that your results held up when you tested the model in a completely different data set. This external validation provides rigorous evidence that your findings are not artifacts.

In the appendix of the paper, you can also provide additional details about the calibration and model fit by adding a calibration plot and modern performance metrics. Avoid using weak goodness-of-fit methods such as the Hosmer-Lemeshow test and instead use modern methods such as the Brier score (mean squared error) and Spiegelhalter calibration test, which are useful metrics to include. The overall proportion classified correctly is an improper scoring rule that should be avoided. This is often displayed as the "Overall Percentage Correct" in a classification table. When an event is rare, a model that predicts that no one will have the event will have a high proportion classified correctly—even though this model is worthless. The c-index or area under the curve (AUC) along with 95% confidence intervals in a receiver-operating characteristics curve (ROC curve) provides more information about the performance of a model. Use a nonparametric calibration curve to assess the intercept.

If your sample size is large, you can randomly split the data into training and validation data sets. With smaller samples, a rigorous internal bootstrap validation is preferred.

PRINCIPLE 90 • Present the results of the multivariate analysis in a clinically useful format and convert into a graph.

Tables of multivariate analysis should provide a balance of clinical and statistical information. These tables are most useful when they are designed jointly by clinical and statistical experts. Tables are discussed in further detail in Chapter 24.

Do not allow multivariate analysis to overcomplicate your paper. Provide a balance of multivariate results to show that you did not subjectively synthesize unseen results with a black box. Present evidence from each major step of the analysis. Otherwise, reviewers may suspect that you created a model that you believed was true and simply used statistics to support your opinion. A paper that does not provide this evidence demands an unacceptable leap of faith from the reader, and much of the science is lost by this apparent subjectivity. Prespecify your analysis in detail and then tell a linear story to be transparent.

VITAL POINT

When you use several multivariate models to choose variables for a scale or an index, clearly describe how you chose the factors for the final model.

The variable selection process should be objective, clear, quantifiable, and reproducible. Use a conceptual (rather than an empirical) basis for selecting variables into the models. For example, do not select variables based solely on prescreening with P values from massive univariate testing (Sun et al., 1996); consider what makes sense clinically. This pretesting inflates the Type I errors. Avoid stepwise variable selection and instead use modern data reduction methods. With these methods, you narrow a list of potential predictors by eliminating those with a large amount of missing data, those that are highly redundant (e.g., hematocrit and hemoglobin), and those that are not biologically plausible predictors.

Group the potential variables into logical, clinically meaningful categories, such as preexisting diseases, injury severity factors, time factors, and treatment factors. Then you can design multivariate models to test groups of variables in stages or blocks, according to a logical ordering system and a hierarchical design. These results will have more practical value than robotically analyzed data. Once you have a model, you can display the results in a forest plot, which is an excellent way to graph the variables in a model.

PRINCIPLE 91 • Learn survival methods: Kaplan-Meier, log-rank, and Cox proportional-hazards regression.

These survival methods are three of the four most commonly used statistical methods in modern medical research (see Table 16.1). The Kaplan-Meier is a method of displaying time to death (or some other event) across time for various groups. The log-rank test provides a P value to assess whether the groups differ. Cox proportional-hazards regression enables researches to assess several predictors of time to death in a multivariate model.

The growing popularity of these methods is due to the fact that they are extremely powerful and enable researchers to use smaller sample sizes by using their time-to data in the most powerful way. These methods are not limited to analysis of time to death. They can be used in many other research situations in which time to some outcome is the end point, and the end point has not occurred for all participants (censored). Think creatively about how to use survival methods in your research to assess factors associated with time to an event, for example, time to next heart attack, time to return to work, time to hospital readmission, etc.

To publish a paper in a high-quality journal, you may have to show that you adjusted for several confounding factors and for varying lengths of follow-up. The tool that you will need is Cox proportional-hazards regression. Although many researchers find it easier to have a biostatistician do this analysis, there are several reasons why you should learn how to use this technique and perform the work in collaboration with a biostatistician. First, you will be able to communicate more effectively if you know the basics of building a survival model. Second, multivariate modeling often requires a clinical judgment based on years of experience to select the optimal variables for analysis.

You must demonstrate that you are aware of the assumptions of the statistical methods that you use and document this in the methods with a statement, such as the following:

"For all Cox models, we plotted Schoenfeld residuals against follow-up time and found no violation of the proportional-hazards assumption."

"Cox proportional-hazards models were used to estimate hazard ratios and 95% confidence intervals. The assumption of proportional-hazards regarding the intervention arm was confirmed by means of the Schoenfeld residuals test; no violations of the assumption were found."

One of the assumptions of the Cox model is the proportional hazards assumption. Usually, we assess the difference between the observed and predicted (residual) to assess model fit. For Cox models, it is a little more complicated. Schoenfeld residuals (or partial residuals) are used to assess the proportional hazards assumption. In your statistical software after running a Cox model, save the partial residual and create a smoothed scatter plot of this variable on y versus time on x and assess the correlation. Also, visually examine a graph of the log of the negative log of the Kaplan-Meier survival function versus the log of time to assess whether this is parallel. One should also test whether the interaction of treatment by log of time is significant in the Cox model. If the interaction is significant and there is evidence of nonproportionality, one can use a time-dependent hazard ratio with the interaction in the model. Work closely with your biostatistician to understand the fine points of this type of analysis.

FOR MORE INFORMATION
See Collett (2014) and Cox (1972).

PRINCIPLE 92 • Become familiar with the modern statistical tools.

Reviewers and editors predict that the statistical techniques shown in Table 19.1 will be increasingly important in the future. One obvious theme was big data. Developing skills in these areas will be a smart investment in self-education. Collaborating with an experienced methodologist can help you incorporate these methods into your research.

Use caution with newer statistical methods that have not been completely developed and rigorously validated. When using a new statistical method, also prespecify that you will also assess the data with well-established statistical techniques (Table 19.2).

TABLE 19.1   Statistical Tools of the Future

- Big data techniques
  - Ever more complex forms of modeling to analyze large observational data sets
  - Continued evolution of dealing with big data from large populations
  - Statistical techniques to assist evaluation of focused information from large databases
  - Rigorous statistics will be increasingly necessary at all levels, but computational skills will be increasingly important to study large data sets.
  - Big data techniques, methods for analyzing high-dimensional data and massive data sets
  - Because we are seeing far more large data base analysis, the statistics need to be appropriate.
  - Those needed for working with large complex data such as whole genome sequencing data and that have yet to be developed
  - Big data and machine learning techniques; need to educate editors and reviewers on how to judge and interpret these
  - Complex regression analysis of existing "big" data
  - Analysis of registry data and big clinical data will need to be revisited.

(continued)

TABLE 19.1	**Statistical Tools of the Future** (continued)

- Bootstrap
- Techniques for cluster randomized trials
- Simulations
- Statistics of molecular genetic analysis
- Approaches and assessment of methods of handling missing data, such as multiple imputation
- Propensity score analysis
- Statistical techniques to help better match comparative populations
- Identification of biases
- Adaptive clinical trials
- Pragmatic trials
- Random forest
- Marginal structural models
- Mendelian randomization (see Burgess & Thompson, 2015)
- Competing risk analysis
- Mediation analysis (i.e., X causes M [mediator] and M causes Y)
- Statistical methods to infer causality using observational data
- Mixed-effects models
- Logistic regression
- Cox proportional-hazards regression
- Data reduction
- Nonparametric methods
- Models for hierarchical data
- Models for longitudinal data
- Path analysis
- Multidimensional scaling
- Semiparametric regression methods
- Self-learning tools imbedded into the electronic health record of a learning health care system
- Automatic phenotyper; tools that identify unusual patterns of a new disease or epidemics built into the electronic medical record
- Statistical data cleaning tools that automatically detect possible errors in data sets, such as transposing hematocrit and hemoglobin
- Methods of conduct and interpretation of formal systematic review and meta-analysis (The jury is split on this one. Some believe it will be more important in the future, and others are skeptical: "Meta-analysis is to analysis, what metaphysics is to physics.")
- Variable clustering
- Sparse principal component analysis
- Ordinal regression
- Recursive partitioning/classification and regression trees (CARTs) (mostly for displaying models and understanding interactions)
- Techniques for qualitative research
- Bayesian analyses
- General linear modeling
- "It is not the technique but applying the appropriate technique."

Based on question 33 in the Peer Review Questionnaire (Appendix B): "What statistical techniques do you think will be more important in the future?"

TABLE 19.2	Comparison of Weak/Outdated Statistical Methods and Strong/Modern Methods

Weak/Outdated Methods	Strong/Modern Methods
Dichotomania	Using continuous variables
Reporting results as $P < .05$	Full P value, for example, $P = .017$
Reporting results as NS (not significant)	Full P value, for example, $P = .89$
Overly simplistic models	Logistic regression with restricted cubic splines and rigorous bootstrap validation
Methods that assume linearity	Flexible nonlinear methods
Stepwise variable selection	Data reduction methods, penalized methods/shrinkage
Parametric methods	Nonparametric methods
Pearson correlation	Spearman
Student's t-test	Mann-Whitney U test
Paired t-test	Wilcoxon signed-rank test
Repeated measures ANOVA	Mixed-effects models/Friedman test
Cohen's effect size to justify sample size	Sample size based on a clinically meaningful end point
Last observation carried forward or single imputation (e.g., mean)	Full maximum likelihood methods or multiple imputation
± SEM (standard error of the mean)	95% CI (confidence interval)
Neural networks	Random forest
No model validation	Bootstrap validation
Dichotomizing ordinal variables	Ordinal regression

ANOVA = analysis of variance.

PRINCIPLE 93 • Draw your conclusions using clinical common sense to interpret your results but do not exaggerate the results.

After you analyze your results, meet with your research team and then carefully draw your conclusions. Drawing conclusions is the sixth and final step in the scientific method. When you and your research team have completed the Observing phase, you can move on to the third phase of the POWER principles: Writing.

REFERENCES

1. *Merriam-Webster's Collegiate Dictionary.* 11th ed. Springfield, MA: Merriam-Webster Inc; 2008.

WRITING

Key Questions to Answer in the Writing Phase and the Section in which to Answer Each:

- Why did you perform the study?   **Introduction**
- What did you do?   **Methods**
- What did you find?   **Results**
- What do your results mean?   **Discussion**

Title Page

PRINCIPLE 94 • Write the sections of your paper in an efficient order.

With the planning and observing phases of your research completed, you should have most of the material you need to write your paper. Few medical manuscripts are, in fact, written in order, from beginning to end. For ease of use, however, the following chapters on writing your paper are presented in the order found in a typical manuscript.

Many experienced medical writers have learned to start their manuscripts by writing the Methods section. The reason is that they can easily sit down at their computer and write three to four pages. Once they get started, the rest comes easier. Often, the hardest part is getting started. You can often write most of the Methods section before the study is completed. This is advisable because you will have the details fresh in your mind and should have the analysis plan prespecified.

Once the Methods section is completed, many researchers create their tables and figures. This will be the meat of the paper and will enable you to write the text of the Results and tell a story. See Table 20.1 for an idea of the order in which sections are often written versus submitted.

TABLE 20.1	Order in Which a Typical Manuscript Is Written versus Submitted	
Recommended Order for Writing a Paper	**Final Order for Submission**	
Methods	Cover letter	
Tables, with titles and footnotes	Title page	
Figures	Abstract	
Figure legends	Introduction	
Results	Methods	
Title page	Results	
Introduction	Discussion	
Discussion	Acknowledgments and support information	
References	References	
Acknowledgments and support information	Tables, with titles and footnotes	
Abstract	Figure legends	
Cover letter	Figures	

TABLE 20.2	Elements of a Good Title

Tells the editor "we have new information and this will be a high-impact paper"
Shows "we know what we are doing"
Interesting
Easy to understand
Accurate promise of the paper's content
Specific concerning the scope of the study
Does not use unexplained abbreviations unless they are widely understood by the target journal's audience. The following are acceptable for most journals: HIV, AIDS, CD4+, DNA, RNA, IQ
Simple, short, concise
10–12 words long
Indicates the study design, for example, "A Randomized Controlled Trial of X"
Eye-catching, a "reader-grabber"
Begins with a key word
Grammatically correct
Worded appropriately for the target journal's audience
States the subject of the article but not the conclusions. Nondeclarative (rather than "X Predicts Y," use "Effect of X on Y")
Not cute, clever, or a question

PRINCIPLE 95 • Give your manuscript a cleverly concise, snappy but professional title to hook the reviewer.

The first words that a potential reader will see are those in your title, so make the title interesting and easy to understand. Be sure your title says "This is new!" and "We know what we are doing!" The title is very important. So, give it more thought. Table 20.2 shows the ingredients for a good title.

If your findings are not broadly applicable, be sure that the title does not suggest otherwise. Does the title explain how your sample differs from the general population? As one editor suggested, "See if your title can show how the study may enhance [or at least apply to] patient care, either now or in the future."

Avoid titles that are cute, clever, questions, or declarative—rather than "Treatment A Is Superior to Treatment B," write "A Randomized Controlled Trial Comparing Treatment A with Treatment B."

Many clinical journals do not allow declarative titles, whereas some basic science journals encourage this. Follow the target journal's guidelines and style on this.

PRINCIPLE 96 • Format the Title Page like an experienced scientist.

The Title Page of your manuscript needs to give the impression that you are an experienced scientist.

While you and your research team are writing the paper, you can use the following technique to avoid coauthorship problems. For the early drafts, list only your name and "et al." on the Title Page—"Smith et al." Let each of your coauthors earn his or her place on the paper and be fair but very specific about what you need from each person and by when. If you list many names on an early draft, some of these people may feel that they do not need to do any additional work on this paper. Some may leave and move onto other jobs. Then you can be in an awkward position of removing someone's name from the final draft of the paper.

For medical research journals, the order of authors is generally as follows: The first author is the person who did most of the work on the paper. The last author is generally this person's mentor, senior person in the group, or head of the lab. The other authors are then in order of the amount of work that they contributed to this paper. Never list a coauthor as a gift or favor. Be sure to include middle initials. See Appendix A (section II.A.2) for criteria for authorship.

Also include the "date last revised" and the name of the target journal on the Title Page. These will be deleted before submission. This information is useful for your colleagues as they give you feedback.

PRINCIPLE 97 • Delete unnecessary words and phrases from your title.

Table 20.3 shows words and phrases that can often be deleted from a title.

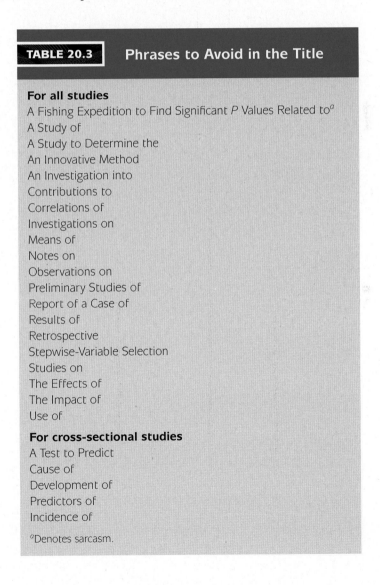

TABLE 20.3	Phrases to Avoid in the Title

For all studies
A Fishing Expedition to Find Significant *P* Values Related to[a]
A Study of
A Study to Determine the
An Innovative Method
An Investigation into
Contributions to
Correlations of
Investigations on
Means of
Notes on
Observations on
Preliminary Studies of
Report of a Case of
Results of
Retrospective
Stepwise-Variable Selection
Studies on
The Effects of
The Impact of
Use of

For cross-sectional studies
A Test to Predict
Cause of
Development of
Predictors of
Incidence of

[a]Denotes sarcasm.

Abstract

WRITING A CRISP ABSTRACT

PRINCIPLE 98 • Take the time to polish the abstract.

Make a good first impression with a well-written abstract to grab the attention of the editors and reviewers. Most people will read only your abstract, so invest plenty of time in writing it. Your abstract should demonstrate that your findings are clinically (or biologically) important and that your study was performed carefully. Ask your colleagues for feedback to identify sentences that need to be refined.

Editors will read your abstract to learn whether it is well written and whether the topic is appropriate for their journal. Many editors will read the last sentence of your abstract as a first step. A good abstract is specific, representative of the article, and structured correctly for the target journal. For example, if the target journal uses a single-paragraph format, obviously, you should as well.

Clearly describe the problem in the first sentence of the abstract. Describe your objective sufficiently, yet simply, and be sure that it is not too broad for a single study to answer. To help the reader understand what you are testing, include the primary null hypothesis in the Methods section of the abstract or make it easy for the reader to understand what your testable null hypothesis is and then include the formal null hypothesis in the statistical analysis section of the Methods section of the paper. Explain how you conducted the study, and finally, describe any notable results and your primary conclusion.

Because a lack of organization often is a problem, many unstructured abstracts can be improved on by using *The New England Journal of Medicine* four-section structure: Background, Methods, Results, and Conclusions. Avoid using the same sentence word-for-word in both the abstract and the body of the paper.

Most researchers write the final draft of the abstract after the manuscript is completed. Some write the abstract first to submit to a conference and use it as a guide for writing the rest of the paper. With either method, remember that preparing a good abstract always requires extensive editing and rewriting.

The abstract must answer these questions for the editor and reviewers:

+ What were these people trying to do—and why?
+ Why is this an important problem to solve?
+ Is this a rigorous, solid study design?
+ Do they have a high-quality data set?
+ Will this be a high-impact paper?
+ Are the conclusions appropriate?

EDITING AND REVISING THE ABSTRACT

PRINCIPLE 99 • Keep the abstract short.

Do not wait for the editor to tell you:

> *The abstract is much too long.*

Most journals have a section on their website that describes the correct format for papers submitted for publication (usually called the "information for authors"). Follow these instructions exactly and compare your format with that of abstracts published in recent issues of the target journal. Usually, structured abstracts (i.e., where a format is specified) are less than 250 words long and unstructured abstracts are less than 150 words long. Some journals (e.g., psychology journals) recommend limiting abstracts to 120 words.

Do not shorten the abstract by excluding key information. The abstract must summarize your study design and briefly state your findings (e.g., $n = X$; the percentage with poor outcome $= Y$). **Do not merely promise that the findings will be described in the full paper.** Put the key data in the abstract. Provide 95% confidence intervals for the primary end point (use the bootstrap method for extra points); do not rely on the P values as the sole evidence and never put the focus on the number of zeros in your P value. Instead, focus on the 95% confidence interval from your clinically meaningful primary end point. The abstract also should briefly describe the clinical relevance of the findings.

Eliminate most abbreviations and all unnecessary words. Do not use abbreviations unless you are certain that the readers of the target journal will understand them. Never cite figures or tables in the abstract. Include key words only if the target journal's instructions request them. During your literature search, you can identify appropriate key words among the MeSH (Medical Subject Headings) terms. In PubMed, change the display format from abstract to MEDLINE. Scroll down to see the MH terms. Place these key words at the end of the abstract.

VITAL POINT

Keep your abstract conclusions specific, conservative and based on your data.

End your abstract with the funding source and ClinicalTrials.gov number (or equivalent reference if outside the United States). For example, "Funded by XXXXXXXX; ClinicalTrails.gov number, XXXXXXXXX."

If your project was supported in any way by an infrastructure grant such as a CTSA (Clinical and Translational Science Award) grant, be sure to cite it. These citations are vital performance measures that document productivity and help your institution renew these important grants. For example:

"The project [publication or poster] described was supported by CTSA Award No. UL1TR000445 from the National Center for Advancing Translational Sciences. Its contents are solely the responsibility of the authors and do not necessarily represent official views of the National Center for Advancing Translational Sciences or the National Institutes of Health."

Cite all grants that supported your research project. Manuscripts do not limit the number of grants that you can cite, and this does not contribute to your word count.

22

Introduction

CAPTURING THE EDITOR'S ATTENTION BY ANSWERING THE QUESTIONS—WHAT'S NEW? AND WHY SHOULD I CARE?

PRINCIPLE 100 • Begin with thunder and wake the reader up from a slumber.

Write a strong introductory paragraph and go right to the essence of the argument to "hook" the reader. The opening sentences of the Introduction and of each section must be original "reader-grabbers" (Baker, 1986). A provocative question, a new perspective, and sometimes a good quotation are useful bait for catching readers.

Sometimes, all you need to do is move a word to improve the cadence, but more often, revising the Introduction takes both time and creative energy. Be imaginative, not imitative. A concise account of the extent, prevalence, or cost of the problem can be effective—if it is well written and interesting.

James Thurber's editor once told him to begin his newspaper articles with a short dramatic lead (Gilmore, 1989). The next day, Thurber's article began:

Dead. That was what the man was . . .

Obviously, a little extreme, but you do need to consider the reviewers' point of view. They may be tired, overworked, and utterly bored with your topic. To interest them, explain why your study is necessary and convey your enthusiasm for the work. Readers are hoping that you answer their question "Why should I read this paper?" Do not exaggerate, however, and never let your tone become emotional or hostile.

The Introduction must also place your paper in the broader context. Link it, diplomatically, to the body of research that preceded it.

PRINCIPLE 101 • Avoid starting the Introduction with short, choppy, overly simplistic sentences.

In the first sentence of the Introduction, you must often provide a definition. This can result in a choppy and unsophisticated opening of your story. Experienced medical writers will start with a more complex sentence that includes a definition as part of the sentence but is not limited to the definition. Here are a few examples:

Before:
"Chronic lymphocytic leukemia (CLL) is characterized by an accumulation of mature B cells. CLL is the most common leukemia among adults in Western countries."
After:
"Chronic lymphocytic leukemia (CLL), the most common leukemia among adults in Western countries, is characterized by an accumulation of mature B cells."
Before:
"Lyme disease is an inflammatory disorder caused by the spirochete *Borrelia burgdorferi*. Lyme disease is the most common parasitic infection in the United States."

After:

"Lyme disease, an inflammatory disorder caused by the spirochete *Borrelia burgdorferi*, is the most common parasitic infection in the United States."

To avoid choppy writing, imagine that you are using a thread and needle to weave an idea from the last sentence to connect it to the current sentence. To learn more about this skill, read Williams' (2013) excellent book *Style: Lessons in Clarity and Grace*. See Table 28.4 for transitional phrases to consider. Consider the old information presented in the last sentence and start the next sentence with a transition that prepares the reader for the new information. If the new information supports the old information, the transition might be "Similarly." If the new information is the opposite of the old information, the transition prepares the reader with "In contrast" or something similar.

PROVIDING ADEQUATE BACKGROUND INFORMATION

PRINCIPLE 102 • Reference and define background information.

Start the Introduction with a general, yet concise, description of the problem that your paper will address. In the next few sentences, reference previous work that supports your assessment of the problem.

Early in the Introduction, define the primary subject of your paper. Define any new, unusual, or vague terms used in the title or Introduction, such as "poor nutritional status" or "preventable death." If other authors have defined these terms differently, help the reader understand the differences between the definitions and explain why you defined the terms as you did.

Anticipate and avoid the following types of criticism:

+ The phrase "high risk" must be applied carefully, defined, and referenced. Otherwise, the reader may wonder, "High risk for what?" "Are all patients at an equally high risk?"
+ Please clarify what is meant by "severe depression."
+ How do we define this condition?
+ Presumably, there is some gold standard against which we measure care. But what is it, and how is it derived?
+ "Uneventful" should be defined.

> **VITAL POINT**
> Define all potentially questionable terms.

You may be convinced that definitions are not necessary because your colleagues will understand the terminology. Today, however, many reviewers may come from outside your subspecialty and may not understand your terminology. Defining unfamiliar terms makes your study easier for them to understand and should improve the ratings of your paper.

PRINCIPLE 103 • Write a concise, focused Introduction.

Reviewers often complain that the Introduction is too long and contains too much history, too many references, and not enough punch. Avoid writing a verbose Introduction that will make reviewers moan, "Who cares?"

You can improve your Introduction by explaining why your research question is important, interesting, or controversial, but do not include paragraphs of information that can be found in a textbook. Although you may have conducted an exhaustive review of the literature, include only the most relevant and significant points in your Introduction. Anticipate criticism such as the following:

+ What sensitivities, specificities, and predictive values have been reported in similar patients?
+ The Introduction needs to reference the literature to show that the reported results are better than a placebo; otherwise, a reader may think, "Maybe neither drug is effective."

+ What is the overall success rate for this treatment in patients with this condition?
+ What is the difference between the complication rates for these groups?
+ What is the evidence that one factor is as important as another in causing the complication?

PRINCIPLE 104 • Use the literature to enrich your Introduction.

Do not over-reference the Introduction. This section, in particular, must be short. On the other hand, if your sample is small or if you do not have an ideal control group, you can strengthen your paper with a few well-selected findings from published studies.

The journalist Philip Ross (1995) wrote, "Flip-flops in the history of health advice are the rule rather than the exception." To avoid this type of criticism, prove that you understand the historical importance of your subject. Within this body of knowledge, position your study. For example, does your study have a larger sample size, better control of confounding factors, longer follow-up, more recent data, or more accurate measurements? Summarize this account as concisely as possible in the Introduction and elaborate on it in the Discussion.

These flip-flops are often the result of inclusion criteria that do not focus on a homogeneous group of high-risk patients. Up until recently, it was difficult to identify high-risk patients in a timely and precise way. Now that it is possible to build real-time predictive models into electronic health records, this is much more feasible. Rather than relying on overly simplistic inclusion criteria or a simplistic scoring system, researchers can assess interventions with modern risk stratification based on probabilities from logistic regression models.

VITAL POINT

Describe the specific shape of the gap in current scientific knowledge and explain how your study fills this gap (Figs. 22.1 and 22.2). Show "This is not already known."

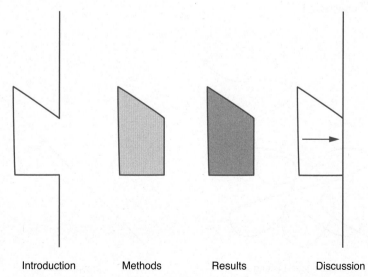

Introduction   Methods   Results   Discussion

FIGURE 22.1. How a paper fills a niche in the literature. The Introduction must demonstrate the specific knowledge gap in the scientific literature. The Methods must show how you will fill that specific shape. The Results show how you filled it. The Discussion shows how you moved the boundaries of science forward.

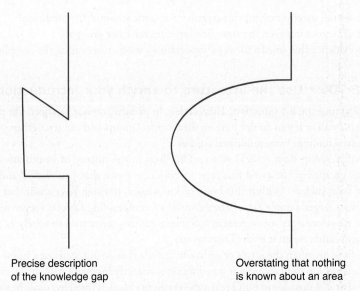

Precise description
of the knowledge gap

Overstating that nothing
is known about an area

FIGURE 22.2. Precise niche versus overstating that nothing is known about an area. Define the knowledge gap in the current scientific literature precisely. Avoid making broad statements about how little is known.

PRINCIPLE 105 • Articulate the prespecified purpose of your study.

The study should not appear to be organized around analysis of a variety of measurements in hope of finding any significant differences. In the Introduction, provide a clear linear map showing the direction of your study, so the reviewer does not interpret it as a "fishing expedition" (Fig. 22.3). A predefined registered analysis plan with a primary end point is the best way to avoid this criticism.

Identify the major point of your paper and write to that point; do not go off on tangents. Deliver what you promise without making the reader hunt for it. The specific aim and hypothesis should be easy to find and understand.

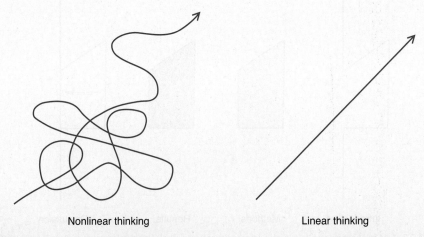

Nonlinear thinking

Linear thinking

FIGURE 22.3. Nonlinear versus linear thinking. A good paper is based on linear thinking and writing. Each section builds on previous sections with the six steps of the scientific method acting as the foundation for this linear thinking.

Be sure that the reasoning in your paper follows a straight line from the purpose (in the Introduction) to the conclusion (at the end of the Discussion). Straying from the hypothesis or the objective of the analysis is a problem with many research papers. A good paper has 1 or 2 main problems to solve but not 14. At the end of the Introduction, be sure to describe the overall purpose of your study but not your conclusions.

If you have trouble deciding where to start, write one sentence for each major section of your paper: Introduction, Methods, Results, and Discussion. For each, answer the question, "What is the most important point of this section?" Identifying these four points can help you to write a focused paper that readers will understand. If this method does not help, remember what Steve Martin said, "Writer's block is a fancy term made up by whiners so they can have an excuse to drink alcohol."

FOR MORE INFORMATION

See the *Publication Manual of the American Psychological Association* (American Psychological Association, 2010) for examples and further details on what is appropriate for the Introduction.

PRINCIPLE 106 • Polish the most important sentence in your paper.

VITAL POINT

The last sentence of the Introduction is the most important sentence in your paper. In it, you must convince the reviewers that the research question that your study addresses is an important question to answer, regardless of the answer. Continue revising the last sentence of your Introduction until it is compelling. The Introduction must build a logical, linear case for this sentence without zigzagging through the history of the field and should funnel from the broad background to your specific question. Study examples of the last sentence in the Introduction from the top journals to develop this skill.

What is the important question that has not already been answered in the literature that you will answer with this study? Invest the time to polish this question until it is precise. Make it easy for reviewers to locate your clearly stated purpose statement by placing it in the last sentence of the Introduction.

Reviewers will be wondering:

+ What is the big question?
+ Where is this going?

One of the most effective ways to help reviewers follow your story is to write one sentence for each of the six steps of the scientific method. The sentence for the first step of the scientific method (state the problem) belongs at the end of the Introduction and should be of this form:

"The problem that this study is designed to address is that from the current medical literature, it is unclear whether treatment A or treatment B is more effective for patients with disease X."

PRINCIPLE 107 • Condense the Introduction.

Writing a good Introduction is a challenge because you must present a great deal of important information in just a few words. How few? Check recently published Introductions in the target journal and make yours slightly less than or equal to the average length. A good rule of thumb is to keep the Introduction to one double-spaced page. To become efficient at writing papers, avoid writing a five-page Introduction and then spending weeks deciding what to delete. If the Introduction is longer than one page, consider moving paragraphs to the Discussion or Appendix.

Sometimes, the best way to write an Introduction is to write one version and then step back from the trees to see the forest. Have someone interview you and challenge you to summarize the Introduction at a higher level. Think hard about what the actual problem is that your study will answer. Then throw your old Introduction away and start with a clean piece of paper to tell this higher level and more insightful but concise story on one page.

VITAL POINT

Nearly all reviewers and editors agreed on the following piece of advice: "Make the Introduction shorter!"

FOR MORE INFORMATION

See Lang (2009).

Methods

PURPOSE OF THE METHODS SECTION

Note: Start the Methods and each major section on a new page. This makes it easier for reviewers to skim.

PRINCIPLE 108 • Provide ample detail in your Methods section to document reproducible research and use supplementary appendices for additional details.

The Methods is the simplest section to write because it simply recounts what you have done. Ironically, however, the leading cause of manuscript rejection is a poor Methods section (Figs. 23.1 and 23.2).

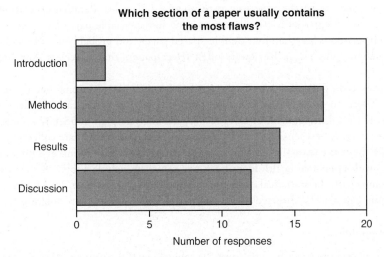

Which section of a paper usually contains the most flaws?

FIGURE 23.1. The manuscript section that usually contains the most flaws. From question 3 of the Peer Review Questionnaire (Appendix B). $P = .010$ based on a chi-square test.

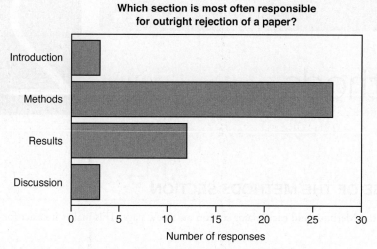

FIGURE 23.2. The manuscript section that is most often responsible for rejection. From question 4 of the Peer Review Questionnaire (Appendix B). $P < .001$ based on a chi-square test.

> **VITAL POINT**
>
> Reproducibility of results is the heart of science, so budget sufficient time to write a complete and accurate Methods section.

The goal in writing the Methods section is to present a clear but detailed exposition of the research design. An exceptional Methods section is an indispensable part of a successful paper. If your Methods section is less than four double-spaced pages, you probably need to add more detail before you submit your paper. Reviewers often reject papers that have less than four pages of Methods.

To avoid exceeding the target journal's word count, include additional details in the paper's appendices. These do not count in the word total. These appendices can include a copy of the study protocol with a description of the prespecified analysis plan, modeling strategy and validation, model diagnostics, sensitivity analyses, a copy of the survey or data collection form, additional details about the statistical analyses and statistical software coding or syntax. For studies that do not involve personal health identifiers, you can even include a table of the raw data from your study along with the statistical coding in the Appendix, for example, see Maron et al. (2011). The Appendix can also be directed at the statistical reviewers who are looking for additional detail.

Example wording:

"Sensitivity analyses were performed to assess the robustness of the primary efficacy analysis (see the Supplementary Appendix)."

"Additional details of the sample size justification and statistical analysis are provided in the Supplementary Appendix."

An excellent example of a researcher who shares raw data and statistical coding online is Jeffrey Leek. See:

http://jtleek.com/papers/

PRINCIPLE 109 • Organize the Methods according to meaningful subheadings.

Table 23.1 shows an example of Methods subheadings. Using subheadings makes it much easier for you to write the paper and for reviewers and readers to understand it. Be sure that you use subheadings that are logical and meaningful and that you have enough text to justify each subheading. A subheading followed by only one or two sentences of text should be avoided.

A new important subheading for the Methods of randomized controlled trials is "Study Oversight." Example wording:

"The study protocol, available along with the most recent version of the statistical analysis plan in the appendix of supplementary material, was approved by the institutional review board at each participating hospital. The study was conducted in accordance with the provisions of the Declaration of Helsinki and International Conference on Harmonisation Guidelines for Good Clinical Practice. All the patients provided written informed consent."

Then describe the data and safety monitor plan and prespecified interim analyses.

Example wording:

"Rules for stopping the study early at interim analyses were prespecified (reference x). The data and safety monitoring board conducted four safety reviews. In addition, two interim efficacy analyses were performed, after 33% and 66% of the required patients had been enrolled; adjustment of the level of significance to account for the two interim analyses was determined by the Lan–DeMets approximation of the O'Brien–Fleming boundaries for group sequential testing, with a final two-sided P value for significance of .0XXX or less."

TABLE 23.1	**Examples of Subheadings to Provide a Framework in the Methods Section**[a]

Study Design
Eligibility Criteria
Randomization and Blinding
Intervention and Compliance
Assessment of End Points
Safety
Study Oversight
Statistical Analysis
****

Patients
Study Design
Study End Points
Statistical Analysis
****

Study Design and Population
Clinical Assessment
Intervention
Outcome Assessment
Statistical Analysis

[a]Mentors can create an outline using headings such as these to help their mentees work more efficiently.

THE STUDY DESIGN

PRINCIPLE 110 • Develop a golden study design and define it with precise terminology.

The Methods section should of course describe the study design and explain how the data were collected. Yet, as Kassirer and Campion (1994) pointed out, many papers are rejected because the authors did not adequately explain the experimental design. This problem also is evident in Figures 23.3 and 23.4.

Part of the problem is simply miscommunication. "Retrospective" is a word that causes much confusion. Retrospective study is the old terminology for case-control study. As described in Chapter 3, the term "retrospective" refers to the act or process of surveying the past and often is based on memory. In a retrospective study, people with and without a specified outcome are compared. Researchers investigate the histories of these two groups to look for the presence of, or exposure to, a particular factor. Then the proportions of subjects with this factor are compared between the two groups.

If you collected your data by surveying the past (retrospectively), explain why this approach was appropriate, despite its limitations. Retrospectively collected information often is of poorer quality than prospectively collected information because the presence or absence of many conditions is not documented consistently in routine medical records. For instance, smoking and drinking histories may be vague or may not be recorded at all. Histories provided by subjects often are inaccurate and biased. In addition, the control group may be a major limitation because it is the potential source of many types of bias.

In both the Methods and Discussion, provide information to help the editor and reviewers see why they should recommend your paper for publication rather than wait for a study with prospectively collected data. Also state whether you included observations that were recorded before the study began.

Example 23–1.

If you reported blood pressures, state whether you obtained the readings from records of previous admissions and office visits or if all readings were observed and recorded after you began the study.

Always explain whether you recorded the study variables before or after the disease or outcome occurred and also whether you assigned the patients to the study groups prospectively or retrospectively. Also state whether you reviewed charts before or after the patients were discharged.

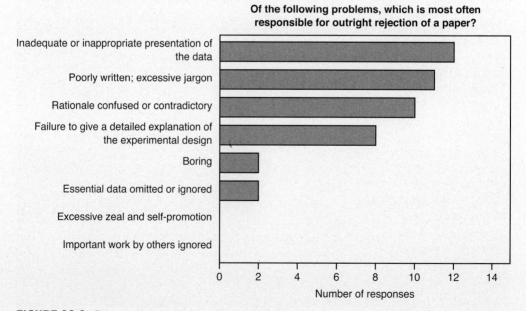

Of the following problems, which is most often responsible for outright rejection of a paper?

FIGURE 23.3. Presentation problems and rejection. From question 13 of the Peer Review Questionnaire (Appendix B). $P = .021$ based on a chi-square test.

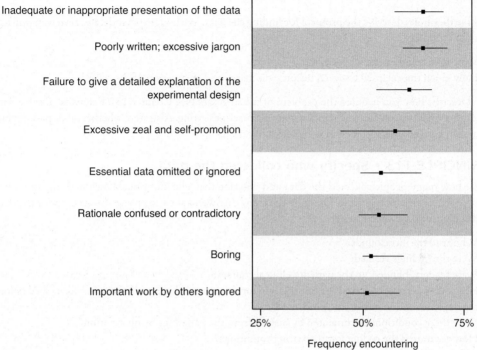

FIGURE 23.4. The frequency of presentation problems. Answers are ranked by the median and boot-strap 95% CI using the sliding scale responses 0% (never) to 100% (always). From question 12 of the Peer Review Questionnaire (Appendix B). $P = .002$ based on the Friedman test.

VITAL POINT

Avoid oversimplifying your study by describing it with vague or outdated study design terminology. Precision is essential for reproducible research.

PRINCIPLE 111 • Use the term "prospective" carefully.

Prospective designs begin with subjects who do not have the outcome under study, for example, people without cancer. The presence of suspected etiologic factors is determined (e.g., smoking), and the subjects are followed up to see in whom the outcome of interest develops. Many medical researchers misuse the word "prospective." Instead of "retrospective" and "prospective," use more specific terms, such as "case–control," "prospective cohort," "retrospective cohort," or "cross-sectional," to describe your study design. A case-control study would identify a group of people with lung cancer and a control group without lung cancer. Then investigators would assess whether these people had a history of smoking.

PRINCIPLE 112 • Describe your data collection methods in detail.

To describe your data collection methods adequately, think like a journalist and answer the following questions:

+ Who?
+ What?
+ When?

+ Where?
+ How?
+ Why?

Furthermore, describe the protocol for finding the data. Without explicit details, reviewers will ask such questions as:

+ Were data complete for all patients?
+ How much time elapsed between hospital discharge and abstraction of the records?

Describe how you handled the problem of missing data (see Chapter 13). Extensive missing data and other quality problems will damage your manuscript's rating. Also state whether all or part of your cohort of patients was included in previous publications.

PRINCIPLE 113 • Specify who collected the data.

State how many people collected the data and describe their qualifications. Document the intrarater and interrater reliability testing. Describe the steps that were taken to ensure the accuracy of the data and coding, or reviewers may ask:

+ Who read the ultrasounds?
+ Were the findings verified?
+ Were readers "blinded" to the patients' clinical courses?
+ How many persons collected the information for this study? Were conditions that developed before the implementation of the study included?
+ Were these conditions documented by history from the patient or by observation?
+ How accurate is the coding for preexisting conditions?

Reporting that "there was no documented history of X" usually is more accurate than claiming that a subgroup of patients "never had X."

PRINCIPLE 114 • Describe the setting of the study.

Explain where the study was conducted and provide relevant information about the institution, such as:

+ What type of population is served by the hospital or institution?
+ Is the setting urban, suburban, or rural?
+ How many beds does the hospital have?
+ Is the facility a teaching hospital?
+ Is it a tertiary care center?

PRINCIPLE 115 • Define your variables to enable replication.

Carefully define important variables, grades of conditions, and criteria for disease severity. Reviewers expect that any potentially confusing terms in the title, abstract, or Introduction will be clearly defined in the Methods. Double-check that you have defined all nebulous terms.

Example 23–2.
Congenital anomalies/malformations and deformations can be defined with International Classification of Diseases (ICD-9) codes: 740.0 through 759.9, or for ICD-10: Q00–Q99. Note how this coding provides a concise, yet unambiguous definition.

The Methods must provide enough detail to enable one of your peers to reproduce your study. To ensure that it does, look for the following types of problems:

+ The diagnoses are not sufficiently rigorous for us.
+ How and when were measurements and determinations for the key variables made?

+ How were the conditions diagnosed or classified?
+ Would most experts in this field agree with these definitions?
+ What protocol was followed for treatment?
+ Were all three variables needed for a positive finding, or any one of the three?
+ A brief description of how mobility and activity were measured is needed.

State the cutoff points for diagnosis of medical conditions. You can avoid lengthy descriptions by referencing laboratory, statistical, and scaling methods to standard works. For the reader's benefit, consider using textbooks or literature reviews rather than highly technical original papers and include page numbers. If you modify a published method, provide enough detail to make your variation reproducible. Finally, reference any previous publication that described your study's database, protocol, or design.

Anticipate reviewers asking, "How much?" "How long?" and "When?" For example:

+ *Give an indication of when the blood was drawn and whether or not the patients were fasting at the time of blood drawing.*
+ *The Methods need to be expanded. Tests were performed twice a week, but it is unclear which tests were included in the final analysis.*
+ *In the Materials and Methods section, the authors describe their use of X. The authors need to be much more precise in describing how X was evaluated. If an abnormal value was detected, did the authors verify it by additional readings? Did the authors take six readings and average them? And so on.*

Reviewers expect details:

+ *How many milligrams of the drug were injected?*
+ *How about the size of the needle?*

How can you provide more detail about the methods used in your study? Imagine that the reviewers are trying to reproduce your study. What additional details will they need to know? Are there definitions that you can include or make clearer? Can you provide more detail about the conditions in the laboratory? Have you provided the manufacturer of the tests used? **The single most important thing you can do to get your paper published is to carefully describe the details of your methods in a manner that would enable another researcher to reproduce it.** Imagine the difference between a cake that was made from a vague recipe and one that was made from a recipe that was complete and included all of the necessary details.

ELIGIBILITY

PRINCIPLE 116 • Describe the source of the study subjects.

In the Methods, present objective inclusion criteria. State the number of patients who met your inclusion criteria. Saying "I deemed 79 patients inappropriate" is both archaic and unreproducible and gives the impression that you selected cases that agreed with your opinion. Keep track of which patients were excluded from the study.

State how many patients were excluded and for what reasons. Also explain how many patients were excluded for more than one reason. If you established any priority for the exclusion criteria, explain your decision. Compare the excluded patients with the study group. In the Discussion, explain how any differences between the groups could alter the interpretation of the findings.

VITAL POINT

Do not include results in the Methods section.

For randomized controlled trials, you can end the Methods with a statement such as this:

Findings from the study are described in accordance with Consolidated Standards of Reporting Trials (CONSORT) guidelines.[x]

Then reference the most recent version of the CONSORT statement, such as this:

x. Schulz KF, Altman DG, Moher D, et al. CONSORT 2010 statement: updated guidelines for reporting parallel group randomized trials. *Ann Intern Med* 2010;152:726–732.

PRINCIPLE 117 • Provide the beginning and ending dates of the study.

Give the dates that were used in your inclusion criteria and explain why you chose these limits. If you later uncover a few more "good cases" that occurred outside these limits, resist the temptation to add them. Remember, your article may be read in many countries, and you can avoid confusion by spelling out the month. For example, 1/12/15 may be read as January 12, 2015, or December 1, 2015.

RANDOMIZATION AND "BLINDING"

PRINCIPLE 118 • Explain your rationale for randomizing.

In the Methods section, state whether the subjects were randomly assigned to receive the treatment and provide reproducible details of the randomization methods that you used. Indicate the type of randomization, how it was implemented, and software used. In the Appendix, include randomization detail, such as the seed used. A seed is a number (such as 1234) used to as a starting point to initialize a pseudorandom number generator that enables one to reproduce the random number table.

Reviewers usually prefer blinded randomization. Yet, according to Fried (1974), " . . . the claims for the RCT [randomized controlled trial] have been greatly, indeed preposterously overstated." Despite reviewers' preference for randomization, randomized studies can have problems.

> *Example 23–3.*
> Suppose, for instance, that as part of a study of educational methods, class sizes were randomly set as large or small. A number of factors might affect the outcome. Teachers might change their teaching methods based on the size of the class. Consequently, the results might be caused not by the number of students in the classroom but by the teaching method.

Reviewers may regard nonrandomized studies as too weak for publication unless you prove that the groups were similar or that you controlled for the differences between the groups.

For many clinical problems, an observational study is the only ethical alternative. These studies often are less expensive, more realistic, and more efficient than experimental studies because they answer the research question quickly. You must build your case, as a lawyer would, for observational studies.

In observational studies, the variables (e.g., class size) are not manipulated; they simply are observed in their natural state, with various conditions and various outcomes. Statisticians often prefer comprehensive observational databases to randomized controlled trials, especially to evaluate potentially lifesaving therapies (Berry, 1989; Royall et al., 1991). As Truog (1992) pointed out, for some clinical research problems, observational studies provide the optimal balance of high-quality treatment and scientific research. The take-away message is to always explain your reasons for selecting your study design.

Having said that, more large randomized controlled trials are needed in clinical medicine. These trials will become a natural part of future learning health care systems. It is easy to quickly dismiss randomization as impossible, but often, with a little thought, there are ethical ways to randomize and answer many important questions. Successful hospital administrators and quality improvement leaders will become more comfortable with randomization to learn what works and what does not work. Health outcomes are often slow to improve because hospital managers rush to fix problems but fail to include an evaluation of what works. Science and randomization do not slow the progress of improving patient outcomes—they speed progress.

PRINCIPLE 119 • Describe the informed consent process used in your study.

For all randomized studies, experimental investigations, and studies that used interviews with human subjects, state whether you obtained informed consent. Demonstrate that you protected the patients' rights. If you did not obtain informed consent, explain why. For example, you may have received a waiver of the informed consent process. Journals will not even consider manuscripts that do not properly address the issue of informed consent. Be careful to avoid saying that "patients were consented." Instead, describe this as patients were informed about the study and then chose to give consent.

Example wording:

"Written informed consent was obtained from all participants prior to enrollment."
"All patients provided written informed consent before study entry."

FOR MORE INFORMATION

See Hulley et al. (2013) for a discussion of informed consent and exemptions.

INTERVENTION AND COMPLIANCE

PRINCIPLE 120 • Provide specifics for any drugs or devices that were tested.

For studies of biomedical devices, enclose unfamiliar engineering terms in quotation marks and define these terms specifically for the readers of the target journal. Capitalize any proprietary names (e.g., trademarks). Describe other competing medical devices and explain why you studied that particular brand and model.

Some journals list the name of the device with the manufacturer's name, city, state, and country in parentheses. The key point to remember is that reviewers and editors will be especially concerned with potential bias and disguised advertising.

For pharmaceutical studies, provide the dosage and route of administration. As always, follow the policy of the target journal for providing drug names. Most journals use the drug's generic, or nonproprietary, name (e.g., aspirin, digitalis) in text. The first time you name each drug, include the proprietary, or trade/brand, name (capitalized) and the manufacturer's name and location in parentheses.

PRINCIPLE 121 • Omit unnecessary details.

Although computer hardware and software specifications may be an important part of your work, avoid providing superfluous details in the Methods section. In most cases, you can simply provide the name and version number of the statistical software. Editors and reviewers should insist that investigators include a statement about the statistical software in the Methods section of every manuscript. This is essential for reproducible research.

Example wording:

"The data analysis for this paper was generated using SAS software, version 9.4 (SAS Institute)."
"Analyses were performed with the use of SAS software, version 9.4 (SAS Institute), and the R statistical package (version 3.2.3).^{x}"

Then in the references, you can include a reference for R, such as:

x. R Core Team. R: a language and environment for statistical computing. Vienna, Austria: R Foundation for Statistical Computing; 2016.

Or

x. R Core Team (2016). R: A language and environment for statistical computing. R Foundation for Statistical Computing, Vienna, Austria. http://www.r-project.org/.

Within the R software, you can type: "citation()" at the command prompt(>) and then cut and paste the citation.

To cite a package, such as the survival package, within R, type: "citation("survival")."

"We performed all analyses using SAS software, version 9.4 (SAS Software), and IBM SPSS software, version 23.0."

"All analyses were performed with the Stata Statistical Software: Release 14 (StataCorp, 2015, College Station, TX: StataCorp LP)."

PRINCIPLE 122 • Provide a full evaluation of the screening tests.

When you compare several clinical tests, state whether the tests were diagnostic, screening, or prognostic according to the following criteria:

+ Diagnostic tests determine the presence of a disease.
+ Screening tests are relatively inexpensive diagnostic tests that detect individuals who need more testing.
+ Prognostic tests predict the outcome of a disease.

If some of your patients underwent more than one test, explain the order of testing and the rationale for this order. If some of the tests were repeated, explain which results were included in the analysis and graphs. Also, explain your institution's testing protocol.

For some conditions, sensitivity is important; for others, specificity is more important. Discuss the relative importance of sensitivity, specificity, positive predictive value, negative predictive value, and overall accuracy for patients with the study condition. Include 95% confidence intervals (CIs). Finally, describe how many patients with an adverse outcome had more than one abnormal test result.

FOR MORE INFORMATION

See Dawson and Trapp (2005); Fletcher et al. (2012); and Haynes et al. (2011).

END POINTS AND OUTCOME

PRINCIPLE 123 • Define your primary outcome in a clear and reproducible way.

End points are the variables that represent the completion of a study interval (e.g., discharge from the hospital or death). The Methods section must include a reproducible, detailed definition of your end points.

When using a variable as a measure of outcome, clearly define your criteria. Even if they seem obvious, define all measures of outcome. If you use a definition that differs from that found in the dictionary, provide your definition. Defining your outcome in detail will improve the odds of publication by avoiding criticism such as the following:

> My major concern continues to be the end point that you used for discharge, the patient's ability to walk independently. You provide us with no indication as to how far the patient should be able to walk, over what surface, and, for instance, if stair climbing is part of this evaluation.

SAMPLE SIZE

PRINCIPLE 124 • Justify your sample size with reproducible detail.

A description of the sample size calculations is a crucial but often neglected part of the Methods section (Figs. 23.5 and 23.6). When reviewing medical manuscripts, statistical consultants frequently ask the editor, "Can the authors provide any rationale or statistical power considerations underlying their choice of sample size?" (Colton, 1990).

In addition, biostatisticians often ask, "Did the negative study have sufficient power to detect clinically meaningful effects, if such effects truly existed?" (Colton, 1990).

Describe the method that you used to calculate the necessary sample size. Provide enough detail and adequate references (e.g., which study the standard deviation was based on) so that others can reproduce your sample size calculations. Also reference the statistical software that you used.

See Chapter 9 for more details.

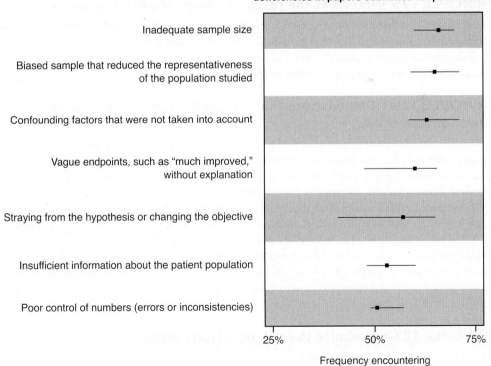

How frequently do you encounter the following deficiencies in papers submitted for publication?

FIGURE 23.5. The frequency of research design problems. Answers are ranked by the median and bootstrap 95% CI using the sliding scale responses 0% (never) to 100% (always). From question 23 of the Peer Review Questionnaire (Appendix B). $P < .001$ based on the Friedman test.

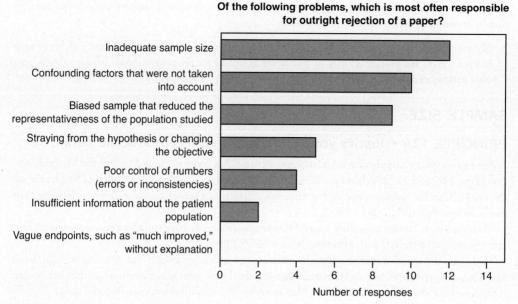

Of the following problems, which is most often responsible for outright rejection of a paper?

FIGURE 23.6. Research design problems and rejection. From question 24 of the Peer Review Questionnaire (Appendix B). $P = .054$ based on a chi-square test.

PRINCIPLE 125 • Interpret the results of small studies cautiously.

If your study has a small sample size, discuss the low power of statistical tests. Do not include this interpretation of your sample size in the Methods section; it belongs in the Discussion. In studies with small samples, anticipate greater variance, lack of statistical power, and large differences that are not statistically significant but nevertheless may be clinically important.

PRINCIPLE 126 • Demonstrate that you understand the statistical power of your study.

Describe the sample size that is necessary to achieve statistical significance for a clinically meaningful end point and provide a statistical basis for the number of patients included in your study. Although most clinical research papers need a complete statement about sample size, many do not include such a statement. These topics are discussed in more detail in Chapter 9.

To estimate sample size, begin with the typical power calculation settings: a power of .90 and a significance level of .05 (the equivalent of a 5% chance of a Type I error and a 10% chance of a Type II error).

Many people are confused by the concept of Type I and Type II errors (Fig. 23.7). A simple way to understand this idea is to consider the null hypothesis "innocent until proven guilty." The four possible outcomes are shown in Figure 23.8. A jury tries to minimize the possibility of convicting an innocent person (Type I error) and minimize the possibility of setting a guilty person free (Type II error). For each clinical research study, you too must balance the risk of these errors.

PRINCIPLE 127 • Minimize the risk of a Type I error.

Table 23.2 shows the features of a Type I error.

PRINCIPLE 128 • Minimize the risk of a Type II error.

Table 23.3 shows the features of a Type II error. In studies with small samples, report and discuss the power and probability of Type II errors. Remember, Type II errors are more common with small samples.

The null hypothesis is:

Decision	True	False
Accept the null hypothesis	No error (1 — alpha) 95%	Type II error (beta) 20%
Reject the null hypothesis	Type I error (alpha or *p*) 5%	No error (1 — beta, power) 80%

FIGURE 23.7. Illustration of Type I and Type II errors. The percentages represent the conventional levels that many researchers use.

The truth is that the assumption of innocence is:

The Jury's Verdict	True (Truly Innocent)	False (Guilty)
Accept the assumption: Acquit	No error 1 — alpha Innocent person acquitted	Type II error Beta error Guilty person acquitted
Reject the assumption: Convict	Type I error Alpha error Innocent person convicted	No error Power Guilty person convicted

FIGURE 23.8. Analogy of a jury's decision illustrating Type I and Type II errors.

TABLE 23.2 Features of a Type I Error

Rejection of a true null hypothesis
False claim of a difference
Common when a researcher is too ready to reject the null hypothesis
Alpha error
Occurs approximately 5% of the time with a *P* value threshold of <.05
Analogous to convicting an innocent person

TABLE 23.3 Features of a Type II Error

The chance of missing a real effect
An acceptance of a false null hypothesis
False claim of no difference when a difference actually exists, but the sample size is too small to prove it
Common when a researcher is too ready to accept the null hypothesis
Beta error (β)
Occurs approximately 20% of the time with a power of 80% (power = $1 - \beta$)
Analogous to acquitting a guilty person

To remember these error types, use the following mnemonic device: A Type I error is an alpha error, and A is the first letter of the alphabet. A Type II error is a beta error, and B is the second letter of the alphabet. Then remember that the alpha threshold corresponds to the P value significance threshold (typically .05).

PRINCIPLE 129 • Rely on the median and bootstrapped confidence interval rather than the mean and standard deviation.

You can maximize the value of small and skewed samples by using the data analysis techniques that professionals use. For example, you can report the median (middle value) rather than the mean for small samples as well as for ordinal variables and for skewed data. In these situations, the median is a more accurate estimate of central tendency. Researchers will often report the interquartile range (IQR)—the 25th and 75th percentile—along with the median. A more sophisticated approach is to report the CIs around the median using the bootstrap method.

Example 23–4.

Group	Length of Hospital Stay (days)	Mean ± SD	Median (bootstrap CI)
1	10, 10, 11, 11, 12, 12, 13, 13, 14, 14	12.0 ± 1.5	12 (10.5 to 13.5)
2	10, 10, 11, 11, 12, 12, 13, 13, 14, 365	47.1 ± 111.7	12 (10.5 to 13.5)

Example 23–4 shows that one number (365) distorts the mean but not the median.

If you decide to report a median rather than a mean, report the median for similar variables throughout the paper. Mixing medians and means for similar variables may confuse readers and make them suspicious.

To compute the median and 95% CI with the bootstrap, follow these steps:

In IBM SPSS: Analyze, Descriptive Statistics, Frequencies . . ., Move variables to the right, under Statistics select Median, Continue, under Bootstrap . . ., check Perform bootstrapping, Set seed for Mersenne Twister = 1234, Continue, OK.

STATISTICAL ANALYSIS

PRINCIPLE 130 • Make the statistical presentation easy to understand.

Show that you understand the statistical methods used and can clearly report the statistical results. Although most reviewers are highly skilled physicians and scientists, many need help understanding some of the advanced statistical analysis used in most modern studies.

Verify that the Methods section describes the statistical analysis adequately. The biostatistician and the primary writer must work together and should check the final draft to ensure that their sections fit together seamlessly. Inconsistencies in the description of the statistical analysis may raise questions about the quality of your work.

Example 23–5.
If, instead of writing "logistic regression," you incorrectly write "logistical regression" or "logistics regression," reviewers may have trouble believing anything else that you say. Minor point-mutation typos can create major concerns, such as writing "Turkey's post hoc test" rather than "Tukey's post hoc test."

Describe with footnotes in tables and the figure legend page exactly where and why you used the principal tests. In addition to using the correct tests, you must interpret each one adequately. If you used any unusual statistical methods, reference them and explain why you decided not to use more common statistical methods. You cannot simply say that you applied matching and logistic regression. Describe them in detail and explain precisely how you used them.

> **VITAL POINT**
>
> Edit the description of the statistical analysis carefully to create a recipe for reproducible research.

Many reviewers lack the necessary skills to evaluate statistics. When editors were asked, "Do you feel that you have adequate skills to evaluate the statistical aspects of most medical manuscripts you are asked to review?" 29% of the editors said "No." In response to the same question, twice as many reviewers (58%) said "No" (Byrne, 2000). Although many of the editors said that they consulted statistical reviewers when necessary, you can help reviewers and editors by revising your description until you minimize the possibility of misinterpretation.

For papers with statistical methods that are beyond the basics, it is wise to have a coauthor who is an experienced biostatistician. This has also been demonstrated to increase the probability of acceptance (Altman et al., 2002).

PRINCIPLE 131 • Define statistical significance intelligently.

Include the word "considered" in descriptions of statistical significance such as "a P value of less than .05 was considered statistically significant."

Example wording:

"A two-sided P value of less than .05 was considered to indicate statistical significance."
"All tests were two-sided, and P values of less than .05 were considered to indicate statistical significance."
"P values were two-sided, and values of less than .05 were considered to indicate statistical significance."
"All tests were two-sided, and exact P values are provided."

Whenever possible, avoid dichotomizing P values into significant or not and provide exact P values for the readers to evaluate. Change the focus away from the P value to the 95% CI for the clinically meaningful end point.

PRINCIPLE 132 • Provide reproducible details of your statistical methods.

Any professional biostatistician given a copy of your data should be able to verify your results after reading the Methods section. Use this criterion to determine how much detail to provide.

You can start the "Statistical Analysis" section of the Methods by clearly stating your null hypothesis and the specific statistical test that you will use to test it, for example:

"The primary null hypothesis was that there would be no difference between randomization groups in the proportion of patients free from cancer at 1 year. We tested this hypothesis in an intention-to-treat analysis using a chi-square test, at a .05 alpha level."

The Methods section should have three sentences each addressing steps 2, 3, and 4 of the scientific method: 2 = formulate the null hypothesis, 3 = design the study, and 4 = collect the data.

PRINCIPLE 133 • Justify your choice of statistical tests.

A common criticism by reviewers is inappropriate use of statistical tests by authors. Without a clear explanation showing that the appropriate statistical methods were applied, reviewers may ask:

+ Who oversaw the statistics?
+ Does a biostatistician agree that the proper tests were done?

From these comments, one can see how including a biostatistician as a coauthor significantly increases the odds of acceptance (Altman et al., 2002). Reviewers tend to be reassured that the statistical analyses were performed appropriately if a biostatistician has his or her name on the paper. Of course, this is no guarantee that the statistics are flawless, but it helps build credibility.

PRINCIPLE 134 • Include your complete prespecified statistical analysis plan in the Appendix.

In the Methods section, describe your statistical analysis plan and explain that is was prespecified. If you also include analyses that were not prespecified, label this as post hoc.

"The power of the study was 80%" is too simplistic. Instead provide reproducible detail.

> *Example 23–6.*
> We calculated that this study would need to assign 476 patients to each of the two study groups for the study to have 90% power to detect a minimally important absolute difference of 10 percentage points between the treatment group and the placebo group with respect to the rate of disease cure after 1 year (from 60% to 70% [reference here]; odds ratio 0.65), at an alpha level of .05. We planned to include a total of 1,058 patients in the study to account for a 10% rate of loss to follow-up.

Then in the Appendix of the paper, you can provide additional detail about the sample size software used, whether this is based on a chi-square or Fisher's exact test, ratio of patients in the two arms, etc.

The next paragraph of the Methods would describe the statistical analysis plan, for example:

"All analyses were performed according to the intention-to-treat principle. We used the chi-square test and Fisher's exact test for categorical comparisons of data. Continuous variables were summarized with medians and bootstrapped 95% CIs. Nonparametric methods were used regardless of the distributions to provide robust comparisons. Differences for continuous measurements were tested by the Mann-Whitney U test. The primary end point of cure at 1 year was analyzed with a logistic regression models in four prespecified subgroups (stages 1 to 4). The data and safety monitoring committee reviewed the interim analysis data twice according to the prespecified plan described in Appendix A. A *P* value of less than .05 was considered to indicate statistical significance; all tests were two-tailed. All statistical analyses were performed with the statistical package SAS and the R software (http://www.r-project.org, version 3.2.3)."

If your paper includes subgroup analyses, be sure this is prespecified and follow the advice in "Statistics in Medicine—Reporting of Subgroup Analyses in Clinical Trials" by Wang et al. (2007). Use a forest plot to illustrate the findings.

Occasionally, when researchers attempt to prove that one treatment is not different from another treatment, they choose overly conservative statistical tests for which it is more difficult to obtain a *P* value of less than .05. Explain your reasons for choosing specific tests, or readers may think that you are trying to fool them. Many prominent journals now have a separate statistical review—all the more reason that your statistical recipe must be complete and match your prespecified analysis plan.

Additional examples of how to word the description of the statistical software:

"Statistical analyses were performed with the use of SAS software, version 9.4 (SAS Institute)."

"The R software program (R Project for Statistical Computing, http://www.r-project.org, version 3.2.3) was used for all analyses."

"We used the Stata statistical software for all analyses (StataCorp, 2015; Stata Statistical Software: Release 14. College Station, TX: StataCorp LP)."

"The statistical software IBM SPSS, version 23.0 (IBM) was used for all analyses."

In general, it is prudent to have two biostatisticians using different statistical software verify each other's results by sharing only the data and the Methods section of the paper as instructions. In the Methods, cite both software packages and mention this replication.

"Analyses were conducted with the use of SAS software, version 9.4 (SAS Institute), and R software, version 3.2.3 (R Project for Statistical Computing). All *P* values are two-sided."

FOR MORE INFORMATION

See Figure 16.1.

PRINCIPLE 135 • Learn statistical shorthand.

Understanding common statistical symbols, acronyms, and abbreviations will help you to interpret medical literature and read statistical books (Table 23.4). Chapter 28 (Principle 218) explains how to print Greek and other symbols.

TABLE 23.4	Commonly Used Statistical Symbols and Abbreviations
Symbol or Abbreviation	**Description**
Greek	
α = alpha	Probability of a Type I error, significance threshold level for the P value, typically $P < .05$, a preset rejection level
β = beta	Probability of a Type II error, $1 -$ power, typically 0.20
μ = mu	Mean, average
π = pi	Population proportion or 3.1415
σ = sigma (lowercase)	Population standard deviation
σ^2 = sigma squared	Population variance, standard deviation squared
χ^2 = chi-square	Chi-square statistic
Σ = sigma (uppercase)	Sum
Φ = phi	Phi coefficient
English	
ANOVA	Analysis of variance
AUC	Area Under the Curve
c	concordance probability = ROC area = AUC
CI	Confidence interval
df	Degrees of freedom
D_{xy}	Measure of discrimination, Somers' D_{xy} rank correlation
e	Base of the system of natural (Napierian) logarithms (e = 2.71828)
F	Variance ratio
H_0	Null hypothesis
H_A	Alternative hypothesis
∞	Infinity
N	Number in entire population, sample or size of finite population
n	Number in a subsample or subset
NS	Not significant
OR	Odds ratio
P	Probability (range, 0–1)
r	Pearson correlation coefficient (range, -1 to $+1$)
RR	Relative risk
r_s	Spearman rank correlation coefficient

(continued)

TABLE 23.4	Commonly Used Statistical Symbols and Abbreviations *(continued)*

Symbol or Abbreviation	Description
R^2	R squared, amount of variation explained
ROC	Receiver operating characteristics curve used to assess the performance of a predictive model
s	Standard deviation of a sample mean
s^2	Variance of a sample mean
SD	Standard deviation of a sample
SEM	Standard error of the mean
t	Student's t-test statistic
Z	Observation X in standard form, standard score, standard normal variate, standard normal variable or distribution

Results

ORGANIZING THE RESULTS

PRINCIPLE 136 • Present your results enthusiastically but professionally.

Most scientists are excited about their results, but many fail to convey this excitement and consequently write dull manuscripts.

Archimedes's reaction may have been extreme—yelling "Eureka!"—when he discovered how to measure the purity of gold. Yet, imparting this spirit of excitement, especially in the first few sentences of the Results, would improve most manuscripts.

After you analyze your data, reflect on what it means. Save your speculations and comments for the Discussion but do not report results robotically. Never start the Results with a page of number-heavy text. Instead, summarize similar types of numbers in tables, and invest the time to create reader-friendly professional graphs. As with the Methods, organize your material with an outline to make the Results easy to read.

Step 5 of the scientific method is analyze the results. Include one sentence in the Results that summarizes this and builds in a logical way from the previous four steps.

A sentence that starts with "Table" or "Figure" is generally weak; for example, "Table 1 shows that the baseline characteristics were similar between the two arms." A stronger sentence moves this information to the end, such as "The baseline characteristics were similar between the two arms (Table 1)."

PRINCIPLE 137 • Present your data in a natural and logical order to tell a story.

Often the most logical way to present your Results is to tell your story in the chronological order in which you discovered the findings but omit the details of your thought process. **Do not overstate the results or repeat in detail information that is given in the tables.** Instead, refer the reader to the tables and shorten the text of the Results. Keep the Results as organized and as simple as possible by moving important but distracting results to the Appendix.

If the order of discovery does not provide an appropriate presentation, consider organizing the Results sequentially from the clinician's perspective (e.g., prepregnancy, antepartum, postpartum) or topically (e.g., maternal, fetal).

Inadequate presentation of the results is a common reason for outright rejection (See Figure 23.3). To avoid this problem, verify that your results and follow-up data are unambiguous, complete, accurate, and presented logically.

Clean messy data sets before submission. For example, when the n (number of patients) changes, explain why. Provide the precise number of incomplete cases rather than vague statements about missing data (e.g., "data were complete for most patients"). Footnotes in tables are a good way to accomplish this without adding to your word count.

Never bewilder the reader with statistics. Instead, translate, summarize, and interpret the results of your analysis. Strive for clarity and brevity. Then obtain a second opinion to verify that the presentation of your results is adequate and well structured and that your rationale is not confused or contradictory.

PRINCIPLE 138 • Start your Results section with the major positive findings to tell a balanced and objective story.

Describe the sample early in the Results. In the first sentence, state how many patients met the inclusion criteria and then state what percentage had the primary outcome under investigation. Although it is very important to explain which patients were excluded or dropped from the study, avoid starting with a long explanation of the various groups that were excluded. A CONSORT flowchart diagram is a convenient way to move this information out of the text and into a figure. If you already have too many figures, move this diagram to the Appendix.

VITAL POINT

Include a table transparently describing the study patients. This will reduce reviewers' concerns about bias between the groups and differences between your sample and larger populations.

Describe the base population at the hospital or clinic from which the study sample was drawn. Make it easy for the reader to understand baseline rates for preexisting conditions and diseases that patients may have had. Avoid overused words, such as "demographics" and "parameters." Instead, use "variables," "factors," or "characteristics." Provide sufficient information about the patient population to avoid comments such as the following:

+ *"More information needs to be provided about the population from which this sample was taken. Were they all seen at one hospital? Does this hospital specialize in high-risk pregnancies?"*
+ *"What percentage had maternal complications?"*
+ *"How does this patient population differ from published studies that have different conclusions?"*
+ *"Table 1 should contain substance abuse, diabetes, hypertension, and so forth."*

> *Example 24–1.*
> Patients randomized to Group I were not statistically different from patients in Group II in terms of age, hypertension, or smoking history.

For randomized controlled trials, Table 1 is typically a comparison of the two arms of the trial. By chance alone, 1 in 20 of the variables will have a P value $<.05$. There is disagreement between biostatisticians and nonbiostatisticians on whether or not to include a column of P values in this table. Statisticians generally favor no P values for Table 1. If the guidelines for the journal recommend not including a column of P values for Table 1, follow this advice. Then in the footnotes for Table 1, report any significant differences; for example, "There were no significant differences between the groups except with respect to baseline weight ($P = .038$)" or "There were no significant differences between the groups in any of the characteristics listed here."

FOR MORE INFORMATION

Knol et al. (2012) discuss this issue in "*P*-Values in Baseline Tables of Randomised Controlled Trials Are Inappropriate but Still Common in High Impact Journals."

PRESENTING STATISTICAL RESULTS

PRINCIPLE 139 • Report the 95% confidence intervals for the key variables.

Although you should report P values for the findings that support your conclusion, the emphasis should be on the 95% confidence interval (CI) for the clinically meaningful end points.

Reviewers pointed out the following common mistakes that investigators make in analyzing data:

+ *"Being very 'P' centered."*
+ *"Reliance on P values to make conclusions."*
+ *"The belief that a P value of <.05 means the finding is important, and P value >.05 means the finding is meaningless."*
+ *"Making analytic decisions based on how it affects the P value rather than on what the correct approach is for the question being asked."*
+ *"Concluding that since the P value from a study is <.05 that the observed effect must the 'true.'"*
+ *"Paying too much attention to P values and not enough to 'The Full Monty.'"*

Relative risk is the ratio of the incidence of outcome in the exposed group to the incidence of outcome in the unexposed group. In addition to giving the outcome percentage for each group, results are often more informative when you report relative risk (or odds ratio) and CI.

> *Example 24–2.*
> One could report, "The complication rate was higher in Group I than in Group II (6.8% vs. 1.7%)." However, reporting that "the complication rate was 4 times higher (relative risk 4.0, 95% CI 2.1 to 6.1)" is more informative.

The odds ratio measures the odds of having the risk factor among people with the disease divided by the odds of having the risk factor among people without the disease.

The odds ratio is typically used for case-control studies. Relative risk, incidence, and prevalence usually are not appropriate for case-control studies because the samples are not representative of the larger population. Report both the absolute and relative risks but avoid percent change.

FOR MORE INFORMATION

For more details, see Fleiss et al. (2003); Friedman et al. (2015); Haynes et al. (2011); Hulley et al. (2013); and Kuzma and Bohnenblust (2004).

A 95% CI for the relative risk (or odds ratio) is crucial. This interval shows readers the variability around the point estimate (Fig. 24.1). Provide CIs for every relative risk, odds ratio, and hazard ratio (Fig. 24.2). Never overestimate the size of an effect by providing only the relative risk without the CI.

Critical readers will want to know whether the 95% CIs include the value 1.0 (the null hypothesis), and if not, how far they are from 1.0. A relative risk of 1.0 suggests there is no difference in the proportion of people with the disease between the exposed and the unexposed groups. A relative risk may be much higher than 1.0, but if the 95% CI overlaps 1.0, you usually can conclude that the increase in risk is not statistically significant and that the P value is >.05.

When one group has no patients with the outcome under study, the exact relative risk cannot be calculated. In this case, report it as infinity (∞) with CIs, as in the following example.

> *Example 24–3.*
> Relative risk = ∞; 95% CI 4.7 to ∞.

In summary, always provide 95% CIs for your primary results. Adding CIs improves most papers, and these values can be displayed graphically in forest plots.

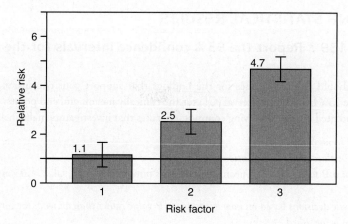

FIGURE 24.1. Example of the relative risk (RR) and 95% confidence intervals (CI) for three risk factors. For risk factor 1, the RR is greater than 1, but the 95% CI (I-shaped symbol) clearly crosses the line at 1.0, which is the null hypothesis. Therefore, you would conclude that risk factor 1 is not a significant factor (assuming that you had sufficient statistical power). Risk factors 2 and 3 have RR and CI values that clearly are greater than 1. Therefore, you would conclude that they are statistically significant risk factors. Similar graphs could be created for odds ratios and hazard ratios.

FOR MORE INFORMATION

See Dawson and Trapp (2005); Kleinbaum et al. (1982); and Mehta et al. (1985). Altman et al. (2000) have written an excellent book on CIs: *Statistics with Confidence: Confidence Intervals and Statistical Guidelines*. This book provides you with a serial number to download the "Confidence Interval Analysis" (CIA) Software from this website:

https://www.som.soton.ac.uk/research/sites/cia/download/

	Exposed?	
	Yes	No
Diseased? Yes	a	b
No	c	d

	Smoker?	
	Yes	No
Lung cancer? Yes	a	b
No	c	d

Relative risk	$\dfrac{a/(a+c)}{b/(b+d)}$	$\dfrac{\text{Incidence among exposed persons}}{\text{Incidence among nonexposed persons}}$
Attributable risk	$[a/(a+c)] - [b/(b+d)]$	Incidence among exposed persons – Incidence among nonexposed persons
Odds ratio (relative odds)	$\dfrac{ad}{cb}$ or $\dfrac{a/b}{c/d}$	$\dfrac{\text{Odds that diseased person was exposed to risk factor}}{\text{Odds that nondiseased person was exposed to risk factor}}$

FIGURE 24.2. Relative risk, attributable risk, and odds ratio.

PRINCIPLE 140 • Use statistical terms skillfully.

1. **Significant** means "probably caused by something other than mere chance." Medical researchers customarily label findings "statistically significant" if the probability of their finding occurring by chance is less than 5% ($P < .05$). Verify that your Results show statistically significant findings when you use the word "significant." Otherwise, later in the Discussion, clarify what may be clinically significant despite the lack of statistical significance, especially with small samples.

   Reviewers may be confused and say:

   For Figure 2, no P values are displayed, nor are they in the legend, even though there is a statement about "significant differences."

2. **Random** refers to the idea that each element in a set has an equal probability of occurrence. Do not use the word "random" to mean "haphazard," "unplanned," or "incidental."
3. A **sample** is "a finite part of a statistical population whose properties are studied to gain information about the whole."[1] "Sample" has this technical meaning in research. Other uses of the term only confuse the reader.
4. A **random sample** is a chance selection in which all members of the base population presumably have the same chance of being selected. Random sampling is commonly used to reduce bias.
5. **Correlation** is a statistical measure of the strength of the linear relationship between two continuous or ordinal variables. The term "correlation" should not be used in a nonstatistical sense, especially in a title. Do not describe the association between categorical variables as a "correlation." Use "correlation" only with two interval-level or ordinal-level variables. For example, if you report a correlation with race, reviewers may think that you are statistically illiterate. Also, when you report the results of a correlation, never confuse the correlation coefficient (r) with R squared (R^2).

   Ambiguous technical writing annoys reviewers, so avoid these five pitfalls and be alert for similar problems.

PRINCIPLE 141 • Present *P* values professionally.

Provide the full P value. Do not use "NS" (not significant) and minimize the use of inequalities (e.g., $P < .05$). Before computers enabled the calculation of exact P values, researchers often were forced to use these vague terms. Researchers looked up the critical values for their sample size in statistics textbooks. These tables provided rough estimates of P values ($<.05$ or $<.01$). Avoid this outdated method of reporting P values.

In the following situations, however, you cannot or should not use an exact P value.

+ If the P value is less than .001, report "$P < .001$." Do not report "$P = .00000621$."
+ If the P value is nearly 1.0, some software packages report "$P > .95$"; this terminology is acceptable.

Use a consistent number of decimal places to report P values. For example, do not report "$P = .1$" in one place and "$P = .00005$" in another. The use of three places ordinarily is sufficient (e.g., $P = .024$, $P < .001$). Provide P values for variables in tables, even if the comparison is 0% versus 0%. Use your statistical software to double check all P values in the final draft of your manuscript. Explain any discrepancies, or reviewers may tell you:

The P value of .1 on line 7 of page 10 should be checked. According to my calculations, the P value is .218.

The New England Journal of Medicine instructs authors to report P values as follows:

"Except when one-sided tests are required by study design, such as in noninferiority trials, all reported P values should be two-sided. In general, P values larger than 0.01 should be reported to two decimal places, those between 0.01 and 0.001 to three decimal places; P values smaller than 0.001 should be reported as

P<.001. *Notable exceptions to this policy include P values arising in the application of stopping rules to the analysis of clinical trials and genetic-screening studies."*

Full or exact *P* values refer to displaying the actual number rather than $P < .05$. Do not confuse this with *P* values from exact test that are provided by Fisher's exact test and the StatXact software.

Do not report *P* values without other pertinent clinically meaningful information (e.g., odds ratio, mean, standard deviation [SD], CI). Avoid orphaned *P* values by stating which statistical tests you selected to compute each *P* value. An orphaned *P* value is one presented without indication of the statistical test used. In the footnotes for tables, specify which statistical tests were used to compute which *P* values. Include detailed footnotes for every table—these do not increase your overall word count. For example, a *P* value in the table of .001[a], might have a footnote: "a—denotes a *P* value based on the Mann-Whitney U test."

Never imply significance when none exists. If the *P* value is not significant, avoid saying that it was "trending toward significance." How do you know the intention of the *P* value? Examples of unprofessional ways that authors describe *P* values just above .05 can be found here:

http://mchankins.wordpress.com/2013/04/21/still-not-significant-2/

Finally, do not use the standard error of the mean (SEM) in place of the SD to mislead readers into believing that the variability is small. Remember that the SEM is calculated by dividing the SD by the square root of the sample size (*n*). The SEM is used to estimate the precision of the larger population mean from the sample mean. The SEM is an intermediate step in statistical analysis and has no clinically meaningful interpretation. Instead, use the SD or CI.

FOR MORE INFORMATION

To learn more about the differences between the SD and SEM, see Bartko (1985).

The relationship among the SEM, SD, and the sample size (*n*) are described below:

$$SEM = SD / \sqrt{n}$$
$$SD = SEM \times \sqrt{n}$$

When reporting CIs, consider using the bootstrap method, which is a more robust and sophisticated method of computing CIs. See Principle 129. The UCLA Institute for Digital Research and Education website provides instruction on how to conduct the bootstrap and many other statistical analyses:

http://www.ats.ucla.edu/stat/

PRINCIPLE 142 • Interpret *P* values intelligently.

Avoid claiming that a small *P* value proves that your findings are strong. A weak association or a small difference in a large study also can produce a small *P* value. Consider evidence beyond the *P* value. Use your clinical judgment to evaluate the magnitude and importance of differences. On the other hand, do not dismiss differences between study groups that fall within the normal range.

Never brag about the number of zeros in your *P* value. Focus the reader's attention on the CI of a clinically meaningful end point, ideally related to quality of life.

FOR MORE INFORMATION

See Bailar and Hoaglin (2009); Salsburg (1985); Ware et al. (2009); and Yancey (1990).

ANTICIPATING PITFALLS IN THE RESULTS

PRINCIPLE 143 • Report results in the target journal's format.

For some journals, especially psychology and psychiatry journals, you must be sure to report the degrees of freedom (df) and the statistic's test value. To speed the submission and review process, include this information in your first draft. The *Publication Manual of the American Psychological Association* (American Psychological Association, 2010) describes the required format in great detail.

> *Example 24–4.*
> The rate of depression was higher in Group I than in Group II, $\chi^2(1, N = 200) = 11.31, P < .001$.

> **VITAL POINT**
>
> Even if the target journal does not require this level of detail, keep all important statistical output organized in a clearly named folder since you may have to submit your paper to another journal that does. At the end of the project and periodically while writing the paper, your biostatistician should send you the latest version of the master data set along with a complete statistical report that includes all of the statistical software coding and syntax.

Keep a copy of the final data file (database or spreadsheet) and the data file for the statistical package in a safe location. Label, document, and organize this material because you may need it years later. For example, an editor may agree to publish your paper if you add the df and the statistic's test values. In this situation, you will need to refer to the statistical output.

The following is an overview of df. The df is a concept used in statistics to determine the most appropriate distribution for calculating the P value for your sample size and number of groups. For the chi-square, you can calculate the df as follows:

(Number of rows $- 1$) $\times$ (Number of columns $- 1$)

Example 24–5.
For the Student's t-test (using the pooled variance method), calculate the df by subtracting 2 from the total sample size ($df = n - 2$).

Also, good science can be easily audited to see how the final data set was obtained from the raw data. For reproducible research, consider including your statistical coding (syntax) in the Appendix of your paper. You might even be able to include deidentified data (or a subset of key variables) in the Appendix. Modern statistical software such as R combined with tools such as sweave and knitr enable researchers to carefully document reproducible research and create dynamic reports.

Use the supplementary appendix to provide the statistical reviewers with the material they might need. Outline your regression modeling strategy and validation, discuss model diagnostics, and describe sensitivity analyses. If there are several methods of analyzing your results, include the prespecified method in the Results and the others in the Appendix.

PRINCIPLE 144 • Describe people sensitively and diplomatically.

When you describe people in your study, avoid all potentially pejorative terms. Providing a general guideline for this principle is impossible, but Table 24.1 shows examples. Regarding your biostatistical collaborators, be sure to build a supportive team environment; one pejorative term to avoid is "MS-level biostatistician." Instead, refer to people by their current title and rank. For example, one would not introduce a police detective as a bachelor-level police officer. We are all extras in other people's plays, but success in science requires excellent people skills.

TABLE 24.1	Pejorative Terms to Avoid

Pejorative Term	Preferred Term
Mental disorders	Impaired cognitive function
Mentally ill person	Person with mental illness
Demented, senile	A person with dementia
SCI patients versus normal patients	Person with SCI versus nondisabled persons
Diabetic pregnancies	Pregnancies complicated by diabetes
Diabetics	Patients with diabetes
Four of the five recurrences died.	Four of the five patients with recurrences died.
Mental retardation	Intellectual disability
Mentally retarded person	A person with cognitive disabilities
	Developmentally disabled
A person afflicted with Down's syndrome	A person with Down syndrome (Note: there is no 's)
Wheelchair-bound people	Persons who use wheelchairs
Paraplegics/paralyzed people	Persons with paraplegia
Among elective THR patients	Among patients who undergo elective THR
Of THR patients	Of patients who have undergone THR
Elective THR patients	Patients who underwent THR
	Patients with total hip arthroplasty
In 43 patients used as controls	For 43 patients who served as controls
Schizophrenics	People diagnosed with schizophrenia
Epileptics	People with epilepsy
The elderly	Older people
MS-level biostatistician	Biostatistician
Autistic children were compared with normal children.	Children with autism spectrum disorder were compared with typically developing children.
Patients were consented.	Patients were informed about the study and gave consent.

A good rule of thumb is to use people-first language. SCI = spinal cord injury; THR = total hip replacement; MS = Master of Science degree.

FOR MORE INFORMATION

See the National Center on Disability and Journalism, headquartered at the Walter Cronkite School of Journalism and Mass Communication at Arizona State University.

http://ncdj.org/style-guide/

During the course of your study, especially during data cleaning and analysis, you must protect the confidentiality of patients by using case numbers rather than names. In your paper, however, be sensitive about using the word "cases" to describe people. Rather than "the patient developed diabetes," write "diabetes developed in the patient." Rather than "complaints," use "symptoms." Rather than "the patient denied (or complained)," write "the patient reported."

Describe the person first and then name the disease or disability. "Patients with diabetes" is appropriate; "people of smoke" is a bit extreme. Table 24.2 shows diplomatic terms that can be used.

TABLE 24.2 Diplomatic Terms to Use

Problematic Term	Preferred Term
Patient denied	Patient reported
Patient developed diabetes	Diabetes developed in the patient
Managed patients	Treated patients
Complained	Reported
Complaints	Symptoms
Patients failed treatment	Treatment failed
Case	Research participant, respondent, man, woman,
45 males	45 male patients, 45 men
67 females	67 female patients, 67 women
Chairman	Chairperson, chair
Patients who developed X	Patients in whom X developed
Two patients developed X.	Two patients had X.
Had surgery	Underwent surgery
Few mortalities	Few deaths
Demise	Death
Expired, succumbed	Died
Primary procedures accounted for 87 patients.	Primary procedures were performed on 87 patients.
Patients have worse outcome.	Patients experience worse outcome.
Patients with complications	Patients who experience complications
None of the 27 patients had a complication.	No complications occurred in the 27 patients.
Had a complication	Experienced a complication
Patients with extended hospitalizations	Patients who stayed in the hospital for extended periods
Fetus was aborted.	Pregnancy was terminated.
Cesarean section, C-section	Cesarean delivery
Cesarean section for fetal distress	Fetal risk requiring cesarean delivery
Intrauterine growth retardation	Intrauterine growth restriction
Motor vehicle accidents	Motor vehicle collisions
Accidents in the home	Injuries in the home
Man and wife	Husband and wife, man and woman
Orientals	Asian people
Senility	Dementia
Compliance	Adherence

Do not label people by their disease—"hypertensive patients." Instead try "patients with hypertension."

Patients report symptoms—they do not complain or have complaints. Likewise, they do not deny having symptoms—they report that they have no symptoms. Patients are treated, not managed. A disease can be managed. Finally, treatments can fail, but patients do not fail treatment.

PRINCIPLE 145 • Write a comprehensive and convincing results section.

In many papers, the Results section is too short (see Fig. 12.1). Do not limit the Results to a few variables significantly related to the primary outcome.

Provide results for the most severe form of outcome. For example, describe the mortality rate overall and for important subgroups. Although it is impossible to define the appropriate length for all papers, if your paper has less than two double-spaced pages of Results, you probably should add more findings before you submit it. If you are not sure what to add, try to anticipate which results researchers will need to include in their meta-analysis. Also, anticipate three reasons that reviewers are likely to reject your paper and add results to address these head-on.

The Results section can often be strengthened by adding results of a survey that you conduct to show a knowledge gap or equipoise among physicians or patients. In this way, you can prove that the information that you are presenting is new and important. Today, it is easy to conduct e-mail surveys using tools such as REDCap.

Show the consistency of your evidence from different angles, or you may give the impression that your data are inconclusive: a common reason for rejection.

Example 24–6.
If you found an association between alcohol use and a certain outcome, do not rely on one P value to convince readers. Analyze drinks per day, drink-years, and subgroups (e.g., nonsmokers). Include all of Hill's Criteria for Causation to provide a more comprehensive Results section. For more information about the consistency of evidence, see Table 24.4.

Especially when reporting the outcome of different treatments, make it easy for the reader to understand that you controlled for the severity of disease. Explain which variables you controlled for and how. Although some of this information is included in your Methods, the Results must show that your methods of controlling for confounding factors actually worked. Provide separate results for patients with a good prognosis and those with a poor prognosis. Report results for patients who underwent primary surgery separately from results for those who underwent revisions. If you omit or ignore important data, reviewers may ask for additional details.

In most rejected manuscripts the Results section is too short (see Fig. 12.1). If the Results are less than two pages, do another literature search and then reanalyze your data to compare with published results. Finally, never write a Results section that leaves the reader with the impression of overanalysis or data dredging. Remember, by chance alone, 1 in every 20 statistical tests will provide a P value of $<.05$. For this reason, reviewers may be concerned that your findings are the result of testing too many variables. This is the reason that you want to have a detailed prespecified analysis plan (including subgroup analyses) registered with ClinicalTrials.gov or elsewhere. Also, master data reduction methods and avoid approaches that are too extreme in letting an algorithm automatically select variables without expert oversight (see Steyerberg, 2010).

VITAL POINT

Make a long Results section easier to write—and read—by including subheadings in your early draft outline, such as the following:

   Baseline Demographic and Clinical Characteristics
   Efficacy Outcomes
   Adverse Outcomes
   Laboratory Abnormalities
or
   Study Patients
   Primary End Point
   Secondary End Points
   Quality of Life
   Adverse Events

PRINCIPLE 146 • Acknowledge that you are aware of small cell sizes.

In an analysis of a binary risk factor (smoking) versus a binary outcome (lung cancer), there are four cells in a two-by-two table. In tables $> 2 \times 2$, with more than four cells, some cells or subgroups presented in the text and tables may be too small to permit any sensible analysis. Combine the categories into cells with larger N values, or explain your reasons for not doing so.

Example 24–7.
In an analysis of pressure ulcer patients grouped by anatomic level of spinal cord injury, certain subgroups may contain few patients. However, for some readers, knowing the number of patients with a lesion at each level may be important. Combining injuries into general categories (e.g., cervical, thoracic, lumbar) would make it impossible for these readers to get the information they need.

In situations such as this one, you can report the results using specific categories and then combine them for statistical analysis when needed. Always record information in as much detail as possible and then, if necessary, combine the values into more general categories for analysis.

PRINCIPLE 147 • Specify a follow-up time frame when reporting rates.

Example 24–8.
Stating that "the recurrence rate of pressure ulcers was 17%" is meaningless without an explicitly defined follow-up period. Instead, state that "during the first postoperative year, the recurrence rate of pressure ulcers was 14.2%."

To calculate a true rate, you need three pieces of information:

1. The number of patients with the study condition
2. The size of the population at risk
3. A time frame

Researchers most often forget to include the third piece of information: a time frame. Table 24.3 shows three examples of rate calculations.

TABLE 24.3   **Formulas for Calculating Rates**

Rate	=	Outcome during a specific period / Population at risk for outcomes during a specific period
Attack rate	=	Number of new cases of a specific disease in the population at risk during a specific period / Number of persons at risk during or at start of the specific period or average populations during the time interval
Neonatal mortality rate[a]	=	Number of deaths of live-born infants (0–27 days of age) in a year / Number of live births in the same year

[a]Often reported per 1,000 live births.

TABLE 24.4   **Hill's Criteria for Evaluating Causation**

Temporally correct association (exposure/cause occurs before the outcome/effect)
Strength of the association (usually a statistic, such as an odds ratio or R^2)
Dose–response relationship/biologic gradient (monotonic/consistent stepwise increase in
   poor outcome associated with increases in exposure)
Consistency of the findings (from different studies and populations)
Biologic plausibility of the hypothesis (consistency with existing knowledge)
Specificity of the association (cause leads to a single effect not multiple)
Coherence between epidemiologic and laboratory findings
Experimental evidence
Analogy (similar diseases have a similar cause–effect relationship)
Strength of the study design

See Hill (1965) and Rothman et al. (2012).

PRINCIPLE 148 • Use the tools of professional epidemiologists to evaluate and report causation.

Many clinical research papers that evaluate cause and effect can be improved by applying the criteria shown in Table 24.4.

FOR MORE INFORMATION

See Haynes et al. (2011); Hill (1965); Kleinbaum et al. (1982); Mausner and Kramer (1985); and Rothman et al. (2012).

PRINCIPLE 149 • Use rigorous scientific methodology to create a new clinical scale or predictive model.

A clinical scale usually is a simple scoring system designed to help health care professionals estimate the risk that an outcome will occur and provide crude risk stratification. The criteria shown in Table 24.5 can help you to design a quality scale. For predictive models, use data reduction methods rather than the outdated stepwise variable selection approach. Data reduction methods refer to taking a list of potential predictors and narrowing it down to a reasonable size by obtaining expert content

---

TABLE 24.5   **Criteria for Evaluating a Clinical Scale**

Consistent statistical evidence from the data in support of each factor
Biologically plausible interpretation for the causal mechanism underlying each factor
Evidence in the literature that each factor was associated with the development of the
   outcome
Improvement in the sensitivity and specificity of the total score caused by the addition of
   each factor

input, eliminating variables with a large amount of missing data and those that are redundant (e.g., hemoglobin and hematocrit). Be thoughtful in selecting variables for a model and avoid having the computer automatically select variables without human input.

Rather than creating a simple clinical scale that sums points for various factors, consider creating a logistic regression model and use the probability of the outcome for risk stratification. The scale method is an outdated and imprecise method that is no longer relevant now that computers are ubiquitous.

To convert the output from a logistic regression model into a probability, take the beta coefficients and intercept and compute a Z score, for example:

$$Z = -5.25738 \text{ (the constant / intercept)} + age \times 0.029524 \text{ (beta coefficient for age)} + male\_gender \text{ (1 = male, 0 = female)} \times 0.923548 \text{ (beta coefficient for gender)}$$

Then the Z value is used in the following formula to compute the probability of complication X:

$$\text{Probability of complication X} = 1 / (1 + e^{-Z})$$

Where e is $= 2.71828$ (base of the natural logarithm).

So, for example, a 90-year-old male would have a 15.7% chance of developing complication X.

$$Z = -5.25738 + (90 \times 0.029524) + (1 \times 0.923548) = -1.67667$$

$$\text{Probability of complication X} = 1 / (1 + 2.71828^{1.67667}) = 0.157 \times 100 = 15.7\%$$

Predictive models such as this are now being embedded into the electronic health record and will become more important for risk stratification and medical research.

FOR MORE INFORMATION

See Dawson and Trapp (2005); Haynes et al. (2011); Salzberg et al. (1996); and Steyerberg (2010).

PRINCIPLE 150 • Make clear what was adjusted for with your multivariate analysis.

When you present the results of the multivariate analysis, explain which factors were controlled for in the model. Although you may have described the analysis in the Methods, in your Results, explain which tests were used. Do not make broad statements (e.g., "After adjusting for preoperative factors …"). For regression models, report the goodness of fit and model diagnostics. Be as transparent as possible and provide enough detail for another researcher to reproduce your results. Use the Appendix to provide the details that a biostatistician would be looking for.

PRINCIPLE 151 • Present numbers for similar variables consistently.

Use a consistent number of decimal places. As a rule, use one decimal place for the mean and SD of whole numbers.

Example 24–9.
The mean age in Group I was significantly lower than that in Group II (42.7 ± 3.3 vs. 53.8 ± 2.6, $P = .014$).

Of course, consult the target journal's instructions for authors and recent issues of the target journal to identify any deviations from these guidelines, but never report numbers to meaningless decimal places (e.g., the average venous pH was 7.42179, the mean age was 27.21 years).

PRINCIPLE 152 • Include only results in the Results section.

Focus on your hypothesis and move any interpretations of the results to the Discussion. Separate the Results and the Discussion—completely. For example, the following sentence is an interpretation and should be moved to the Discussion: "This finding is not entirely unexpected."

> **VITAL POINT**
>
> The Results section rarely requires references. A sentence that requires a reference probably belongs in another section.

Sometimes investigators expect to find certain results, but the data do not agree with their preconceived notions. Do report this at the end of the Results, but discuss it in the Discussion section. These surprising findings certainly will interest many of your peers.

TABLES

PRINCIPLE 153 • Design reader-friendly tables and avoid dichotomania.

Well-designed tables and figures are more important than most medical researchers realize because reviewers often read them first. As with your title and abstract, make a good first impression with your tables, but remember that editors often object to the inclusion of more than a few tables; redundant tables and graphs add unnecessary length and cost. Dichotomania refers to the poor practice of dividing continuous variables into two categories (body mass index [BMI] becomes obese vs. not, hematocrit becomes anemic vs. not). Although it is acceptable to dichotomize occasionally, excessive use of this technique is poor science.

Some readers have trouble interpreting tables, so make your tables clear and focused. Anticipate how the reader will mentally sort rows and consider revising your table to reflect that order.

In tables, include only pertinent data and avoid redundancies. A person who skips the text and reads only your tables should be able to draw conclusions similar to yours.

Often, you can make your tables easier to read by adding the percentage for each row.

Example 24–10.
Tables often show the column percentage of men and women, forcing readers to mentally calculate the row percentage for the mortality rates among men and among women.

	Survived (n = 870)	Died (n = 63)	Row Percentage	P Value
Sex				< .001
Male	22.1%	42.9%	12.3%	
Female	77.9%	57.1%	5.0%	

PRINCIPLE 154 • Do not repeat information in the tables and text.

Many writers repeat the exact information in the text and tables. This mistake irritates both reviewers and editors. Make sure, however, that the text agrees with the tables and figures.

For example, are the inclusion criteria inconsistent between the Methods and the tables? If so, verify that the data are correct and add a footnote to the table to explain why the information is correct but appears inconsistent.

Explain any significant differences between the tables and the text. Describe the medical diagnoses in the text or a table but not both.

Avoid most abbreviations and acronyms in tables. If you must use abbreviations, define each one in the table's footnotes. For example, "⁺BMI denotes body mass index, which is the weight in kilograms divided by the square of the height in meters."

TABLE 24.6	Checklist for Creating an Appealing Table

Simple and self-explanatory—can stand alone
Formatted for the target journal
Not a repetition of the text
Double-spaced
Units provided for each variable
± Values identified as either a standard deviation or a standard error of the mean
Full P values included (rather than * = P < .05; and NS = not significant)
Values rounded appropriately, not mean age was 56.218
Format consistent with the other tables
No vertical lines; avoid excessive boxing
Extensive footnotes to define all abbreviations and acronyms
Footnotes identify which statistical test was used for each P value.
Confusion eliminated from prereview feedback

Explain in the text the numbers presented in the tables. If the number of subjects changes, explain the change. If some patients have more than one condition, add a footnote to the table explaining why the percentages do not total properly. Keep the tables simple but not informal. For example, all tables need easy-to-understand column headings.

PRINCIPLE 155 • Create high-quality transparent tables.

Table 24.6 shows a checklist of the components of a quality table.

PRINCIPLE 156 • Cite and summarize all tables and figures in the text.

Many reviewers highlight the citation for each table and figure in the text (e.g., "see Table 1") to verify that all citations are complete. In the text of the Results, emphasize the key point of each table and graph.

> **VITAL POINT**
>
> Remember to place the tables, figure legend pages, and figures *after* the text and the references (see Table 20.3).

PRINCIPLE 157 • Present adverse outcomes perceptively and transparently.

Report all complications and side effects objectively and in detail. Comparing complication rates between study groups requires thoughtful analysis and organization. In some reports, investigators attempt to obscure the truth by overwhelming the reader with tables of results. If, however, you wish to publish your findings, remember that reviewers expect a realistic comparison to answer the question: Do the benefits outweigh the adverse effects of this treatment? Complex tables are not a substitute for intelligent analysis of the findings.

Reviewers expect an accurate and honest account of the side effects of therapy in your study population and the limits of follow-up for side effects. Some of the top journals do not want authors to decide whether adverse events are drug related.

If your study was not a randomized clinical trial, be careful when you interpret data or outcome as "caused by" different therapies. Causality is difficult to prove for many reasons. Treatment protocols change over time, and patients with more severe disease often are given more aggressive treatment (or combinations of treatment) than patients with less severe disease. If your study was not designed to compare treatments and yet shows differences in outcome for different treatment groups, you have three choices:

1. Do not focus on the outcome analysis.
2. State the limitations of your interpretations and describe the indications for each treatment.
3. Use propensity score analysis.

PRINCIPLE 158 • Add a simple table to solve anticipated criticisms.

If your paper does not have too many tables, adding a table may make it easier for the reviewer to understand your conclusions. Ask yourself: Would another table or graph avoid any anticipated criticism or confusion? If your manuscript has more tables than average, you may be able to combine some of the information into a summary table.

PRINCIPLE 159 • Give the reader ample results in tables.

Show all the data. For small studies, you can often list the raw data in a table. This transparency goes a long way with reviewers. For larger studies, include as much raw data in an appendix. This is not only good for science but improves your odds of publication and increases the citations for your paper (Piwowar et al., 2007).

Using a table will avoid the following type of comment:

"With only 20 patients, a table of the raw data for the most important variables would enable the reader to verify these findings."

You can help the reader by providing not only the number of patients but also the number of hospitals, observers, clinicians, and days of follow-up. You can provide this information in the text or tables of the Results.

Researchers who continue with this line of research will often look to your paper for information needed to estimate the sample size and power. An important detail that is often omitted from publications is the SD of the difference from paired analyses. Think about the information that you can include to make it easier for the next researcher to compute the sample size.

FIGURES—DESIGN GRAPHS THAT WILL SELL YOUR CONCLUSION

PRINCIPLE 160 • Use graphs and other figures to illustrate the major points after you have conducted the statistical analyses.

Visual displays can help readers understand your findings. Many readers prefer to read a graph rather than a page of numbers or text. Consider using a variety of types of figures (e.g., graphs, diagrams, a CONSORT flowchart, screen shots of computer displays, photographs, radiographs, micrographs, anatomic drawings, family trees) to illustrate different points. Anticipate what reviewers might prefer to see in a graph:

+ *"A survival graph for the comparisons on pages 9 and 10 would make it much easier to understand the differences among the groups."*

If you include superfluous or repetitive figures, reviewers may respond as follows:

+ *"Neither Figure 1 nor Figure 2 is needed."*
+ *"I do not think that illustrations 6 and 7 add anything, and they should be omitted."*

For each figure, ask yourself: Would a table present this finding more clearly? Figures show trends and multiple comparisons more effectively than tables. Tables are more effective for presenting a mixture of variables that cannot be displayed on the same scale.

Ask a colleague who is experienced in creating scientific graphs to review your paper and tables and suggest more sophisticated ways of graphing the major points.

If you have several graphs with the same horizontal axis label, you often can combine them into one figure by stacking them in panels. This paneling technique helps the reader and allows you to use more graphs without exceeding the journal's limit.

PRINCIPLE 161 • Create a professional figure legends page.

Provide a detailed, easy-to-understand legend (caption) for each figure that clearly explains each graph. These legends are placed together on one page after the tables and *before* the figures. Because the figure legends do not count in your overall word count, you can add additional details here that reviewers will be interested in.

> **VITAL POINT**
> Obtain written permission for any figures or tables that you include from published work.

PRINCIPLE 162 • Spend a lot of time on your figures and pay attention to the details.

Label each axis clearly. For example, the y-axis label should be perpendicular to the text and parallel to the y-axis. Use thick lines and text that is large enough to read when the figure is reduced to fit on a journal page. When your graph is reduced to fit in a column, the axis labels should be similar in size to the printed text. You can reduce your graph with your graphics software or on a photocopier to see how it will look. Edit the graph until it is as uncluttered and professional as possible. Use *The New England Journal of Medicine* as a style guide.

Use a sans serif typeface (e.g., Helvetica) and do not automatically accept the defaults in your graphics software. For example, software packages often will place legends in inappropriate places; move them as necessary.

You can customize you graphs with the R software and packages such as ggplot2. Journals will often import your file and edit to their style with Adobe Illustrator. Medical journal graphic artists will also often use Adobe Photoshop, Poser (Smith Micro Software), Cinema 4D Studio (MAXON Computer), and Adobe Flash Professional to create and edit illustrations and graphics. Although most researchers would have little need for these products, it is wise to consider aspects of a paper that might be appropriate for an online interactive graph or video for the journals website. As journals move from paper to online, these interactive graphics, data-driven graphics, and videos are becoming more important to journals. See the interactive graph and animation in the following examples:

http://www.nejm.org/doi/full/10.1056/NEJMsa0805646

http://www.nejm.org/doi/full/10.1056/NEJMsa066082

Avoid imposing three-dimensional effects on two-dimensional graphs. Default settings for graphs are often cluttered with background lines and too many axis numbers. Delete all unnecessary lines and numbers to maximize the information to ink ratio.

For each graph, identify the number of patients in each subgroup. For example, in each bar graph, each bar should indicate the number of cases (e.g., 9/17). Each bar also should have a percentage to help the reader understand the point of the figure. In addition, clearly indicate the overall sample size for the graph.

FOR MORE INFORMATION

If you have trouble with graphs, figures, slides, or conference posters, seek help from a professional. If you need a referral, the Association of Medical Illustrators can recommend a freelance medical artist. Briscoe's (2013) book *Preparing Scientific Illustrations: A Guide to Better Posters, Presentations, and Publications* is also a good source for more information. Tufte's (2001, 2006) books *The Visual Display of Quantitative Information* and *Beautiful Evidence* are thought-provoking books. An excellent graphical software package for R is ggplot2 (Wickham, 2010). Shiny is a web application framework for R, which provides a method of displaying graphs online (http://shiny.rstudio.com/). Finally, Bertin (1981, 2010) has two excellent books on graphics—one a classic and one more modern.

PRINCIPLE 163 • Use spline graphs to show nonlinear relationships.

A spline graph is a sophisticated method of illustrating nonlinear relationships. Because few biomedical measurements are linear, it is best to avoid assuming linearity (Fig. 24.3).

A spline graph (nonlinear line graph) that illustrates an important interaction is a perfect example of this point. An exploding pie chart that shows the percentage of men and women included in a study is the mark of an amateur and could be replaced with one number (Fig. 24.4). As with tables, figures should agree with, but not repeat, information in the text.

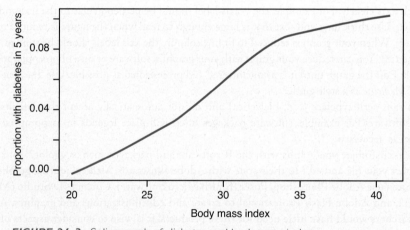

FIGURE 24.3. Spline graph of diabetes and body mass index.

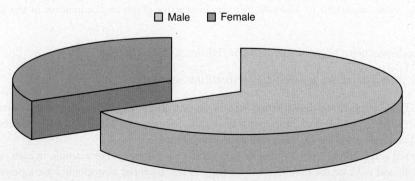

FIGURE 24.4. Exploding pie chart showing percentage of male and female. Avoid this type of amateur graph.

PRINCIPLE 164 • Use a CONSORT diagram/flowchart to make clinical trials easy to understand.

A flowchart is a diagram of boxes and connecting lines that shows the steps in a system, such as a study protocol. For randomized clinical trials, you should use a flowchart to illustrate the number of patients at each stage and in each arm or branch of the study. One flowchart often can replace a drab paragraph of text in your Results. A good flowchart provides a clear picture of the patients at each phase. See Ewigman et al. (1993) and Noto et al. (2015) for examples of how effective a flowchart can be.

Because many reviewers like to sketch out a flowchart as they read, anticipate this need. Providing a flowchart will make it easier for reviewers to read your paper. If you leave it up to reviewers to create their own flowcharts, they may become annoyed if their numbers do not agree with yours. Flowcharts also can illustrate the study protocol, testing scheme, and pattern of decisions.

See the following website for a "CONSORT Diagram Generator" from the University of Washington:

https://depts.washington.edu/hrtk/CSD/

This website also has a number of templates that you can start with. For those who use Microsoft Office, the Visio software module can be used to create flowcharts. Another option is Lucidchart (https://www.lucidchart.com/). More basic flowcharts can be created in Microsoft Word using autoshapes.

PRINCIPLE 165 • Use scatter plots to interpret and display the distribution of two continuous variables.

A scatter plot, also called a "scatter diagram," or an "X–Y graph," is a two-dimensional graph of two continuous variables (Fig. 24.5). A scatter plot of the results can help you to identify more appropriate ways to analyze the data. You can use statistical software to create scattergrams quickly so that you can examine the data visually.

Consider including a scatter plot of the primary point in the Appendix of your paper. Plot the individual points (with one continuous variable on the x-axis and the other on the y-axis) to show the distribution of the individual points and how they fit a regression line. Use different symbols to identify the groups.

In R, scatter plots can be created with the command:

plot(age,bmi)

In IBM SPSS, scatter plots can be created with the menu commands:

Graphs, Legacy Dialogs, Scatter/Dot, Simple Scatter, Define, move one variable to the X Axis and one to the Y Axis, OK.

Any superimposed points must be marked in some way or jittered (moved slightly), or a reviewer may count the points on the scattergram and complain about any discrepancies.

To create high-quality figures for publication, transfer your data to a graphics package or the R software program. You can edit these graphs to produce a professional image. Then you can save the file as a pdf.

VITAL POINT

When your results differ from published studies, try to create graphs and tables similar in format to those that have been published to make it easier for readers to compare them. Interpret your graphs with an open mind. Ask yourself what the authors of the contradictory studies would conclude from your graphs.

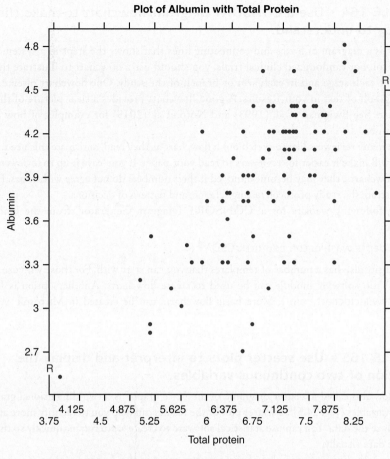

FIGURE 24.5. Scatter plot of serum albumin concentration and total protein.

For showing agreement between two continuous variables, use the Bland-Altman method (see Bland & Altman, 1986; Fig. 24-6). A Pearson correlation is not the correct method of showing agreement.

PRINCIPLE 166 • Use histograms to understand the key distributions.

For the most important continuous variable in your study, explain the histogram's distribution in the text of the Results. For example, is it normal or skewed? If it is skewed, how severely is it skewed, and in which direction? Is it bimodal? Figure 24.7 shows an example of bimodal data. To illustrate the histograms for two groups, consider creating a back-to-back histogram. This can be done in R with the ggplot2 package or in the Hmisc package with the command "histbackback." In R, once the package is installed and loaded, you can use a question mark before the command to obtain help, for example, "?histbackback."

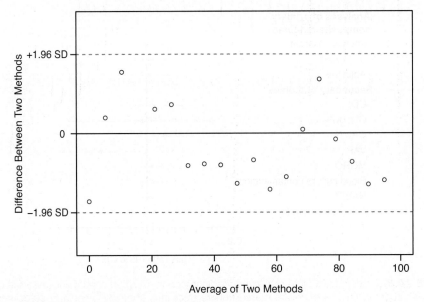

FIGURE 24.6. Example of a Bland-Altman plot.

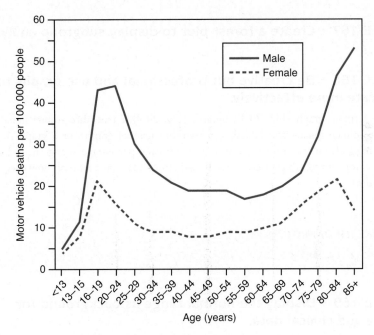

FIGURE 24.7. Example of a bimodal distribution. (Data from the Insurance Institute for Highway Safety. *Status Report of the Insurance Institute for Highway Safety. Vol. 30.* Arlington, VA: Insurance Institute for Highway Safety; 1995.)

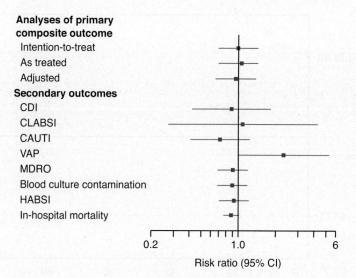

Analyses of primary composite outcome
- Intention-to-treat
- As treated
- Adjusted

Secondary outcomes
- CDI
- CLABSI
- CAUTI
- VAP
- MDRO
- Blood culture contamination
- HABSI
- In-hospital mortality

Risk ratio (95% CI)

FIGURE 24.8. Forest plot. CDI, *Clostridium difficile* infection; CLABSI, central line–associated bloodstream infection; CAUTI, catheter-associated urinary tract infection; VAP, ventilator-associated pneumonia; MDRO, multidrug-resistant organisms; HABSI, health care–associated bloodstream infection. (From Noto, et al. Chlorhexidine bathing and health care-associated infections: a randomized clinical trial. *JAMA*. 2015;313[4]:369–378.)

PRINCIPLE 167 • Create a forest plot to display subgroup analyses.

See Figure 24.8.

PRINCIPLE 168 • Be creative but professional and use graphs to communicate more effectively.

You can use a spline graph (Fig. 24.3), ngrams (Fig. 24.9) a true three-dimensional graph (not simply a three-dimensional effect added to a two-dimensional graph), or a graph that illustrates the relative change from the control group but avoid using percentage change from baseline as an end point. Scan top journals to get fresh ideas. Keep in mind that some journals now encourage the use of color in figures.

FOR MORE INFORMATION

See Briscoe (2013).

PRINCIPLE 169 • Display the normal range as background for laboratory and clinical data.

For major findings, especially the results of laboratory tests, provide the normal values. When you graph your findings, add the normal range (e.g., shaded as a band in the background). Providing a normal range specific to the study population is even better.

PRINCIPLE 170 • Graph the performance of predictive models and new cutoff points on ROC curves.

When you are presenting a new predictive model and comparing with alternative methods of predicting, receiver operating characteristics (ROC) curves are informative ways of displaying these data

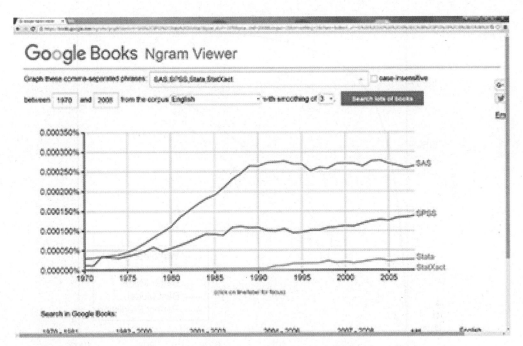

FIGURE 24.9. Google Books Ngram Viewer.

(Fig. 24.10). On the y-axis, plot the sensitivity. On the x-axis, plot the value that is 100 minus the specificity. The statistical software will calculate the sensitivity and specificity at various cutoff points and connect the points with a line.

In IBM SPSS, the commands are as follows:
    Analyze
    ROC Curve . . .
    Select the predicted probability variable (Pre-1)
    Move it into Test Variable
    Select the outcome variable (such as died) and move it into State Variable
    Enter 1 for Value of State Variable (assuming 1 = died, 0 = survived)
    Check with diagonal reference line
    OK

In R, you can use the ROCR package.

ROC curves are also useful for selecting the most appropriate cutoff point for screening tests. Draw a diagonal line from the top left corner to the bottom right corner. The intersection of this diagonal line with the curved plotted line provides an objective cutoff point that maximizes sensitivity and specificity. Be sure that your graph has a frame that is square, not rectangular. You usually can see the "elbow" of the line clearly as the point that is closest to the upper left corner.

Whenever you suggest a new cutoff point, provide an ROC curve. Show that you examined the data carefully to determine this new cutoff point. Include sufficient raw data to show that you chose the single best cutoff point. Do not expect anyone to take your word for this type of finding.

FOR MORE INFORMATION
See Fletcher et al. (2012); Haynes et al. (2011); and Lang (2009).

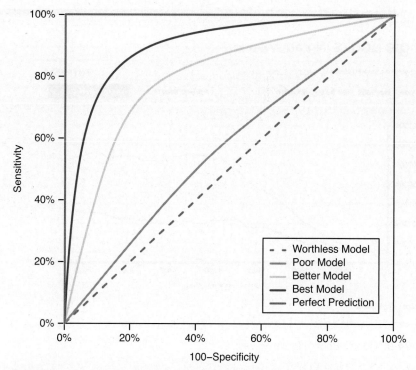

FIGURE 24.10. Example of a Receiver Operating Characteristics (ROC) curve.

PRINCIPLE 171 • Keep graphs simple but scientific.

Make your graphs eye-catching but simple. On the other hand, do not eliminate important details. For example, for survival curves, include the number of patients at risk during each interval of follow-up below the x-axis and indicate that the scale reflects probability, not actual percentage of outcome.

PRINCIPLE 172 • Distinguish among "percent," "percentage," and "percentile."

When you graph a change, be sure that you understand the meanings of the terms "percent," "percentage," and "percentile." A change from 80% to 40% is a decrease of 40 percentage points but a 50 percent decrease. Unless it appears in a table's column heading, "percent" usually is preceded by a number (e.g., 20.7 percent, 100 percent). Otherwise, use "percentage" (e.g., "A large percentage of patients . . . "). "Percent" is not used as a noun in most medical writing.

Percentile is "a value on a scale of one hundred that indicates the percent of a distribution that is equal to or below it (a score in the 95th percentile).[1] Percentile is not a smarter way of saying percent.

FOR MORE INFORMATION

See section 16.2.4 of the *AMA Manual of Style* (American Medical Association, 2007).

PRINCIPLE 173 • Master the elements of a high-quality figure.

Table 24.7 shows a checklist for creating a quality figure, and Table 24.8 shows a comparison of outdated and modern graphical methods.

TABLE 24.7	Checklist for Creating an Appealing Figure

Self-explanatory and can stand alone without the author's narration
Tested and refined for clarity with prereviews to eliminate confusion
± Values defined (SD, SEM, or CI)
95% CIs included (avoid SEM)
Created with modern scientific software (e.g., R and the ggplot2 package)
Clear, detailed figure legend
Information that is not included in the text
Numbers displayed for each subgroup
Easy-to-understand axis labels
Meaningful use of shading and cross-hatching
Thick lines (≥ 1 point)
Large text, Helvetica or Arial font
Full exact P values
Transparently displays individual patients in a dot plot or line graphs for small studies rather than hides the data with a dynamite plot
Avoids three-dimensional effects, such as an exploding pie charge for male/female
High information to ink ratio
Does not assume linearity and allows for nonlinear splines, etc.
pdf Format (avoid bitmaps and screen shots)
Saved in a vector format so journals can edit with Adobe Illustrator
Legible for color-blind readers
Number at risk for each group displayed across time below the x-axis for survival graphs
Code/syntax for the graph is provided in the appendix for reproducible research.

SD = standard deviation; SEM = standard error of mean; CI = confidence interval.

TABLE 24.8	A Comparison of Outdated and Modern Graphical Methods

Weak/Outdated	Strong/Modern
Dynamite plot (bar + plunger)	Dot plot, box plot, line graph
Linear regression line (for nonlinear data)	Lowess spline
Stacked bar graph	Line graphs
3-D exploding pie chart	Anything
3-D bar graphs	Box plot
—	Spaghetti plot
Correlation matrix	Heat map
Static graph	Interactive graph, animation, video
Scatter plot	Animated bubble graph
Cluttered bar graph	Radial graph, radar chart

REFERENCES

1. *Merriam-Webster's Collegiate Dictionary.* 11th ed. Springfield, MA: Merriam-Webster Inc; 2008.

Discussion

> *"The society which scorns excellence in plumbing because plumbing is a humble activity and tolerates shoddiness in philosophy because it is an exalted activity will have neither good plumbing nor good philosophy. Neither its pipes nor its theories will hold water."*
>
> —JOHN W. GARDNER

FOCUSING THE DISCUSSION

PRINCIPLE 174 • Start the Discussion with your most important finding.

Your Discussion should start with one sentence that clearly shows that your paper contains new information. Either accept or reject your original null hypothesis. If you are unsure how to start, you can always begin with "We found that . . ." then describe your primary finding and explain the importance of this discovery. This first sentence must show that you learned something by answering an important question that was not already answered in the current medical literature. Alternatives for starting your Discussion are:

"Our data show that . . . [your primary finding] and this is clinically important because . . ."
"The trial demonstrated that . . ."
"The results of this randomized clinical trial show that . . ."
"The results of our analysis indicate there is . . ."
"This prospective cohort study showed that . . ."
"These studies confirm that . . ."
"In this study, we determined whether . . ."
"Our findings support the use of . . ."
"In our randomized trial of x versus y . . ."

Never start with a dull history lesson, as in the following examples:

"In 1962, Smith et al. showed that . . ."

Who cares? This is a paper about your findings!

"Smoking results in significant morbidity and mortality."
"For the past three decades, the obesity rate has been rising."
"Disease X was first identified in 1943."

Remember to end the first sentence of the Discussion with "and this is clinically important because . . ." or some variation on this. Editors are often annoyed by "having to work to figure out what the point of the manuscript is."

Reviewers at high-impact clinical research journals will want you to answer questions such as the following early in the Discussion:

1. Is this novel?

2. Is it really good science?

3. Is it a strong data set?

4. Is it well powered?

5. Is it analyzed correctly?

6. Is it going to move the field forward?

7. Does this change clinical practice?

8. Will it have high impact?

PRINCIPLE 175 • Confine the Discussion to your results and comparisons between other publications and your results.

The Discussion is completely different from the Results. The Discussion is the place to discuss the implications of *your* findings, not simply repeat them. In the Discussion, do not discuss any findings that you did not present in the Results. Confine the Discussion to the data that your study generated.

When asked "How do you define a good article?", one reviewer wrote:

> *"Everything builds and integrates with prior section: Introduction, Methods, Results, Discussion including implications."*

ANTICIPATING PITFALLS IN THE DISCUSSION

PRINCIPLE 176 • Provide practical information.

In the Discussion, distill useful information from your data by interpreting the results and drawing conclusions. Most readers prefer pragmatic, "how-to" knowledge. To provide it, separate the science from the rhetoric. Also, remember that obvious leaps of logic will annoy editors.

The Institute of Medicine estimated that it takes an average of 17 years for new knowledge from randomized controlled trials to be implemented into practice. Therefore, editors and reviewers are interested in practical information that can be applied to improve patient outcomes.

PRINCIPLE 177 • Discipline yourself to stick to your subject and keep the Discussion focused.

Use a structured outline to avoid going off on tangents. Good papers have a targeted Discussion. They are not rambling. Many Discussion sections are too long (see Fig. 12.1) and tend to recapitulate information given in the Results. Ask yourself: "Is all of the Discussion relevant?" Tell a story about your findings and how they fit into the niche you identified in the literature—once upon a time we had this research question . . .

In telling your story, move the references to the background by changing sentences from "In 2009, Smith et al. showed that X causes Y" to "X causes Y (Smith et al., 2009)."

PRINCIPLE 178 • Describe the new information that your paper provides.

Anticipate and avoid the most common reviewer criticism, *"This is nothing new!"* For example, researchers were writing a paper about a hospital readmission predictive model. They anticipated a reviewer criticism that physicians and nurses could already identify which patients would be readmitted. To address this concern, they added a section in the Discussion describing a study that demonstrated that from experimental evidence, this was untrue.

VITAL POINT

Unoriginal, predictable, or trivial results guarantee rejection.

PRINCIPLE 179 • Compare your study with previous studies.

Ask yourself, "What comparisons and contrasts do the experts in this field want to see?" Discuss how your results compare with landmark papers. Try to critique—concisely—the major studies most similar to yours.

If your conclusion differs dramatically from published reports, explain why. Do not dismiss earlier studies flippantly; those authors might be asked to review your manuscript. When you contradict published work, be honest but diplomatic.

VITAL POINT

Say what you mean, mean what you say, but don't say it mean.

Write the Discussion as if you are talking with the reader. Imagine that the authors of the landmark papers on your subject are sitting around a table, listening as you discuss your findings and their publications with a sophisticated level of diplomacy. If necessary, explain how your measuring method differed from theirs. Can you present your results in the same units of measurement to allow comparison? How were your methods an improvement over previous studies? Rather than attacking other researchers, describe how you are building on what they discovered. Success is more likely with a win-win philosophy.

Reviewers provided the following comments on this topic:

"Contains no historical perspective"
"Authors are clearly biased and cherry pick data to support their views."
"Selective reviewing of the literature, i.e., U.S. researchers tend to only include other U.S. research (even if there is international research that is relevant)"
"Incomplete review of prior literature (especially older papers)"

PRINCIPLE 180 • Overcome reviewers' initial negative reactions.

Reviewers often start with the assumption that your paper does not add anything new. You can use subheadings to present your story in logical sections that anticipate the reviewer's response, "This work has been done before." This type of organization will help prove that it has not. Remember that the peer-review process has a "tendency to select against novel work" (Olson, 1990). Because many reviewers strongly resist new ideas, novel or controversial findings need extra support. Use Hill's criteria for causation for this extra support (see Table 24.3).

Reviewers also may wonder about confounding factors that are not mentioned (e.g., nutritional status, socioeconomic status, the hospital's level of care). Anticipate the major concerns of reviewers and address them in the Discussion. If some of these factors could skew your data and affect your results, explain why you did not measure them. Moreover, from your experience, identify important variables for future study.

PRINCIPLE 181 • Offer only specific criticism of other papers.

Making a sweeping critical statement is like throwing a boomerang, so be prepared. Study the literature carefully and make specific factual statements.

PRINCIPLE 182 • Keep the Discussion short and structured.

Reviewers and editors report that the Discussion typically is too long and often flawed (see Figs. 12.1 and 23.1). Do not force the reviewer to say:

The Discussion should be shortened.

According to reviewers, wordiness is the most common writing problem (see Fig. 32.1). Rewrite, using the fewest words possible. To produce crisp writing, find and delete unnecessary words. For example, many sentences begin with unnecessary words. Many sentences can be improved simply by deleting the words "a," "the," and "that."

If you have trouble deleting any of your hard work, save the deleted sections in another file. You may be able to use these sections for another paper, possibly a literature review.

DISCUSSING IMPLICATIONS

PRINCIPLE 183 • Discuss the interrelation of key variables.

Explain how the different measures of poor outcome are interrelated. Show how the cause and effect relations are biologically plausible. Describe whether the key variables are correlated or independent.

Most statistical software packages can create a correlation matrix, which is a grid that shows the interrelation among variables. Although this usually is much too detailed for publication, you should refer to it when you write the Discussion.

In IBM SPSS, the steps are Analyze, Correlate, Bivariate . . . , select the variables, check Spearman, OK.

In R, use the Hmisc package and type rcorr(variable1, variable2).

In Stata, use Statistics, Summaries, tables, and tests, Nonparametric test of hypotheses, Spearman's rank correlation, select the variables, OK.

PRINCIPLE 184 • Explain your rationale for research judgments.

Describe any unusual methods or analyses that you used and explain why you deviated from the usual methods. For example, explain your motivation for deciding on the sample size, the definitions of outcome, and the statistical tests. Can you provide any support for these decisions?

PRINCIPLE 185 • Discuss the financial implications of your findings.

In the past, many medical research papers were written without any mention of money. Now, however, with the changes in health care financing, most reviewers expect to see some discussion of the financial ramifications (e.g., a cost–benefit analysis). If possible, compare and discuss the cost and duration of hospital stay, especially for the important subgroups. What are the costs of various types of treatment? How do your results relate to current issues in health care financing? How is this topic important at a time when health care dollars are shrinking? Explain the financial implications of the outcome and trends that you report. One exception: PCORI (Patient-Centered Outcomes Research Institute) does not support formal cost-effectiveness analysis.

PRINCIPLE 186 • Speculate intelligently.

State what is speculation. Avoid gross speculation. If you cannot provide evidence to support your opinion, expect a reviewer to tell you to delete the sentence. As one editor suggested, "Keep the

Discussion lively, related to the results, but speculate with intelligence." Ask your internal reviewers and coauthors to consider whether the speculative sections of your Discussion are appropriate. As Vivian Siegel, the former editor of *Cell*, says, "Within the Discussion section only, you can and should speculate, but don't speculate on your speculation."

PRINCIPLE 187 • Consider alternative explanations for your Results.

In the Discussion, consider the opposing point of view by taking a devil's advocate position. Do not wait for a reviewer to play this role. Identify the strengths and note the weaknesses of your study. Most papers are improved by adding a few paragraphs under a subheading such as "Limitations of the Study." Address these questions: What problems occurred during your study? If you had to repeat the study and had unlimited funding, what would you do differently? What are the weaknesses in your Methods? As experienced researchers know, you cannot believe all analysis at face value. Often, waiting for corroboration before acting on data is the best policy. Provide a biologically plausible explanation of how your findings could be associated with the outcome reported.

PRINCIPLE 188 • Be skeptical of published work.

One reviewer identified the following common mistake in analyzing data: failure to consider the "null" hypothesis. Most clinicians assume that any published report is true and, after reading an article, unconsciously add their own name to the author list. This is especially true for younger doctors and students. It is safer to assume that the author is wrong and then see if he or she can overcome your skepticism.

Another reviewer said that a common problem occurs when people read only the conclusions, and not the body of the paper, or do not compare the results with published reports.

In your Introduction and Discussion, do not simply summarize published papers: critically evaluate their methodology, findings, and conclusions. For example: Are their conclusions based on recent data and a large sample size? Are the data drawn from a population that is appropriate for your needs?

DISCUSSING POTENTIAL PROBLEMS

PRINCIPLE 189 • Recognize and discuss selection bias.

Explain how the people who were selected for the study differ from those who were not selected. For example, during your chart review, were you missing more private patients than clinic patients? Do not misinterpret your results and present flawed information. In the Methods, you should have stated which subjects were excluded and when they were excluded. In the Discussion, explain why you excluded patients with other severities of the study condition. If your point has been proven for other populations, justify why the population that you studied is different and required to further prove the point.

Example 25–1.
People with depression might be particularly willing to respond to a questionnaire on depression, but then obviously, the results would suffer from this selection bias.

PRINCIPLE 190 • Discuss the implications of analyzing only respondents.

For questionnaires, explain how your sample of valid respondents differed from those who did not respond. For example, a problem would occur if 50% of the potential respondents were men and only 25% of the actual respondents were men. If you surveyed a local group, explain how your sample differed from subjects more broadly distributed across the country or even the world. Provide some data on the direction and strength of this bias.

PRINCIPLE 191 • Discuss prediction cautiously.

For cross-sectional studies, explain that you understand that correlation does not equal causation. With this type of study design, avoid making strong conclusions regarding prediction and the development of conditions. Carefully interpret findings about risk factors that you assume antedated conditions. Collaborate with an experienced methodologist for papers about prediction and causal inference.

PRINCIPLE 192 • Be modest.

When you describe your study or a finding with the words "the first," "only," or "largest series," modesty requires that you add "known to us." Alternatively, you can write, "We are aware of no published reports that describe . . ." To convince the reader that your statement is true, explain how you conducted your literature search.

PRINCIPLE 193 • Describe your findings with appropriate balance.

Use words such as "proves" cautiously; "indicates" usually is more appropriate. Also, phrases such as "solves an important problem" are too enthusiastic and therefore inappropriate. Do not overstate the importance of your findings. Show the evidence and discuss it but remain understated and objective. Your prose should be bland and studious. Be direct and honest about the results of your study. **Include 95% confidence intervals in your Discussion (as well as in your Results) to show that you are aware of the variability of your findings.**

PRINCIPLE 194 • Describe the strengths and limitations of your follow-up.

Reviewers often are interested in long-term follow-up data. For journals that require long-term follow-up, give the minimum and median follow-up times in the Results. Also, compare your follow-up with that of published studies. If reviewers think that the follow-up is too short, they may reject the paper. In the discussion of the paper's limitations, explain how your sample differs from the general population or the ideal sample. Reviewers may wonder whether the findings are skewed because your sample has a disproportionately high or low incidence of the risk factor.

PRINCIPLE 195 • Identify a "control group" in the literature.

If your study does not have an ideal control group, you may be able to use information from published studies to strengthen your Discussion. Although a control group from the literature is not a substitute for an actual study control group, it is better than no comparison at all. For example, in our paper (Byrne et al., 2011), we compare our results of 7-year trends in employee health habits from a workplace health promotion program with national and state figures and goals. We contrasted our trends over time with those of the Centers for Disease Control and Prevention's Behavioral Risk Factor Surveillance System, the National Highway Traffic Safety Administration's National Occupant Protection Use Survey, and Healthy People 2010 goals. These studies provide reliable benchmark data that is publically available on their websites.

PRINCIPLE 196 • Discuss any surprising findings.

Point out any results that readers will find striking, even if the result was not intended or the variable was not important. If you do not address unusual findings, reviewers may give your Discussion a poor rating.

PRINCIPLE 197 • Discuss the problems associated with small sample size.

Tables often show large differences that are not statistically different. These differences might be caused by large variations in the measurements or by the inclusion of too few subjects. Discuss any limitations caused by a small sample size. If you did not find statistically significant differences because the sample size was small or the incidence was low, be sure that you understand the detectable limits of your study. Also discuss the rationale for your sample size. Addressing these issues is far better than waiting for an editor to point them out in a rejection letter.

THOUGHTFUL CONCLUSIONS

PRINCIPLE 198 • Conclude the Discussion with a "bolt of lightning."

The body of a good paper is a thunderbolt in reverse: It begins with thunder (the Introduction) and ends with lightning (the conclusions). Quality papers end with strong, clear conclusions.

Clearly state your recommendations so that reviewers do not ask:

"What do the authors recommend?"
"No recommendations are made as to what the clinician is to do with this information. It is interesting that differences in X exist, but how are we to alter management of these patients based on this?"

Your summary statement, usually the final sentence in the Discussion, must capture what is important about your study. Do not end your Discussion with weak statements. Remember that most people read the Abstract, the conclusions, and then the Introduction—in that order. The last paragraph should begin "In conclusion" or "In summary . . ."

PRINCIPLE 199 • Provide cautious conclusions that are fully supported by your data.

Many writers give inadequate attention to their conclusions. As a result, they often are the weakest link in a manuscript. The sixth and final step of the scientific method is draw conclusions. Write one sentence for this step that builds on the previous five steps.

Unsupported conclusions are one of the most common and severe problem with interpretation (Figs. 25.1 and 25.2). The conclusions must be drawn from the data presented in the manuscript. Any conclusions that are drawn from the statistical analysis must be justified in plain English, so polish your conclusion statement to avoid the following type of critique:

"The main weakness of this paper is that the authors neither consider nor control for many confounding factors. Therefore, the conclusion needs to be more conservative."

Answer the following questions: Are the conclusions correctly derived from the data presented? Can the conclusions be improved by narrowing the statement? Are the recommendations too general? Will the editor think that the conclusions are unwarranted?

Remember, even if your conclusions are correct, if they are not consistent with the evidence in your Results, your paper probably will be rejected. Anticipate reviewers saying that your conclusions:

+ Are inappropriate for the data
+ Do not follow from the data
+ Contradict the data and ignore important literature

Do a complete literature search and include relevant information, even if it does not support your conclusion or the novelty of your work. Editors and reviewers will do their own literature search, and omitting these publications will prove difficult to overcome.

Many researchers analyze their data incorrectly and then believe their interpretation. For example, they selected a unit in their hospital with a high rate of complication X, implemented a bundle of interventions, used a before–after design with no randomized control group, and were fooled by regression to the mean that their intervention improved outcomes. A stronger study design would have selected six units in the hospital with high rates of complication X and randomly assigned three to the intervention and three to the control group. As long as the control group continues to receive the current

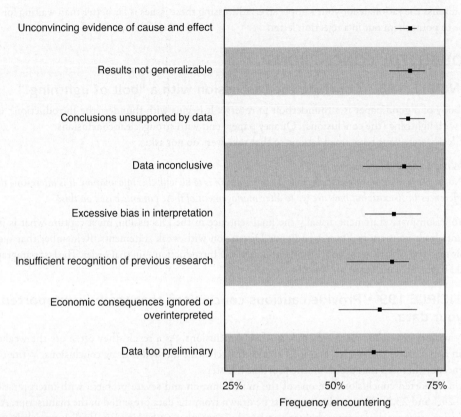

FIGURE 25.1. The frequency of interpretation problems. Answers are ranked by the median and bootstrap 95% confidence intervals using the sliding scale responses 0% (never) to 100% (always); from question 8 of the Peer Review Questionnaire (Appendix B). $P = 0.049$ based on the Friedman test.

standard of care, most institutional review boards (IRBs) will approve this. This is how learning health care systems will test interventions and publish papers in the future—the conclusions will be fully supported by the data.

PRINCIPLE 200 • Answer the question: "Who cares?"

What are the clinical implications of your findings? If you do not discuss the clinical implications of your paper, it probably will be rejected. To avoid this problem, offer precise, concrete suggestions. Include data and references to show that your suggestions could improve outcome. Otherwise, reviewers may say:

"Why is this research question important? The Introduction and the Discussion need more detail about the clinical applications of these findings."

Consider adding a section under the subheading "Practical Considerations and Future Implications." In this section, answer the following questions: Can you think of more interesting ways to look at your results? If you were a patient with the condition under study, how could these findings be useful? Of course, also explain how your study can help clinicians who treat patients with the condition under study.

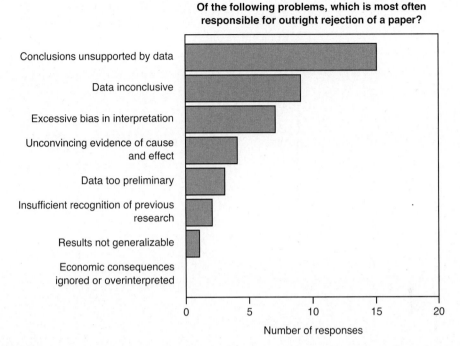

FIGURE 25.2. Interpretation problems and rejection. From question 9 of the Peer Review Questionnaire (Appendix B). $P < .001$ based on a chi-square test.

PRINCIPLE 201 • Tone down the conclusions to match the data.

Limit conclusions to the boundaries of the study. Conclusions drawn from uncontrolled retrospective data must be conservative. Will the reviewer think that your conclusions are sound based on the design of the study? For example, if no patients in your study died, reviewers might wonder how you can draw conclusions about morbidity and mortality. If your study was not a randomized clinical trial, interpret your findings carefully, especially those regarding treatment and outcome and cause and effect.

PRINCIPLE 202 • Describe precisely what further research is needed.

If you recommend additional research, explain why and provide detail about the type of study needed. For example, if you conclude that a larger sample is needed, explain why your paper makes a contribution despite this problem. Otherwise, the reviewer might agree with you, send the manuscript back, and encourage you to enlarge your own sample. Rather than "More research is needed," specify the next research project needed: "A randomized controlled trial with a 5-year follow up of at least 450 patients with Stage I tumors is needed."

The conclusions should be written with an understanding of the big picture and provide a bridge to the future.

References

CREATING A HIGH-QUALITY REFERENCE SECTION

PRINCIPLE 203 • Allow enough time to create a flawless reference section.

Many authors do not realize the importance that editors place on an accurate reference section. Present the reference section properly for the target journal. Use full-length articles from peer-reviewed journals. Papers that are submitted for publication, but not officially accepted, are not allowed as references by most journals. For many journals, conference abstracts are not allowed unless they are published in a journal.

A paper that is accepted for publication, but not yet published, may be cited as a reference. Add "in press" in parentheses in place of the volume and page numbers. Update this reference before your paper is published.

When you are writing early drafts of your paper, be sure that the reference citations are 100% correct the first time. Including sloppy or incomplete references, such as "Smith 2015," in these early drafts creates unnecessary work later. Do not add a reference and then wait until the final draft to decide how to use it. Include the statement for the reference in the body of the manuscript.

An all-encompassing broad bibliography is viewed as a major flaw in a clinical research paper. Limit references to key citations and avoid citing every publication on the subject. Look for appropriate, recent, or review references in journals with large circulations. Including 40 references usually is adequate for clinical research papers (Halsey, 2012), but some journals limit the number to 20.

Double-check your paper for statements that require references, especially statements that do not agree with the work of most investigators. Otherwise, reviewers may say:

> *"The bibliography does not cite many important papers."*

Reference any statement that might make a reviewer ask "How does the author know that?"

Reviewers are often annoyed by "excessive citation of authors' previous publications" and not citing important international papers and not citing important older publications. Avoid "self-promoting language with reference to own work only."

PRINCIPLE 204 • Place reference citations properly.

For most journals, place the citation number directly after the name of the cited author, not at the end of the sentence. When you report the work of several authors without naming them, however, place the citation number at the end of the sentence (e.g., "Previous reports have shown an incidence of 50%.[13,24,29]"). In the text, superscript the reference numbers or place them in parentheses or square brackets, depending on the journal's style.

REFERENCING SYSTEMS

PRINCIPLE 205 • Learn the differences among the major referencing systems.

The three major systems are:

1. **Vancouver System**, Citation Order, or Citation-by-Reference: References are numbered and listed in the order in which they are cited in the text. For medical journals, this system is the most common.
2. **APA**, Author–Date, Name and Year, or Harvard System: References are cited in the text with the last name of the primary author and the year of publication. The reference list is arranged alphabetically by the authors' names. This system is also called the "APA" (American Psychological Association) system.
3. **Alphabet–Number System**: References are listed in alphabetical order according to the primary author's last name and cited by numbers in the text.

FOR MORE INFORMATION

The details of these systems vary from journal to journal, so as always, follow the guidelines for the target journal. Refer to the *Publication Manual of the American Psychological Association* (APA, 2010) for legal references or journals that follow the APA system.

Appendix A describes standard methods of referencing various sources. Researchers sometimes call these Uniform Requirements the "Vancouver style"—the Committee first met in Vancouver.

PRINCIPLE 206 • Format references for the target journal.

If you submit a paper with references that follow the format of another journal, the reviewers and editors may think that your paper was rejected by another journal. Avoid this.

For references that are difficult to obtain, you can direct the reader to the source (e.g., "available from . . ."). Include a scanned image of the table of contents of a book or first page of a paper if it will be difficult for the manuscript editor to find online.

REFERENCING SOFTWARE

The statistical software used in your study should have been described in the Methods as in the following examples. With most software, you can click on "Help" and then "About" to obtain the version number.

Example 26–1.
1. All data analyses and statistical computation were conducted with the use of the SAS software (version 9.4) and R (version 3.2.3, http://www.r-project.org, R Foundation for Statistical Computing).
2. We performed all analyses using SAS software (SAS Institute), version 9.4, and IBM SPSS, version 23.0.
3. Analysis was conducted with the statistical program Stata/SE, Version 14 (StataCorp, College Station, TX).
4. SAS software, version 9.4 (SAS Institute), and the R programming language (R Foundation for Statistical Computing) were used for statistical analyses.

In the past, authors would also reference software manuals in the reference section. The more modern way to address this is to add a detailed statistical appendix and a statement at the end of the methods such as the following:

"Additional details of the statistical analysis are provided in the Supplementary Appendix."

Occasionally, it can be important to have a more traditional reference for the statistical software. Within the R software, you can type "citation()" to obtain the appropriate citation to cut and paste, such as:

"R Core Team. (2014). R: A language and environment for statistical computing. R Foundation for Statistical Computing, Vienna, Austria. http://www.r-project.org/."

In addition, you can obtain the citation for the specific R package used with the following command: citation("package"), for example, citation("survival").

The R software can also be referenced as follows:

"R: a language and environment for statistical computing. Vienna: R Foundation for Statistical Computing, 2016."

For sample size justifications, you can reference the sample size software in the Methods or the Appendix as in the following examples:

+ Sample-size calculations were made with the use of nQuery Advisor, version 7.0 (Statistical Solutions).
+ The PS program (version 3.1.2) was used to compute the sample size.

Then in the references add:

Dupont WD, Plummer WD: "Power and Sample Size Calculations: A Review and Computer Program", Controlled Clinical Trials 1990; 11:116–28. (http://biostat.mc.vanderbilt.edu/wiki/Main/PowerSampleSize)

Modern reproducible research also requires that you reference your data collection methods, for example, if you used REDCap, include a description such as:

"Study data were collected and managed using REDCap electronic data capture tools hosted at [YOUR INSTITUTION].[1] REDCap (Research Electronic Data Capture) is a secure, web-based application designed to support data capture for research studies, providing (a) an intuitive interface for validated data entry; (b) audit trails for tracking data manipulation and export procedures; (c) automated export procedures for seamless data downloads to common statistical packages; and (d) procedures for importing data from external sources."

And then a reference:

1. Paul A. Harris, Robert Taylor, Robert Thielke, Jonathon Payne, Nathaniel Gonzalez, Jose G. Conde, Research electronic data capture (REDCap) - A metadata-driven methodology and workflow process for providing translational research informatics support. J Biomed Inform. 2009 Apr;42(2):377–81.

POLISHING THE REFERENCES

PRINCIPLE 207 • Check the references to ensure that minor details are correct.

Use PubMed to double-check all references for accuracy of citation, attribution, format, and completeness. Also be sure that each reference is cited correctly in the text. If your time is limited, consider hiring someone to check that your references are 100% correct.

FOR MORE INFORMATION

See the American Medical Writers Association for freelance help.

http://www.amwa.org/jobs_freelance_directory

Verify each reference with the pdf of the paper and be sure that the cited references say what you think they say. Many errors are found in the reference section. Editors and reviewers cannot determine how carefully you conducted your research; therefore, many will look at the details of your references to assess the quality of your work and attention to detail.

When citing online journals or websites add "(Accessed [date] at [website])."

Make sure that you have enough references from the current and previous year. Often, a project will sit on a back burner and the references are not updated for the final draft. Do include references from the target journal and from any recommended or anticipated reviewers.

PRINCIPLE 208 • Use modern reference management software to help organize references.

The software programs that organize and reformat your references have become quite sophisticated and can save time especially if you must resubmit your paper to a journal with a different reference style.

FOR MORE INFORMATION

See EndNote, Reference Manager, RefWorks, Zotero, Mendeley, and Wizfolio.

PRINCIPLE 209 • Remember to cite coauthors.

When you name an author in your text, give the coauthors credit, too. If you are discussing the work of one author, use "he" or "she"; if the study has two or more authors, use "they."

Example 26–2.
One author:

> Lathers-McGillan[1] described Y. She reported that . . .

Two authors:

> Jones and Wagner[2] reported X. They found that . . .

Three or more authors:

> Smith et al.[3] found Z. They reported that . . .

The term "et al." means "and others." It is an abbreviation for two Latin terms: et alii (masculine) and et aliae (feminine). Journal style for citing multiple authors varies. Some use "et al.," which may or may not have a period and may or may not be italicized. Other journals avoid "et al." and alternate among the following (Halsey, 2012):

+ Smith and associates
+ Smith and colleagues
+ Smith and coworkers
+ Smith and coinvestigators

CHAPTER

27

Industry Publications

PRINCIPLE 210 • Have the scientists write the paper, not marketing.

If a manuscript looks like a marketing language, it will get killed. So avoid "Industry Style" in which the paper concludes "Drug X was effective and should go forward in development." The title should not state the conclusion. The paper must be an unbiased, objective evaluation of the results that demonstrates intellectual curiosity about the mechanism and related science. The paper must also show how this new knowledge fits into the existing literature.

Those who work in the pharmaceutical industry are trained to produce FDA submissions (for the U.S. Food and Drug Administration), but publishing a paper requires a different set of skills. A paper must tell an interesting story—not simply a robotic, dry report with a large number of tables. Partner with academic scientists and biostatisticians who can change it from bulleted lists that prove "our drug is better" to a story that links to previous findings, ties together the current findings, discusses mechanism, and provides a vision of the future.

For an FDA submission, the analysis is prespecified—cut and dry with little to no creativity. For a publication in a medical journal, the analysis and primary end point should be prespecified, but it must go beyond this to examine other potential explanations of the findings. The analysis also needs to assess for various forms of bias.

Industry papers sometimes use outdated statistical methods that were used previously with a conservative but successful FDA submission. For example, many still use last observation carried forward rather than multiple imputation to address missing values. Many still use analysis of variance (ANOVA) and other parametric methods rather than more robust regression and nonparametric methods. Also, there is a tendency to rely too heavily on univariate methods rather than regression models.

Avoid describing P values as "narrowly missing statistical significance" or "trending toward."

Avoid the practice of having ghost authors write a manuscript and search for academic authors to put their names on it. Instead, add a section to the Methods, such as the following:

"The study was designed by the senior (last) author and the first author. The data were collected by the Diabetes Center at Hospital X and analyzed by the lead statistician (the third author) in collaboration with the remaining four authors, all of whom vouch for the completeness and accuracy of the data, analyses, and study protocol. The manuscript was written entirely by the five listed authors. Pharmaceutical Company Y provided funding for the study but did not provide the study drug, which was purchased commercially and the cost paid for by Hospital X. The full protocol is available at NEJM.org."

PRINCIPLE 211 • Create transparent and informative tables of the drug's side effects.

For a manuscript, you need to limit the number of tables and present the information in a way that would be of interest to clinicians and scientists. Some journals are concerned about having authors decide if a complication was drug-related or not. Avoid minimizing the side effect—"patients vomited nonstop for 10 days but the drug was well tolerated."

Include a CONSORT diagram with an honest and complete accounting of all patients and dropouts.

FOR MORE INFORMATION
See Senn (2003, 2008).

EDITING

Key Questions to Answer in the Editing Phase:

- Have you said what you intended to say?
- Are you asking too much of the reader?
- Did the trial work as planned?*
- How do the findings compare with those from other studies?*
- What are the clinical implications of the findings?*

---

*Friedman et al. (2015).

Preparing Your Manuscript for Submission

SEEKING INTERNAL PEER REVIEW

PRINCIPLE 212 • Have your manuscript peer reviewed internally.

One editor advised: *"Have an experienced author of manuscripts read the paper before submitting it."*

A reviewer wrote: *"Review other papers to understand how to thoughtfully write a paper. Be humble and listen to the advice of your senior authors who should be critical enough to make a paper better and avoid rejection."*

Let us assume that you have finished the **P**lanning, **O**bserving, and **W**riting phases. At this point, many unsuccessful medical researchers submit their manuscripts for publication. Successful writers find the patience and determination to complete the remaining two phases of the POWER principles: Editing and Revising.

Reading takes energy. Your job is to write a paper that takes less energy to understand.

> **VITAL POINT**
>
> Before you submit your paper to a journal, ask several colleagues to review it, especially those who are experienced in journal publishing. Also, be sure that you have several researchers outside your group read the paper and then revise according to their suggestions before the first submission.

At Vanderbilt University, we developed a successful formal expert feedback program, called "Studios," to make it easier for researchers to obtain this type of internal review. Investigators fill out a brief online manuscript Studio request form and then a Studio manager invites a multidisciplinary team of experienced experts to attend a 1.5-hour meeting to provide constructive feedback on how to improve the manuscript. "The Clinical and Translational Research Studios: An Interdisciplinary Model" won the 2012 Association of American Medical Colleges (AAMC) Award for Innovations in Research and Education. Details of the Studio program are described in a paper published in Academic Medicine (Byrne et al., 2012); the appendices of the paper provide the details for other universities interested in duplicating it. See:

https://victr.vanderbilt.edu/pub/message.html?message_id=141

Find unbiased colleagues who can provide rigorous, honest, and insightful reviews. After your colleagues read your manuscript, ask them to summarize what they learned. Revise the manuscript to make it easier for the reader to come away with the story you are trying to tell. E-mail the manuscript for comments and a copy of the internal peer review form (Fig. 28.1) to each coauthor, several colleagues, and your biostatistician for critical review.

The purpose of this form is to help medical researchers to critique
their colleagues' manuscripts before submission.

General instructions:

With track changes or a red pen, mark the sections that require clarification.
Highlight areas in which the wording or numbers are confusing or incorrect.

Describe the three major weaknesses of this paper:

I.

II.

III.

Check any of the following areas that are weak and require additional work before submission:

_____ Importance and originality of the subject for the target journal

_____ Adequacy of the study design/appropriateness of the approach

_____ Adequacy of the patients or materials studied

_____ Accuracy of the interpretation of the results

_____ Statistical analysis

_____ Relevance of the Discussion section

_____ Soundness of the conclusions

_____ Appropriateness of the references

_____ Appropriateness, clarity, and adequacy of the tables/figures

_____ Clarity of the presentation

_____ Accurateness and adequacy of the abstract

What additional information would you need to reproduce this study?

How would you strengthen the Discussion and analysis?

(Circle all that apply.)

Which sections are too long?	Abstract Introduction Methods Results Discussion
Which sections are too short?	Abstract Introduction Methods Results Discussion
Which tables would you delete?	1 2 3 4 5 6 7 8+
Which figures would you delete?	1 2 3 4 5 6 7 8+

FIGURE 28.1. Internal peer review form.

What conclusions would you draw from these results?

Which sections of this manuscript could be misunderstood?

What flaws are evident in the execution of this study?

How could the title be improved?

	No	Yes
Did this study raise and resolve an important question?	____	____
Does this manuscript follow the target journal's standard format?	____	____
Is the writing clear and concise?	____	____
Are the paragraphs organized to allow for intelligent skimming?	____	____
Are the units of measure included and abbreviated consistently?	____	____
Is this study interesting?	____	____

FIGURE 28.1. *(Continued)*

Ironically, many people are offended by how they are thanked in the acknowledgments. For this reason, give a copy of the acknowledgments to everyone you thanked (to be sure that they are happy with the way you characterize them, their job title, and their contribution to the paper). Obtaining written permission from all persons named in the acknowledgments is a wise step—even if it is not required by the target journal.

When you ask colleagues to review your manuscript, indicate where you are planning to submit your paper and ask your colleagues to do the following:

1. Mark any sections that are difficult to understand. Did they have to rearrange sentences to understand them?
2. Summarize their reactions to the paper with comments in track changes or in the margins.
3. Mark where they stopped reading and any sections that they skipped.

Address your colleagues' concerns and also edit your paper to avoid the following types of comments:

+ I found the manuscript somewhat difficult to follow in places.
+ I am uncertain as to how you arrived at the numbers X, Y, and Z in the Results. They do not correspond to the tables. I am confused. Please explain.

Explain any apparent discrepancies between the text and the tables. Reread the Results and delete any information that appears in the tables.

Do not rush to submit your paper. Remember, journals often spend months reviewing manuscripts. To increase the chance that your paper will be accepted, spend more time editing your writing to avoid the problems listed in Figures 28.2 and 28.3. Consider having your manuscript professionally edited, especially if your primary language is not English.

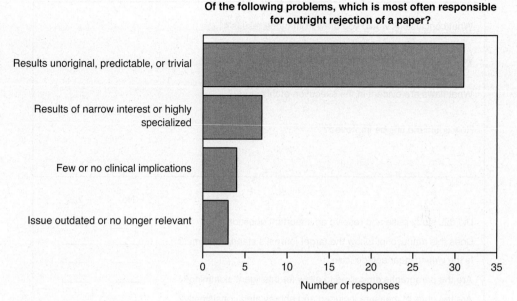

Of the following problems, which is most often responsible for outright rejection of a paper?

FIGURE 28.2. Topic problems that are responsible for rejection. From question 11 of the Peer Review Questionnaire (Appendix B). *P* < .001 based on a chi-square test.

FOR MORE INFORMATION

See the American Medical Writers Association for writing or editing assistance:

http://www.amwa.org/jobs_freelance_directory

As you may remember from Figure 12.1, a priority during editing is to make each section the correct length.

VITAL POINT

A good rule is shorten the Introduction and Discussion and lengthen the Methods and Results.

PRINCIPLE 213 • Ask a friend or colleague outside your specialty to critique your paper before you submit it to a journal with a general audience.

Your manuscript may be too specialized or complicated for many readers. To anyone other than you and your coauthors, your writing may be impossible to understand.

Half of the manuscripts submitted to the *British Medical Journal* are quickly rejected for one of three reasons:

1. Lack of originality
2. Serious scientific flaws
3. Lack of importance to a general medical audience

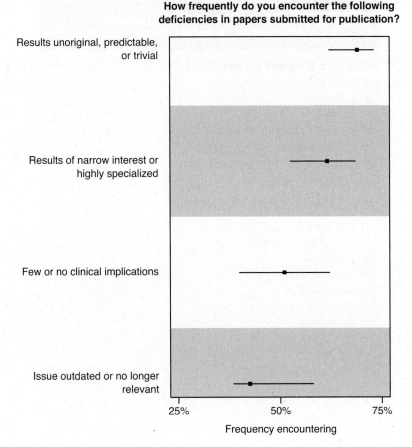

How frequently do you encounter the following deficiencies in papers submitted for publication?

FIGURE 28.3. Frequency of topic problems. Answers are ranked by the median and bootstrap 95% confidence intervals using the sliding scale responses 0% (never) to 100% (always); from question 10 of the Peer Review Questionnaire (Appendix B). $P < .001$ based on the Friedman test.

Consider these points and rewrite any sections that people outside your field may not understand. Although at this point in the process some flaws cannot be eliminated, you must edit your paper until your message is clear and direct.

EDITING FOR BREVITY AND CLARITY

PRINCIPLE 214 • Eliminate all jargon.

Jargon is obscure, often pretentious, language with long or unnecessary words. Jargon in medical research papers causes countless problems and should be avoided. Within each specialty, medical researchers use distinctive words or phrases. The trouble occurs when authors must communicate with those outside their specialty, geographic area, or generation. The specialized terms then become gibberish.

When you must use a phrase that could be considered jargon, enclose the term in quotation marks and define it. After the initial explanation, do not repeat the quotation marks. Also avoid colloquialisms, clichés, and euphemisms (Table 28.1).

Avoid clichés like the plague. They are a dime a dozen.

When you are editing, ask yourself: "Can I express my idea in a shorter, more direct, or less technical way?" Careful editing can change writing from turgid, bombastic, and pompous to plain English.

TABLE 28.1	Examples of Colloquialisms, Clichés, Euphemisms, and Slang

Colloquialisms and clichés
- First and foremost
- Crystal clear
- In a nutshell
- Landed a patient in the ICU
- State of the art
- Kept in mind
- On top of this
- By a wide margin
- Does this have legs?
- One off
- The common thread
- Level set
- Low-hanging fruit

Euphemisms
- Nonsurvivors
- Passed away
- The rat was sacrificed.

Slang
- Lab
- Prepped, bowel prep
- Temp
- Passed out

Poor English is a common criticism and highly annoying to reviewers, so aim for clear, jargon-free writing.

As Martin Fischer (Daintith, 1989) said, "You must learn to talk clearly. The jargon of scientific terminology which rolls off your tongues is mental garbage."

PRINCIPLE 215 • Use simple declarative sentences but thread them together to tell a story that flows.

Longer sentences are not harder to read but they are harder to write. Try to reword sentences that begin with the phrases shown in Table 28.2. This rewording should make your writing more professional. Some words and phrases are overused as sentence beginnings. Table 28.3 lists suggestions for simplifying or improving sentences.

Sometimes two sentences are closely related but cannot be combined. In this situation, you may be able to edit the first few words of the second sentence to provide a transition from the first sentence. Table 28.4 shows some examples of transitional phrases. Provide context to link old information from the last sentence to the new information in the current sentence.

An example of threading:

"Animal experiments have demonstrated X, Y, and Z. On the basis of these preclinical data, we performed a Phase I trial."

TABLE 28.2	Sentence Beginnings to Avoid

100 patients underwent (add "A total of" before this)
As a matter of fact
Based on the fact that (change to "Because")
Due to (try "Because")
Given the fact that
Hopefully
In a very real sense
In light of the fact that (try "Because")
In order to (try "To")
In other words
In the event that (change to "If")
It follows then, that
It goes without saying
It has been reported by Smith that (change to "Smith reported that")
It has been shown
It is important to note that
It may be
It was found that
More importantly (change to "More important")
Note well that
Of course
Past and present research has outlined
Prior literature suggests that
That is to say
There (change to an active statement)
Whether it be
Yet
Y'all[a]

[a]Denotes sarcasm.

TABLE 28.3	Sentence Beginnings to Use Sparingly

However (move in a few words with commas on either side)
In addition
In general (try "Overall")
It (replace with the phrase that "it" stands for)
Therefore (move it to the middle of the sentence)

TABLE 28.4	Transitional Phrases

Although previous reports have shown X
From this number
For these reasons
Further
In contrast
In addition
In the other trial
Moreover
Similarly
These included
This decrease suggests
This relationship can be
This uncertainty has led to
These results contradict the findings from X
Thus

Avoid starting a sentence with a numeral. Even if the number is written out, the sentence probably will be awkward.

Example 28–1.
"One hundred ninety-seven patients . . ." is a bad way to start any sentence.
"A total of 197 patients..." is better.

PRINCIPLE 216 • Eliminate superfluous commas and dashes.

Reading a sentence is like taking a mental breadth, but do not insert a comma every time the reader needs to, inhale. Most manuscripts can be improved by deleting several commas; however, commas are often needed after a beginning transitional word or phrase (e.g., "Conversely," "In fact,").

Insert a comma before "and" in a series of three or more items, such as A, B, C, and D. The same rule applies to "or."

Use semicolons, not commas, to separate numbered items in a series. For example:

The inclusion criteria were as follows: (1) _____; (2) _____; and (3) _____.

In medical writing, a comma usually is preferred in place of a dash. Save the dash for setting off words that require special emphasis.

FOR MORE INFORMATION

The Gregg Reference Manual by Sabin (2010) is an excellent writing reference book that is both well organized and easy to understand. Norris's (2015) book *Between You & Me: Confession of a Comma Queen* provides an entertaining account of her experience as an editor at *The New Yorker*.

PRINCIPLE 217 • Recognize when to use "that" and "which."

Restrictive clauses are phrases that do not limit the reference of a modified word or phrase. They do not require commas and usually are preceded by "that" rather than "which." Restrictive clauses are essential to the meaning of the sentence. For example: The antibiotic that was most effective was ampicillin. In this sentence, "that" introduces an essential clause. Without the clause, the meaning of the sentence is changed: The antibiotic was ampicillin.

Nonrestrictive (descriptive) clauses are phrases that are set off by commas. They usually are preceded by "which." Nonrestrictive clauses are not essential to the meaning of the sentence; they provide additional information. For example: Amoxicillin, which was used in Group II, was most effective. In this sentence, "which" introduces a nonessential clause. Without the clause, the basic meaning of the sentence is not changed: Amoxicillin was most effective.

Compare the meaning of the following sentences:

1. Surgery is required for Stage II tumors, which do not respond to chemotherapy.
2. Surgery is required for Stage II tumors that do not respond to chemotherapy.

PRINCIPLE 218 • Use professional symbols.

You can use Greek letters, foreign accents, and mathematical and other symbols in your manuscript, even if they are not displayed on your keyboard. These symbols can make your paper look more professional (e.g., $\pm$ rather than $+/-$). To use these symbols on most computers, follow these steps:

1. Hold down the alternate (Alt) key.
2. Type the corresponding three-digit (ASCII) code on the numeric keypad (e.g., 241 for $\pm$).
3. Release the Alt key.

Table 28.5 shows symbols that you can use in your manuscripts. In Microsoft Word, Insert, Symbol, More Symbols (or Advanced Symbols on a Mac), select, Insert will do the same.

TABLE 28.5	Additional Symbols and Codes
Symbol	**Alt + Three-Digit Code**
½	171
¼	172
α	224
β	225
Σ	228
σ	229
μ	230
∞	236
±	241
≥	242
≤	243
÷	246

TABLE 28.6	How to Use the Word "Data"	
Problematic Usage	**Preferred Usage**	
This data	These data	
Less data	Fewer data	
Much data	Many data	
Data was	Data were	

PRINCIPLE 219 • Use the word "data" as you would use the word "numbers."

The following point is minor, but a favorite of many reviewers: "Data" is the plural form of the rarely used word "datum." To determine whether your sentence is correct, replace the word "data" with the word "numbers." In some cases, you can substitute another word to avoid awkwardness. For example, a sentence that begins "Little data is available . . ." can be rewritten as "Little information is available . . ." Table 28.6 shows how to use the word "data."

PRINCIPLE 220 • Submit a professional-looking manuscript.

Most journals prefer that authors avoid using boldface, italics, or underlining. Also, avoid using quotation marks unless you are quoting someone directly or using a word or phrase in an unusual sense (e.g., Preoperative "fine-tuning" consisted of . . .).

Never submit a single-spaced manuscript. Most journal editors prefer double-spaced papers.

Do not right-justify the text and do not break words at the end of a line. Use a type size of 12 points.

Be sure that you are submitting a complete package. Finally, verify that the final manuscript meets all of the requirements listed in the guidelines for authors.

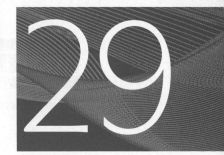

CHAPTER 29

Small but Significant Points to Consider

PRINCIPLE 221 • Follow the target journal's style.

Each journal has its own style. Check the target journal's format for style points (e.g., whether to use "percent" or "%"). For most journals, numbers less than 10 are written out, unless they appear with percentages or units of time or measure. Within each sentence, however, be consistent, regardless of whether a number is less than 10.

> *Example 29–1.*
> Group I had a mean score of 25, and Group II had a mean score of 7 (not "seven").

Be alert to stylistic differences among journals. For example, uppercase P is preferred for P values in most journals but not all. Before you submit your paper, check the relevant style points. These points may seem trivial, but journals are looking for papers written in their style.

FOR MORE INFORMATION

Check a recent issue of the target journal, and refer to *The Gregg Reference Manual* (Sabin, 2010) for specific style points.

Table 29.1 shows differences in house style among journals. Some of the style points suggested in this book are not followed by all journals.

TABLE 29.1	Examples of House Style Differences among Journals

%	percent
$P < .001$	$p < .001$
less than 3.9	<3.9
orthopaedic	orthopedic
Figure	Fig
vs.	versus, v
Grams	g
in-hospital	inhospital
6-year	6-yr
Table 3	Table III
5	five
et al.	et al

Some journals provide information on their house style, for example, BMJ has this website:
http://www.bmj.com/about-bmj/resources-authors/house-style
Wikipedia has a List of style guides:
https://en.wikipedia.org/wiki/List_of_style_guides

TABLE 29.2	Rephrasing from the First Person to the Third Person

First Person	Third Person
Our objective	The authors' objective
Our results	The current study
We analyzed	The authors analyzed
We are indebted to, We thank	The authors thank
I showed that	This study shows that
I used a chi-square test	A chi-square test was used

Example 29–2.
A paper was published in which the outcome was defined in the manuscript as $\leq X$; however, the copyeditor changed it to "greater than or equal to X." Following the target journal's style can minimize the errors introduced during the editing phase.

Some journals do not allow text written in the first person. For these journals, make the types of changes shown in Table 29.2 before you submit your paper. The use of the first person is not wrong, but to improve your odds of acceptance, you will want your paper to match the journal's style as closely as possible.

PRINCIPLE 222 • Create a professional-looking title page.

Appendix A indicates the general information that should be included on the title page, but title pages are very journal-specific. The following are a few additional points:

+ List only coauthors who meet the full criteria for authorship.
+ Include each author's highest academic degree.
+ Provide each author's current job title and institutional affiliation at the time the study was performed.
+ Include the details of where and when the paper was presented.
+ Provide the full name (not just an acronym) of any funding agency for your project and include the grant number.

VITAL POINT

Your goal is to make the editor think "we can publish this paper without an inordinate amount of work."

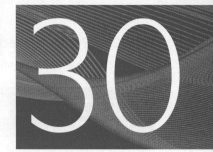

Improving Your Writing

> *"The responsibility of communication lies with the writer, not the reader. Write with your readers in mind."*
>
> —JUDITH SWAN

LEARNING FROM THE EXPERTS

One reviewer advised: *"Read good studies, take them apart, understand them, find a good editor or colleague."*

PRINCIPLE 223 • Study George Orwell's rules.

Orwell (1970) provided the following six rules for writing:

1. Never use a metaphor, simile, or other figure of speech which you are used to seeing in print.
2. Never use a long word where a short one will do.
3. If it is possible to cut a word out, always cut out.
4. Never use the passive where you can use the active.
5. Never use a foreign phrase, a scientific word, or a jargon word if you can think of an everyday English equivalent.
6. Break any of these rules sooner than say anything outright barbarous.

   Many medical researchers ask about the use of the passive versus the active voice. In most cases, medical writing is improved with the active voice, as Orwell advised. In some sentences, however, especially in the Methods section, the passive voice is preferred because it emphasizes what was performed rather than who performed it.

   It is a myth that active is always better. The active is not better—it is just different. Changing all passive to active is not the solution. Scientists do not care about the who, but they care about the what. With good science, it should not matter who did the laboratory experiment or ran the analysis. The results should be the same if another qualified person followed the same methodology.

PRINCIPLE 224 • Apply the guidelines that Ernest Hemingway followed.

Hemingway reported that the following guidelines were "the best rules I ever learned in the business of writing":

1. Use short sentences.
2. Use short first paragraphs.
3. Use vigorous English.
4. Be positive, not negative.

PRINCIPLE 225 • Take Thoreau's advice.

"Simplify, simplify, simplify," advised Thoreau. This advice certainly would improve most medical manuscripts, although it is ironic that Thoreau didn't follow his own advice and write "Simplify."

PRINCIPLE 226 • Heed the advice of medical journal editors.

Table 30.1 provides advice from editors.

TABLE 30.1	Advice from Editors and Reviewers[a]

- Keep it simple!
- Read and follow the instructions for authors.
- Read the instructions to authors, and read several recent articles to get a feel for the "house" style and expectations.
- Make sure your article is a good fit.
- Be straightforward and get to the point. Discuss methods clearly; avoid excessive variables.
- Search the literature before deciding on topic and approach. Review articles in the journal and note tone, approach, level of detail.
- Spend more time reviewing published literature and more time revising your manuscript.
- Stay brief, to the point, focused, clear, simple, use clear tables, use nice illustrations, if possible, use great language.
- Emphasize what is new and why a clinician would care.
- Work harder on writing a punch introduction, even (unbiased) tone, don't overstate results, more thorough discussion of implications.
- Read the journal and see what our standards are, the form to write the manuscript in, and what readers want, who they are, and the focus of the journal.
- Assure the clinical relevance and validity of the study.
- Think it out before.
- Strive for rigorous design and execution; present findings clearly, acknowledge strengths and limitations.
- Present findings in perspective.
- Select only essential information to include.
- Put in all the information needed to make your case.
- Write it clearly. Write carefully and thoughtfully.
- Be original and concise.
- Ask a respected neutral party to review your paper prior to submission.
- Have your paper professionally edited for English grammar.
- Shorten by one-fourth.
- Don't write an article unless you have a clear rationale for it in advance—what is its purpose, what will you present, and why is it important? Use a reporting checklist (e.g., CONSORT, STROBE) to make sure you have included all the important information readers need to assess the research. Don't ignore relevant international research or well-established findings in the field.
- Explicit, logical, clear description of rationale, hypothesis, methods, data losses, analysis and conclusions
- Consult with or collaborate with seasoned writers willing to mentor, use publications from high-impact journals as examples.
- Ask many others to proofread for content and grammar.
- Make sure each section contains appropriate information.
- Get the advice of experts in the methodology of the specific area of interest before designing the project and allocate enough time to complete the project.
- Have a sound a priori rationale before doing the research and let the resultant data speak for itself.
- Pay attention to the design and methods and analysis of the research project.
- Understand that the manuscript should be written with the reviewer in mind.
- Write, rewrite, set it aside, and review. You should review your work with a critic's eyes.
- Be honest.

[a]From question 31 of the Peer Review Questionnaire (Appendix B).

PRINCIPLE 227 • Read (or reread) The Elements of Style.

No matter how experienced a writer you are, rereading this classic book by Strunk and White (2009) is worth your time.

PRINCIPLE 228 • Read Style: Lessons in Clarity and Grace.

This book by Williams (2013) is a readable, informative guide to grammar and writing. Williams provides details and examples to help authors follow vague guidelines such as "Omit needless words" and "Be concise."

EDITING YOUR PAPER FOR A MEDICAL JOURNAL

PRINCIPLE 229 • Include interesting examples.

Whenever appropriate, provide interesting anecdotes to *show* readers rather than *tell* them. In a medical manuscript, examples are appropriate if they are handled professionally.

Can you get your next door neighbor excited about your research?

PRINCIPLE 230 • Edit, edit, edit! Cut, cut, cut!

Table 30.2 shows specific words and phrases that often can be cut to make your paper more professional.

TABLE 30.2	Words and Phrases to Delete
a lot	
additionally	
and/or	
as to	
basically	
case (referring to a research participant)	
he/she, s/he, his/her	
known to be	
literally	
needless to say	
paradigm shift	
rather (adjective)	
really	
seem	
so that	
so as to/in order to (substitute "to")	
that have been	
utilized	
very	
whilst	

TABLE 30.3	Examples of How Sentences Can Be Improved by Deleting the Word "There"

Original:	There has been an increase in the number of patients . . .
Improved:	More patients are . . .
Original:	There were no pulmonary emboli or deep wound infections.
Improved:	No pulmonary emboli or deep wound infections occurred.
Original:	There were 603 patients with . . .
Improved:	A total of 603 patients had . . .
Original:	Because there can be . . .
Improved:	Because X can exist . . .
Original:	There were seven pregnancies . . .
Improved:	Seven infants had . . .
Original:	There was a significant increase in adverse outcome . . .
Improved:	Adverse outcome increased significantly . . .
Original:	There is evidence to suggest that those who cease smoking . . .
Improved:	Those who cease smoking may . . .

PRINCIPLE 231 • Find and remove problem words and phrases.

Use CTRL+F or command+F to find the word "there." Delete it. Rewrite the sentence with an active verb (Payne, 1987). Make sure that the reader understands who did what. These steps improve most sentences. See Table 30.3 for examples of sentences that are improved by deleting the word "there."

If you are submitting your paper to an English language publication, you often can improve your writing by following the suggestions shown in Tables 30.4 through 30.14.

TABLE 30.4	Usage Problems

Problematic Usage	Preferred Usage
while most studies	whereas most studies
whilst 20.2% of those	whereas 20.2% of those
Since this was	Because this was
In this country	In the United States
Half the patients	One-half of the patients
reproducible methodology	reproducible method
analysis was done	analysis was performed
There are several limitations	This study has several limitations
over a short period	for a short period
similar to those above	similar to those used earlier
the above-listed criteria	the previously listed criteria
mentioned above	mentioned previously
prior to	before
parameter	characteristic

(continued)

TABLE 30.4	Usage Problems *(continued)*

Problematic Usage	Preferred Usage
an SCI patient	a patient with spinal cord injury
the albumin was	the albumin concentration was
5-minute Apgar score <7	5 min Apgar score of less than 7
delivered before 37 weeks	delivered before 37 weeks of gestation
White's classification	the White classification
Out of 55 patients	Among the 55 patients
amongst cancer patients	among patients with cancer
Center for Disease Control	Centers for Disease Control and Prevention
mucus membrane	mucus (noun), mucous (adjective) membrane
data was utilized	data were used
investigator, who was blinded to	investigator, blinded to
This demonstrates	This shows
Data were collected on	Data were collected concerning
have good outcome	experience a good outcome
came to the identical conclusion	agreed
All chart data	All data from the charts
data established before	data collected before
a group of MD's	a group of M.D.s
seven PhD's	seven Ph.D.s
Table 1 compares the risk factors.[a]	A comparison of the risk factors is shown in Table 1.

[a]Tables and figures cannot compare.

TABLE 30.5	Describing Results from the Literature

Problematic Usage	Preferred Usage
has been shown to be	is
was found to be	was
In the X report, it was found that	The X report showed that
Smith et al looked at	Smith et al. examined
One of the few studies on X is a paper by Smith et al.	Smith et al. conducted one of the few studies on X.
The current study confirms previous results that indicate	The results of the current study agree with those from previous studies that indicated
X has been well studied showing	X has been studied extensively. Results have shown that
This finding is in contrast to reports for	This finding differs from those reported regarding
There have been studies comparing	Previous studies have compared
The literature reports	Several reports in the literature describe
It would appear that	It appears that

TABLE 30.6 Diction Problems

Problematic Usage	Preferred Usage
This method came about	This method was developed
due to	attributable to
get	(use a more specific verb, such as "become infected with")
The percent with X goes up	The percentage with X increased
like	analogous to, similar to, such as
We felt	We believe

TABLE 30.7 Capitalization Problems

Problematic Usage	Preferred Usage
Chi-Square	chi-square
class IV	Class IV
fishers exact test	Fisher's exact test
Level 1 Trauma Center	level I trauma center
medicare and medicaid	Medicare and Medicaid
pearson correlation coefficient	Pearson correlation coefficient
social security number	Social Security number
students t test	Student's t-test

TABLE 30.8 Phrases to Transpose

Problematic Usage	Preferred Usage
with what is traditionally	with what traditionally is
independently able to walk	able to walk independently
has also been	also has been
as the source of data	as the data source
outcome has usually been	outcome usually has been
should also be examined	also should be examined

TABLE 30.9   Problems with Numbers

Problematic Usage	Preferred Usage
(range 28–92).	(range, 28 to 92 days).
(44/87)	(44 of 87)
Using an estimate of $1,000 per day	With an estimate of $1,000 per patient per day of hospitalization
3 million a year	3 million per year
7 days	a stay of 7 days
stay beyond 11 days	stay in the hospital for longer than 11 days
one percent	1 percent, 1%
an albumin <3.4	an albumin concentration of <3.4
Patients were between 18–65 years of age.	Patients were between 18 and 65 years of age.
Of the 155, 79 patients had	Among the 155 patients, 79 had
There were over 70 million injuries.	More than 70 million injuries occurred.
1,600,000,000 dollars	$1.6 billion[a]
very few	only two patients
quite a small percentage	4%
practically all	98%

[a]One billion in the American system is 1,000,000,000 (10^9); however, in the British system, one billion is 1,000,000,000,000 (10^{12}). Be sure that the reader understands which system you are using.

TABLE 30.10   Hyphenated Terms

Problematic Usage	Preferred Usage
beta blockers	beta-blockers
Cox proportional hazards model	Cox proportional-hazards model
do not resuscitate orders	do-not-resuscitate orders
dose response effect	dose-response effect
double blind study	double-blind study
double check	double-check (verb)
end expiratory pressure	end-expiratory pressure
end stage renal disease	end-stage renal disease
finetuning	fine-tuning
fluid containing cysts	fluid-containing cysts
follow up	follow-up (noun or adjective)
halflife	half-life
health care costs	health-care costs
high risk group	high-risk group
in depth study	in-depth study
intraabdominal surgery	intra-abdominal surgery
intraobserver	intra-observer

(continued)

| TABLE 30.10 | Hyphenated Terms *(continued)* |

Problematic Usage	Preferred Usage
lactose containing food	lactose-containing food
little known study	little-known study
long term care	long-term care
low grade fever	low-grade fever
metaanalysis	meta-analysis
needlestick	needle-stick
noninsulin dependent diabetes mellitus	non–insulin-dependent diabetes mellitus
over a two year period	during a 2-year period
part time employee	part-time employee
S/D ratio	S/D or S-D ratio
short term	short-term
six month review	6-month review
small bowel resection	small-bowel resection
small cell carcinoma	small-cell carcinoma
triple blinded	triple-blinded
third trimester values	third-trimester values
two sided t test	two-sided t-test
one tailed t test	one-tailed t-test
up to date report	up-to-date report
well established efficacy	well-established efficacy
Xray	X-ray (adjective or verb), X ray (noun)
The X ray indicated	The radiograph showed
An X ray was made	A radiograph was made
A X ray reading	An X-ray reading
a 8 hour procedure	an 8-hour procedure
a 80 year old patient	an 80-year-old patient
a 25 fold increase	a 25-fold increase

| TABLE 30.11 | Prefixes and Numbers That Generally Require a Hyphen |

✔ **Prefixes**
- all-
- cross-
- ex-
- high-
- low-
- quasi-
- self-

✔ **Numbers**
- twenty-one through ninety-nine

✔ **Fractions**
- one-half
- two-thirds
- six-tenths

TABLE 30.12 Terms That Do Not Require a Hyphen

Problematic Usage	Preferred Usage
African-American respondents	African American respondents
At base-line, X was 10.	At baseline, X was 10.
case-mix	case mix
check-list	checklist
co-author	coauthor
double-check	double check (noun)
fault-finding	faultfinding
follow-up	follow up (verb)
germ-free	germ free
died in-hospital	died in the hospital
health-care reform	health care reform
high-risk for pneumonia	high risk for pneumonia
home-care	home care
inter-observer	interobserver
life-saving therapies	lifesaving therapies
multi-center	multicenter
non-compliant	noncompliant
non-fatal	nonfatal
non-operative	nonoperative
non-orthopaedic	nonorthopaedic
non-parametric	nonparametric
non-smoker	nonsmoker
non-white	nonwhite
post-operative	postoperative
pre-existing	preexisting
proof-read	proofread
seat-belt	seat belt
set-up	set up (verb), setup (noun)
state-wide	statewide
step-wise	stepwise
straight-forward	straightforward
a ten-fold increase	a tenfold increase
vaccinations were up-to-date	vaccinations were up to date

TABLE 30.13	Words for Which the English Plural Is Preferred

Singular Form	Plural Form
amoeba	amoebas (not amoebae)
analysis	analyses
apparatus	apparatuses
cannula	cannulas
cranium	craniums
crisis	crises
focus	focuses
formula	formulas
hypothesis	hypotheses
index	indices (relating to mathematics)
	indexes (relating to a book)
matrix	matrices (relating to mathematics or medicine)
	matrixes (relating to other subjects)
myoma	myomas
schema	schemas
vortex	vortexes

TABLE 30.14	Words for Which the Non-English Plural Is Preferred

Singular Form	Plural Form
alumna, alumnus	alumni
bacterium	bacteria
criterion	criteria
datum (rarely used)	data
decubitus	decubitus
erratum	errata
medium	media
minutia	minutiae
nucleus	nuclei
ovum	ova
phenomenon	phenomena
radius	radii
stigma	stigmata
stimulus	stimuli
stratum	strata

FOR MORE INFORMATION

If you have questions about hyphenation, remember to hyphenate anything that could be misread. Consult a comprehensive dictionary, such as *The American Heritage Dictionary of English Language* (2012) or *Merriam-Webster's Dictionary* (2016) for guidelines on hyphenation. For medical words, see section 6.12 of the *AMA Manual of Style* (American Medical Association, 2007). For general rules, *The Gregg Reference Manual* (Sabin, 2010) and Table 6.1 of the *Chicago Manual of Style* (2010) are helpful. Many journals use *Dorland's Illustrated Medical Dictionary (2011)* as their standard for style. O'Connor's (1992) book *Writing Successfully in Science* and the *Thesaurus of Alternatives to Worn-Out Words and Phrases* by Fiske (1994) are useful references.

31

Fixes for Problematic Terms

PRINCIPLE 232 • Learn the proper use of problematic word pairs.

Table 31.1 shows pairs of words that cause problems for many medical writers. Avoid using "while" unless you mean "at the same time." "Compared with" usually is preferred to "compared to" for analysis of differences or similarities (Sabin 2010). "Disinterested" means "unbiased, impartial, or fair," whereas "uninterested" means "not interested in, bored, indifferent, or unconcerned."

TABLE 31.1	**Problematic Word Pairs to Master**
while	whereas
compared to	compared with
disinterested	uninterested
since	because
that	which
complimentary	complementary
affect	effect
assure	ensure
each	every
varying	various
lay	lie
principle	principal
efficacy	effectiveness
efficiency	effectiveness
defuse	diffuse
loathe	loath
forgo	forego

FOR MORE INFORMATION

See Chapter 9 of the *AMA Manual of Style* (American Medical Association, 2007).

PRINCIPLE 233 • Use few abbreviations or, better yet, none.

Before you circulate for review a new draft of your paper, use your spelling checker to find abbreviations and acronyms. Also consider using an electronic medical dictionary, such as Stedman's Plus Medical/Pharmaceutical Spellchecker. These tools can help you determine whether you are using too many abbreviations. Most abbreviations and acronyms within the text, tables, and figures should be deleted and the full term given. Limit abbreviations to chemical compounds and standard units of measurement. Do not invent new abbreviations. If you must use abbreviations, define each one the first time it is used.

VITAL POINT

Papers that contain too many abbreviations are difficult to read, and papers that are difficult to read usually are rejected.

Many journals provide a list of approved abbreviations, but even these must be used consistently. If you use a term only once or twice in your paper, do not abbreviate it.

Example 31–1.
The New England Journal of Medicine allows the following abbreviations: AIDS, ANOVA, DNA, ELISA, HDL, HIV, NIDDM, SD, and RNA. It does not allow BUN, CI, CNS, CSF, EKG, MI, OR, qid, or RBC.

PRINCIPLE 234 • Rewrite sentences that begin with the word "it."

Compare the following sentences:

1. It was important to freeze the blood samples to ensure accurate measurements.
2. Freezing the blood samples was important to ensure accurate measurements.

Rather than starting with "it," try to guide readers through your paper by providing orientation at the beginning of sentences. For example, "In 2016, . . ." or "Among the 19 patients, . . ."

Many sentences can be improved by moving the key information to the end of the sentence. When possible, end sentences with a "thump" or a "bang." The last word in the sentence—and the reader's mind—receives the emphasis.

Change from:

Sepsis cost the US healthcare system more than $20 billion, making it one of the most expensive hospital complications with prolonged stays in the intensive care unit.

to:

Sepsis, one of the most expensive hospital complications, cost the US healthcare system more than $20 billion.

PRINCIPLE 235 • Use readable language.

Clarity is competing with the need to sound "scientific."

Through experimentation, Oppenheimer (2006) showed that " . . . contrary to prevailing wisdom, increasing the complexity of a text does not cause an essay's author to seem more intelligent. In fact, the opposite appears to be true."

Buy and use a good thesaurus. The online thesaurus visualthesaurus.com is also useful for finding the precise term. Also be sure that you have an up-to-date dictionary. *Merriam-Webster's Collegiate Dictionary* is a standard used by many medical journals. *The American Heritage Dictionary of the English Language* also is helpful; it contains usage notes for problematic words (see Table 31.1 and Table 31.2). Many medical journals use *Dorland's Illustrated Medical Dictionary* as the main reference.

Finally, as you edit your paper, check for phrases that could confuse readers.

As Lorraine Loviglio, who was the manager of manuscript editing at *The New England Journal of Medicine*, said, "Elegant variation has no place in medical writing. Clarity is more important." Therefore, do not alternate between "placebo group" and "control group." Use one term and make

TABLE 31.2	Common Problems That Copyeditors Correct
Problematic Usage	**Preferred Usage**
ageing	aging
appears to be	may be
ascertained	found
cancelled	canceled[a]
data base	database
determine	detect, learn, find out
die from	die of
do	perform
EKG	ECG, electrocardiogram
implementing	starting
inducement	induction
Kaplan Mier method	Kaplan-Meier method
labelling	labeling
magnitude	size
many persons	many people
neurological deficit	neurologic deficit
obtundation	obtusion
of insufficient magnitude	too small
prior to	before
referred to	called
refractive	refractory
regardless of	despite
relative to	compared with
remittive	remissive
questionable utility	questionable use
the main results	the primary results
towards	toward

[a]Often two spellings are acceptable. One method of assessing which is more popular in modern usage is to create a Google Books Ngram Viewer graph of the terms such as cancelled and canceled.

https://books.google.com/ngrams

Enter the two terms separated by a comma. Change the second year to the current year.

http://grammarist.com/spelling/cancel/

your manuscript consistent. For example, a paper about pressure ulcers should not use the synonyms "pressure sores," "decubitus," or "bed sores" simply to mix it up and make it more interesting.

VITAL POINT

Writing does matter, and rewriting is the key. As Joseph Garland said, "There is no good medical writing—just good rewriting" (*Familiar Medical Quotations*, 1968).

Now that you have finished the Editing phase, you are ready for the final phase: Revising.

REVISING

Key Questions to Answer in the Revising Phase:

- What needs to be improved for this paper to receive a high rating from reviewers?
- Is the writing accessible to nonspecialists?*

---

*Note: Even if the manuscript will be submitted to a specialty journal, revising in a way that permits nonspecialists to understand is important.

32

Revising the Final Draft

PRINCIPLE 236 • Proofread the final copy of your paper—several times.

In the Revising phase, you should ensure that your manuscript is ready for peer review. After you finish writing and editing the final draft, read it aloud—word for word—as if someone unfamiliar with the specific subject were reading it. Be certain that your manuscript says exactly what you want it to say. For example, check that nonessential clauses, for which you lower your voice, are set off by commas. Reading your manuscript aloud helps you to evaluate the punctuation, diction, and general flow of your paper. Look for inconsistencies, such as changing from "Class" to "Stage" to "Grade."

When you proofread your manuscript, be sure that you have not plagiarized anyone. Researchers sometimes copy sections of the Methods and Discussion sections from related reports and borrow examples from colleagues. If you use information from another source, rewrite the material in your own words or reference your sources. Avoid self-plagiarism by obtaining permission from editors where your work was previously published and citing that source.

PRINCIPLE 237 • Watch your tenses.

You can describe information from published work in:

+ the **present tense** (e.g., "X is a risk factor for Y")
+ the **past tense** (e.g., "Jones demonstrated X")
+ the **past perfect tense** (e.g., "Investigators have demonstrated X")

Describe your methods and findings in the past tense (e.g., "We found that X") but describe your conclusions in the present tense. "We conclude that Z is a risk factor for Y, independent of X."

FOR MORE INFORMATION

For a discussion of the logic and examples of the use of tenses in medical writing, see Day and Gastel (2011) or the *Publication Manual of the American Psychological Association* (American Psychological Association, 2010).

PRINCIPLE 238 • Eliminate redundant sentences and needless words.

Use "Track Changes" or take a red pen and see how many useless, superfluous, redundant, extra, pointless, supplementary, extraneous, additional, senseless, and excessive words you can eliminate. Also delete inappropriate or redundant sentences that were identified during your internal peer review.

For example, rather than repeating a long description of your inclusion criteria, refer to "the aforementioned criteria." Table 32.1 shows words that often can be eliminated.

In an article in *The New England Journal of Medicine*, Crichton (1975) described the most common problems with medical writing. The frequency of these problems is displayed in Figures 32.1 and 32.2. As you can see, verbiage and wordiness top the list.

TABLE 32.1	Unnecessary Words

Problematic Usage	Preferred Usage
an excessive number of	excessive
as the result	because
at a high risk	at high risk
at this moment in time	now
before beginning the study	before the study
Between the period of 1/1/2015 and 6/30/2015	Between 1/1/2015 and 6/30/2015
data for all of the variables	data for all variables
in order to	to
in terms of	in, of, for
is able to	can
is known to be	is
it would appear that	apparently
Many studies have been done which support	Studies support
on the basis of	by
one of the	a
over a period of time	over time
prolonged hospital course	prolonged hospitalization
so that	so, to
that have been reported	reported
The general consensus is	The consensus is
The majority of	Most
The nutritional status	Nutritional status
small number of	few
the subsequent postoperative course	postoperative results
There are, however, no reported studies where the potential use of X has been evaluated.	We are not aware of any studies in which X has been evaluated.
this time interval	this interval
those who had given up smoking	former smokers
total number	total
was calculated by arithmetically adding	was calculated by adding
We were also able to discern a trend of higher risk of X	The risk of X was higher
which is known to be	still

Pay particular attention to these problems in the Discussion to avoid the following type of comment:

"Much of the Discussion was rambling, repetitive, and somewhat conjectural."

PRINCIPLE 239 • Place the tables and figures in the correct positions.

Place each table title at the top of the table. Place the captions for all of the figures on a single page (the Figure Legend page) after the tables and before the figures. In the captions, explain the figures and

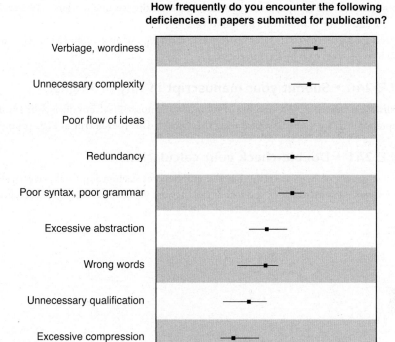

FIGURE 32.1. Frequency of writing problems. Answers are ranked by the median and bootstrap 95% confidence intervals using the sliding scale responses 0% (never) to 100% (always); from question 27 of the Peer Review Questionnaire (Appendix B). $P < .001$ based on the Friedman test.

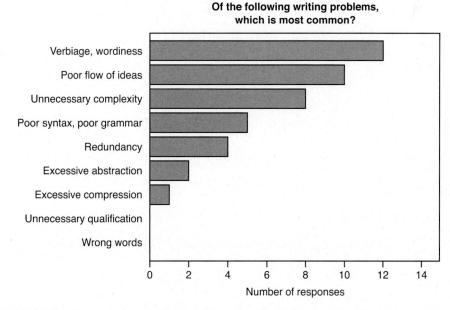

FIGURE 32.2. The most common writing problems. From question 28 of the Peer Review Questionnaire (Appendix B). $P = .009$ based on a chi-square test.

define all abbreviations. Do not put the tables and figures in the Results section; reviewers expect to find them at the end of the manuscript (see Table 12.1).

Never insert graphs in the text; reviewers consider it the sign of an amateur. Similarly, do not use a variety of fonts (typefaces) or type sizes in the text.

PRINCIPLE 240 • Submit your manuscript in July or August.

Journals publish year round, but the number of submitted manuscripts drops during the summer. Your odds of acceptance increase if you submit during this period. This is even true at high-profile journals.

PRINCIPLE 241 • Double-check your calculations.

Use a calculator or spreadsheet to verify that the numbers for each group total correctly. Reviewers often catch obvious mistakes this way, and if they do, they are unlikely to recommend acceptance.

The Cover Letter

PRINCIPLE 242 • Write a persuasive cover letter.

One editor was most annoyed by:

> *"Lack of a cover letter that provides more than a statement of submission, exclusivity, and authorship—i.e., doesn't explain why the manuscript is worth reviewing."*

The cover letter is much more important than many authors realize. This letter usually is your first contact with the editor, and the editor will make some important decisions about your paper based on the contents and professionalism of your cover letter. Note: The cover letter is the only section of the manuscript that is single-spaced.

The purpose of the cover letter is to explain—politely—what you are submitting and why. State the title and length of your manuscript and indicate the number of tables and figures. Explain why you decided to submit your manuscript to that particular journal. Why would your paper be of interest to the readers of that journal? What are the strengths of your paper? Explain which section of the target journal would be most appropriate for your manuscript (e.g., Original Articles, Brief Communications, or Reviews). In the salutation of the cover letter, make sure that you use the current editor's name—and spell it correctly. Avoid writing "Dear Editor." Avoid using the name of the editor of the journal that you submitted to on your first try.

The editor must believe that your paper will increase the impact factor for that journal. The editor must be able to easily understand what is new in your paper and why they should care. Therefore, you must subtly articulate how your paper will provide important information that will be referenced by other researchers in the next few years.

Vivian Siegel stressed the following lessons on interacting with professional biomedical journal editors. Treat editors as a senior colleague or mentor but in a professional and diplomatic way. Help the editors appreciate the significance of your work. Explain what is already known about this area and the advance in your paper. Summarize what is new and why the editor should care. The important question that is answered in this paper is X and this is important because of Y. Describe any related papers that you have submitted or will submit soon. Help the editor identify appropriate reviewers, especially for papers that use unusual methodologies or have a limited number of qualified experts.

Presubmission inquiries allow you to ask several editors from different journals at the same time whether your paper might be something they would be interested in seeing. Although it is unethical to submit your paper to multiple journals simultaneously, this is allowed for these inquiries. This can save you time by having editors tell you that this is not a subject that they would publish, and for the one with the most positive feedback, you have them anticipating your submission, which can make it stand out from the competition. The presubmission inquiry should summarize your study in one or two pages; include the abstract and why you think that your paper would be appropriate for that journal. You can and should do this before the paper is finished.

Some journals such as *The New England Journal of Medicine* have an online Presubmission Inquiries website:

https://cdf.nejm.org/misc/authors/PresubmissionInquiries.aspx

Editors and associate editors often attend scientific meetings. Introduce yourself to them and develop a professional relationship. Offer to review for them and explain why you are a good reviewer for specific topics. Tell them about your research and invite them to your talk or poster. Tell them what you like about their journal and ideas for making it stronger. To quote Vivian Siegel, "Treat editors as your colleagues and they will become your advocates."

FOR MORE INFORMATION

Chapter 13 of *The Gregg Reference Manual* (Sabin, 2010) is an excellent reference for writing a professional letter.

PRINCIPLE 243 • Recognize how editors define a good article.

Table 33.1 shows editors' definitions of a good article. If you can, include a few of these elements in your cover letter.

TABLE 33.1   Editors' Definitions of a Good Article[a]

- One that elicits a Eureka response when one is finished reading it
- Tells a good story, doesn't need the readers to do a lot of outside literature research to understand meaning
- Simple, clear, logical, explicit
- Short, rich on methods, truncated discussion
- Important contribution to a real problem
- A good article clearly reports the findings of a well-designed and rigorously conducted investigation. It clearly explains the question being addressed, why it's important, the extent to which the findings address the question, and what remains to be elucidated in future research.
- Clear, concise, but sufficiently comprehensive to have explained all the main parts of the study, background, and analysis
- Well conceptualized, well designed, relevant, timely, advances knowledge or practice in a meaningful way
- Significant importance, adequate data to support conclusions, and strong intro and discussion to support the importance
- A clearly written, logical piece of work that presents new ideas and supports them with strong experiments, adequate controls, and good experimental design
- Identification of the problem to be addressed; low, to no, bias; meaningful results, both statistically and clinically
- Well-written, good scientific design, clinical importance
- Clinically impactful, focusing on a well-defined problem which offers scientific significance; employs an incisive and informative approach; provides well-controlled data derived from validated or established experimental systems; includes appropriate statistical powering of the data enabling the possibility of a valid interpretation; scholarly integration with other work in the field that illustrates the nature and extent of the advance offered
- Important question addressed with appropriate methods and addresses current gaps

(continued)

TABLE 33.1 Editors' Definitions of a Good Article[a] *(continued)*

- One that provides sound evidence to prove a hypothesis and in turn change and improve the way medicine is practiced
- One that has the potential to change clinical practice
- Written in a straightforward manner, proceeds logically, accurate with appropriate sourcing, has clinical implications, and is on a topic that readers will care about

✔ **Good Study Design**
- Clean methodology
- One that develops a creative or original problem derived from a strong theoretical base; clear hypotheses, adequate sample size, with conclusions drawn specifically from the findings
- Well designed
- Good statistics (fitted to problem type and size)
- Strict adherence to scientific and statistical methodology
- Adequate data sets with clinical correlation
- One that reports clearly and in sufficient detail on a well-designed and well-conducted research experiment or an important question

✔ **Original and Important Results**
- New information
- Clinically useful
- Broad clinical application
- Well designed, addressing a new idea, not too long, incisive, and informative Discussion
- Exciting, new, well-supported data
- Original study, with well-defined aims; well-conceived, executed, and presented
- Newness, trueness, and timeliness

✔ **Strong Presentation of the Data**
- Clearly presented
- Targets readership
- Organized, logical, clearly written, with good Methods
- Well referenced
- One that conforms to the journal's information for authors and contains new, important, well set out information that is likely to really interest readers; refers to up-to-date, relevant references in the world literature

✔ **Conclusions Supported by Data**
- Results not over interpreted
- Appropriate interpretation of results

✔ **Well-Written and Concise**
- Short, concise, clean methodology
- A concise, well-written report of a well-designed study
- Good writing
- One that has content that meets the journal's purpose and is well written (readable)
- Good flow of ideas; easy to follow
- Useful information that is well written

[a]From question 30 of the Peer Review Questionnaire (Appendix B).

PRINCIPLE 244 • Recommend several reviewers.

A. H. Sulzberger of the *New York Times* said, "I believe in keeping an open mind, but not so open that my brains fall out." Similarly, most reviewers try to keep an open mind. Naturally, however, some reviewers will be biased against your study, and getting a fair evaluation from them would be difficult.

Many journals permit—even encourage—authors to submit the names of potential reviewers, and obviously, the editor will screen out colleagues at your institution and your previous coauthors.

If possible, recommend a reviewer who understands your point of view, keeps an open mind, and is qualified to evaluate your paper. Remember, the first thing that some reviewers look for is whether you referenced their previous publications and whether you commented favorably on their findings. You can avoid insulting the recommended reviewers by including their relevant publications in your references but stay within ethical boundaries. Recently, authors were caught recommending themselves and colleagues as reviewers for their own paper using fake e-mail addresses.

You can also recommend a very specific type of expert who would be qualified to review your research without naming someone.

Further, let the editor know whether there is anyone you do not want to review your paper. Editors usually honor these requests. You simply enter the person's name and check a box labeled something like "Designate as Non-Preferred Reviewer."

You and your coauthors should discuss the list of preferred reviewers at least several days before you begin the online submission.

PRINCIPLE 245 • Be candid about what information in your paper has been published or presented before.

Reassure the editor that the information in your paper has not been published before. Also state that you will not submit the manuscript to another journal until the review process is complete. Be sure to describe and submit a copy of any part of the research that has been published (e.g., the abstract). Also tell the editor about any closely related papers but then explain what NEW information this paper provides.

PRINCIPLE 246 • Provide a contact person.

On the title page and in the cover letter, identify the author who is responsible for manuscript negotiations. Provide the corresponding author's full name and full mailing address, all pertinent telephone numbers, and an e-mail address. Make sure that the address is clear and complete, especially if it is outside the country of the target journal.

PRINCIPLE 247 • Introduce yourself and your coauthors to the editor—politely.

Although few authors do this, you should be aware that providing information about yourself and your coauthors can be helpful at some journals; at others, it makes no difference. In your cover letter, you can briefly provide information, such as your credentials and the experience that makes you uniquely qualified to write this paper. Although you may have explained in the Methods section where the study was conducted, in the cover letter, you can explain the advantages of conducting a study there.

Explain that each coauthor has seen and approved the final draft of the manuscript. See the section in Appendix A, Section II.A.2.

Although a well-written cover letter is helpful, a more important concern, as one expert said, is "to have the correct format and ordering of contents of the manuscript."

34

Responding to Peer Reviewers' Comments

| *"That reviewer was an idiot. He did not understand what I meant to say."*
| —The Unsuccessful Medical Researcher

PRINCIPLE 248 • Recognize how the journal review and decision-making process works.

Peer reviewers often spend considerable time and effort evaluating manuscripts. Ordinarily, they are not compensated for this work. Most reviewers give extensive thought to improving the papers that are submitted for publication, so be diplomatic and demonstrate your knowledge of how the system operates.

If your manuscript is returned with comments from reviewers, make those changes that will improve the paper. It is essential to address <u>all</u> the comments, in one way or another, in your revised manuscript.

During the final phase of publishing a paper, do not let your feelings get hurt by the editing process. Manuscript editors have years of experience. Let them help you. Often, they are improving your paper so that a wider audience can understand it.

> **VITAL POINT**
>
> If the reviewers recommend some changes that you disagree with, explain your reasons for disagreement in the cover letter. Do not simply say "I disagree." In general, you should be agreeing with about 90% of the reviewers' recommendations.

Good reasons for not making recommended changes include invalid criticisms and unavailable data. If you strongly disagree with a reviewer's point, do not make the change but do add an explanation or clarification in your paper for the many readers who will ask the same question. Also, explain this in the cover letter to the editor.

Return a copy of the reviewers' comments, with each point addressed. Detail the changes that you made (e.g., "Reviewer 1, Comment 3—NS was changed to '$P = .06$.' on page 6, line 17").

An invitation to resubmit your paper does not guarantee that it will be accepted. You must address the concerns of the reviewers to their satisfaction. Do not cavalierly ignore their suggestions and imply that they are beneath you.

Some reviewers may ask you to obtain more information or perform more detailed analysis. Carefully consider all of the reviewers' comments, and as long as the recommended changes do not detract from your paper, follow their suggestions.

TABLE 34.1	Suggestions for Resubmitting Your Revised Manuscript

1. Follow the suggestions of the reviewers and editors and make all (or most) of the suggested changes.
2. Do not make changes that are simply cosmetic.
3. Obtain approval from each coauthor for all changes.
4. Explain in detail what you have done. Answer each point of the critique and include the page, paragraph, and sentence number for the original and revised manuscripts in the answer.
5. Label, date, and return both the original and the revised manuscripts.
6. Include the manuscript number in your letter and on the revised version.
7. Respond promptly.

Editors understand that reviewers may be biased and that authors may be unresponsive to their comments. Sometimes you can ease the situation simply by talking directly with the editor. Editors are reasonable people with whom you can discuss your concerns. Remember, editors want to help you publish a clear, concise, and accurate paper.

PRINCIPLE 249 • Follow the suggestions for resubmitting your paper.

Table 34.1 shows suggestions for resubmitting a paper.

It is natural to become offended and angry at reviewers' criticisms. To become successful at publishing paper, you must overcome this—or at least "fake it 'till you make it." You can learn something from nearly all criticism. Even if the reviewer asked for something that was already in your paper, you can learn how to make important points more prominent and clear. Take an enlightened approach and be respectful. Never let the tone of your response be one of anger and frustration.

One reviewer provided this advice:

"Taking consideration of reviewer comments is critical—don't be defensive in response. If reviewer didn't understand something or misread it, it was probably not well written. Share your drafts with colleagues early—the more feedback you get, the better. Almost all research is publishable these days—finish those papers that are 95% completed and resubmit those papers which have been rejected."

PRINCIPLE 250 • Do not be discouraged by criticism.

Nearly every published manuscript has been revised based on peer reviewers' comments. Of course, articles invited by the editor have a high probability of publication, but unsolicited manuscripts rarely are accepted outright by several reviewers and an editor.

"It is not the critic who counts; not the man who points out how the strong man stumbles, or where the doer of deeds could have done them better. The credit belongs to the man who is actually in the arena, whose face is marred by dust and sweat and blood; who strives valiantly; who errs, who comes short again and again, because there is no effort without error and shortcoming; but who does actually strive to do the deeds; who knows great enthusiasms, the great devotions; who spends himself in a worthy cause; who at the best knows in the end the triumph of high achievement, and who at the worst, if he fails, at least fails while daring greatly, so that his place shall never be with those cold and timid souls who neither know victory nor defeat."

—THEODORE ROOSEVELT

PRINCIPLE 251 • Revise your manuscript before you submit it to another journal.

If your manuscript is rejected, revise it promptly and submit it to another journal—before you lose your momentum and your research team. Although many prestigious medical journals reject more than 90% of submitted manuscripts, 80% of the rejected manuscripts are published elsewhere. Of the papers that are published elsewhere, 20% of authors make the mistake of never changing the flaws that were pointed out by the first journal's reviewers. Find the energy to avoid being among this 20% of authors.

Remember that you are responsible for finding and correcting the flaws in your paper. Your paper may contain some information that led reviewers to misunderstand your study and criticize it unfairly. However, the next journal that you submit your paper to may send your paper to the same reviewer as the first journal. If you do not make any of the recommended changes, you may receive the same critique and rejection.

If your manuscript was rejected, remember that unless the editor has given you some real encouragement, in most cases, you are wasting your time by sending your manuscript back to the editor for reconsideration. Even if you make all of the changes suggested by the reviewers, they are unlikely to change their minds, and your project may be delayed for months.

If you do appeal a rejection, avoid hitting reply and sending a hasty e-mail or immediately calling the editor. Discuss the appeal carefully with your colleagues and respond with calmness and a logical argument that sticks to the science. For example, if your study was rejected because it was a negative study but the trial had a rigorous study design and answered an important question, you would have grounds for appeal. Some journals do not want to publish negative trials because it hurts their impact factor. Treat the editor as a respected senior colleague—not your enemy.

PRINCIPLE 252 • Understand how publishing decisions are reached.

Many inexperienced medical researchers mistakenly believe that peer reviewers decide whether to accept or reject a manuscript. Many reviewers also believe that they have this authority. For most journals, however, the editor-in-chief makes the final decision. This distinction is important; reviewers and editors often give numerical scores to different features of a paper (see Fig. 28.1). These scores are weighted and summed, to rank potential manuscripts. Papers with the highest scores are considered for publication. The rating system often includes categories such as those shown in Table 34.2. Some journal editors ask reviewers to complete a simple evaluation form, such as that shown in Figure 34.1. Whichever system is used, your chances of acceptance increase if you consider the perspective of reviewers and editors.

TABLE 34.2 Typical Elements in a Priority Rating System

✔ **Some journals use a 1–5 rating system such as the following:**
Scientific accuracy
Originality
Interest to broad readership
Composition (This enables reviewers to indicate that the writing was poor but the science was good.)

✔ **Other journals use a rating system such as the following:**
Clinical and scientific quality
Timeliness of the subject matter
Perceived reader needs
Peer reviewer comments
General editorial requirements

1. Quality
- ☐ Superior
- ☐ Good
- ☐ Fair
- ☐ Poor

2. Recommendation for publication
- ☐ Accept
- ☐ Accept with minor revision
- ☐ Major revision; reconsider
- ☐ Reject because of
    - ☐ Unimportant topic
    - ☐ Unwarranted conclusions
    - ☐ Adequate coverage of subject in the literature already
    - ☐ Poor organization

3. Recommended priority for publication if major criticisms are satisfied
- ☐ Highest priority
- ☐ Intermediate priority
- ☐ Lowest priority
- ☐ Criticisms probably cannot be satisfied.

FIGURE 34.1. Typical reviewer's evaluation form.

Journals receive between 2 and 20 times as many manuscripts as they can publish. Although many papers represent sound work, they are rejected because they do not receive a high enough ranking. Many trivial errors can lower a paper's score to below the threshold for acceptance. Many researchers believe that their paper will not be rejected because of minor imperfections. This is simply not true.

PRINCIPLE 253 • Recognize problems inherent in the peer review process.

As one reviewer observed:

> "The peer review process is imperfect and only works because nobody has a better way. I've had some incredibly stupid reviews indicating the reviewer hadn't read or hadn't understood the thrust of the paper. Another frequent problem is when reviewers ask for conflicting changes. What can you do about that? The whole process is rather complicated, often leading to unwarranted rejection of important, but negative, results and innovative, but unorthodox, reports."

THE FINAL STEPS

PRINCIPLE 254 • Check the page proofs carefully.

If your paper is accepted, carefully proofread the version that the publisher sends to you. Also insist that each coauthor check the proof carefully. Depending on your institution, you also may need to show a copy to the public relations department.

Never make major changes at this point.

Send your changes to the editor promptly. Editors often ask authors to return proofs within 48 hours. Despite the time limitations, devoting enough time to check for typographical errors, incorrect P values, and spelling and grammatical errors is a crucial part of producing a quality paper. Because tables often require substantial reformatting, check the tables in the proofs against your originals. If you used any "in press" papers as references, update them by providing the volume, year, and page numbers. If you used any abstracts as references, determine whether they have been published as full papers, and if so, update your citations.

Communicating with the copyeditor is essential at this point. Always return the proofs, even if you do not wish to make any changes. If you do not understand any marks or queries, call the copyeditor to resolve the problem.

PRINCIPLE 255 • Study "ideal" papers.

Because the focus of this book is avoiding problems, I want to end with some positive models. Editors and reviewers provided the responses and examples of "ideal" papers shown in Table 34.3. Another source of positive models is the book *One Hundred Years of JAMA Landmark Articles*, available from the American Medical Association (AMA).

TABLE 34.3	Examples of Ideal Papers

- Papers published in *NEJM*, *JAMA*, *AJPH*, or *Nature*
- Brown MS, Goldstein JL. Familial hypercholesterolemia: defective binding of lipoproteins to cultured fibroblasts associated with impaired regulation of 3-hydroxy-3-methylglutaryl coenzyme A reductase activity. *Proc Natl Acad Sci U S A*. 1974;71(3):788–792.
- Watson JD, Crick FH. Molecular structure of nucleic acids: a structure for deoxyribose nucleic acid. *Nature*. 1953;171(4356):737–738.
- Jemal A, Siegel RL, Ma J, et al. Inequalities in premature death from colorectal cancer by state. *J Clin Oncol*. 2015;33(8):829–835.
- Most articles by Leonard Seeff (e.g., Seeff et al., 1992)
- Some of the work by Haynes and Sackett (e.g., Haynes et al., 2011; Sackett, 1979)
- "Strategies for the Analysis of Oncogene Overexpression: Studies of the Neu Oncogene in Breast Carcinoma" (Naber et al., 1990)
- "A Controlled Trial of Antepartum Glucocorticoid Treatment for Prevention of the Respiratory Distress Syndrome in Premature Infants" (Liggins & Howie, 1972)
- "The Effect of Vitamin E and Beta Carotene on the Incidence of Lung Cancer and Other Cancers in Male Smokers" (The Alpha-Tocopherol, Beta Carotene Cancer Prevention Study Group, 1994; Marantz, 1994)
- "Standardized Nerve Conduction Studies in the Lower Limb of the Healthy Elderly" (Falco et al., 1994)
- Hoberman A, Greenfield SP, Mattoo TK, et al. Antimicrobial prophylaxis for children with vesicoureteral reflux. *N Engl J Med*. 2014;370(25):2367–2376.
- "Hemodynamic Changes in the Early Postburn Patient: The Influence of Fluid Administration and of a Vasodilator (Hydralazine)" (Pruitt et al., 1971)
- Stamler J, Wentworth D, Neaton JD. Is relationship between serum cholesterol and risk of premature death from coronary heart disease continuous and graded? Findings in 356,222 primary screenees of the Multiple Risk Factor Intervention Trial (MRFIT). *JAMA*. 1986;256(20):2823–2828.

(continued)

| **TABLE 34.3** | **Examples of Ideal Papers** *(continued)* |

- Von Hoff DD, LoRusso PM, Rudin CM, et al. Inhibition of the hedgehog pathway in advanced basal-cell carcinoma. *N Engl J Med*. 2009;361(12):1164–1172.
- Girard TD, Kress JP, Fuchs BD, et al. Efficacy and safety of a paired sedation and ventilator weaning protocol for mechanically ventilated patients in intensive care (Awakening and Breathing Controlled trial): a randomised controlled trial. *Lancet*. 2008;371(9607): 126–134.
- Grant RM, Lama JR, Anderson PL, et al. Preexposure chemoprophylaxis for HIV prevention in men who have sex with men. *N Engl J Med*. 2010;363(27):2587–2599.
- See Cynthia Dunbar or Arthur Nienhuis: Nienhuis AW, Dunbar CE, Sorrentino BP. Genotoxicity of retroviral integration in hematopoietic cells. *Mol Ther*. 2006;13(6):1031–1049.
- Pandharipande PP, Girard TD, Jackson JC, et al. Long-term cognitive impairment after critical illness. *N Engl J Med*. 2013;369(14):1306–3016.
- Needleman J, Buerhaus P, Pankratz VS, et al. Nurse staffing and inpatient hospital mortality. *N Engl J Med*. 2011;364(11):1037–1045.
- The LIFE Study results: Pahor M, Guralnik JM, Ambrosius WT, et al. Effect of structured physical activity on prevention of major mobility disability in older adults: the LIFE study randomized clinical trial. *JAMA*. 2014;311(23):2387–2396.
- Sui X, Golczak M, Zhang J, et al. Utilization of dioxygen by carotenoid cleavage oxygenases. *J Biol Chem*. 2015;290(51):30212–30223.
- We are still searching for the "ideal" paper!

NEJM, *The New England Journal of Medicine*; JAMA, *The Journal of the American Medical Association*; AJPH, *American Journal of Public Health*.

PRINCIPLE 256 • Know when to stop.

Finally, remember that a good paper "has a definite structure, makes its point and then shuts up" (Lock, 1991).

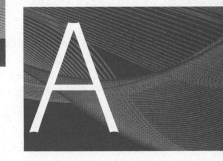

Recommendations for the Conduct, Reporting, Editing, and Publication of Scholarly Work in Medical Journals[1]

Updated December 2014

---

[1]Reprinted with permission from the International Committee of Medical Journal Editors. The official and most up-to-date version is to be found at icmje.org.

I. ABOUT THE RECOMMENDATIONS

A. Purpose of the Recommendations

ICMJE developed these recommendations to review best practice and ethical standards in the conduct and reporting of research and other material published in medical journals, and to help authors, editors, and others involved in peer review and biomedical publishing create and distribute accurate, clear, reproducible, unbiased medical journal articles. The recommendations may also provide useful insights into the medical editing and publishing process for the media, patients and their families, and general readers.

B. Who Should Use the Recommendations?

These recommendations are intended primarily for use by authors who might submit their work for publication to ICMJE member journals. Many non-ICMJE journals voluntarily use these recommendations (see www.icmje.org/journals.html). The ICMJE encourages that use but has no authority to monitor or enforce it. In all cases, authors should use these recommendations along with individual journals' instructions to authors. Authors should also consult guidelines for the reporting of specific study types (e.g., the CONSORT guidelines for the reporting of randomized trials); see http://equator-network.org.

Journals that follow these recommendations are encouraged to incorporate them into their instructions to authors and to make explicit in those instructions that they follow ICMJE recommendations. Journals that wish to be identified on the ICMJE website as following these recommendations should notify the ICMJE secretariat via e-mail at icmje@acponline.org. Journals that in the past have requested such identification but who no longer follow ICMJE recommendations should use the same means to request removal from this list.

The ICMJE encourages wide dissemination of these recommendations and reproduction of this document in its entirety for educational, not-for-profit purposes without regard for copyright, but all uses of the recommendations and document should direct readers to www.icmje.org for the official, most recent version, as the ICMJE updates the recommendations periodically when new issues arise.

C. History of the Recommendations

The ICMJE has produced multiple editions of this document, previously known as the Uniform Requirements for Manuscripts Submitted to Biomedical Journals (URMs). The URM was first published in 1978 as a way of standardizing manuscript format and preparation across journals. Over the years, issues in publishing that went well beyond manuscript preparation arose, resulting in development of a number of Separate Statements on editorial policy.

The entire Uniform Requirements document was revised in 1997; sections were updated in May 1999 and May 2000. In May 2001, the ICMJE revised the sections related to potential conflicts of interest. In 2003, the committee revised and reorganized the entire document and incorporated the Separate Statements into the text, and revised it again in 2010. Previous versions of this document can be found in the "Archives" section of www.icmje.org. This version, now renamed "Recommendations for the Conduct, Reporting, Editing, and Publication of Scholarly Work in Medical Journals" (ICMJE Recommendations), was released in 2013.

II. ROLES AND RESPONSIBILITIES OF AUTHORS, CONTRIBUTORS, REVIEWERS, EDITORS, PUBLISHERS, AND OWNERS

A. Defining the Role of Authors and Contributors

1. Why Authorship Matters

Authorship confers credit and has important academic, social, and financial implications. Authorship also implies responsibility and accountability for published work. The following recommendations are intended to ensure that contributors who have made substantive intellectual contributions to a paper are given credit as authors, but also that contributors credited as authors understand their role in taking responsibility and being accountable for what is published.

Because authorship does not communicate what contributions qualified an individual to be an author, some journals now request and publish information about the contributions of each person named as having participated in a submitted study, at least for original research. Editors are strongly encouraged to develop and implement a contributorship policy, as well as a policy that identifies who is responsible for the integrity of the work as a whole. Such policies remove much of the ambiguity surrounding contributions, but leave unresolved the question of the quantity and quality of contribution that qualify an individual for authorship. The ICMJE has thus developed criteria for authorship that can be used by all journals, including those that distinguish authors from other contributors.

2. Who Is an Author?

The ICMJE recommends that authorship be based on the following 4 criteria:

1. Substantial contributions to the conception or design of the work; or the acquisition, analysis, or interpretation of data for the work; AND
2. Drafting the work or revising it critically for important intellectual content; AND
3. Final approval of the version to be published; AND
4. Agreement to be accountable for all aspects of the work in ensuring that questions related to the accuracy or integrity of any part of the work are appropriately investigated and resolved.

In addition to being accountable for the parts of the work he or she has done, an author should be able to identify which co-authors are responsible for specific other parts of the work. In addition, authors should have confidence in the integrity of the contributions of their coauthors.

All those designated as authors should meet all four criteria for authorship, and all who meet the four criteria should be identified as authors. Those who do not meet all four criteria should be acknowledged—see Section II.A.3 below. These authorship criteria are intended to reserve the status of authorship for those who deserve credit and can take responsibility for the work. The criteria are not intended for use as a means to disqualify colleagues from authorship who otherwise meet authorship criteria by denying them the opportunity to meet criterion #s 2 or 3. Therefore, all individuals who meet the first criterion should have the opportunity to participate in the review, drafting, and final approval of the manuscript.

The individuals who conduct the work are responsible for identifying who meets these criteria and ideally should do so when planning the work, making modifications as appropriate as the work progresses. It is the collective responsibility of the authors, not the journal to which the work is submitted, to determine that all people named as authors meet all four criteria; it is not the role of journal editors to determine who qualifies or does not qualify for authorship or to arbitrate authorship conflicts. If agreement cannot be reached about who qualifies for authorship, the institution(s) where the work was performed, not the journal editor, should be asked to investigate. If authors request removal or addition of an author after manuscript submission or publication, journal editors should seek an explanation and signed statement of agreement for the requested change from all listed authors and from the author to be removed or added.

The corresponding author is the one individual who takes primary responsibility for communication with the journal during the manuscript submission, peer review, and publication process, and typically ensures that all the journal's administrative requirements, such as providing details of authorship, ethics committee approval, clinical trial registration documentation, and gathering conflict of interest forms and statements, are properly completed, although these duties may be delegated to one or more coauthors. The corresponding author should be available throughout the submission and peer review process to respond to editorial queries in a timely way, and should be available after publication to respond to critiques of the work and cooperate with any requests from the journal for data or additional information should questions about the paper arise after publication. Although the corresponding author has primary responsibility for correspondence with the journal, the ICMJE recommends that editors send copies of all correspondence to all listed authors.

When a large multi-author group has conducted the work, the group ideally should decide who will be an author before the work is started and confirm who is an author before submitting the manuscript for publication. All members of the group named as authors should meet all four criteria for authorship, including approval of the final manuscript, and they should be able to take public responsibility for the work and should have full confidence in the accuracy and integrity of the work of other group authors. They will also be expected as individuals to complete conflict-of-interest disclosure forms.

Some large multi-author groups designate authorship by a group name, with or without the names of individuals. When submitting a manuscript authored by a group, the corresponding author should specify the group name if one exists, and clearly identify the group members who can take credit and responsibility for the work as authors. The byline of the article identifies who is directly responsible for the manuscript, and MEDLINE lists as authors whichever names appear on the byline. If the byline includes a group name, MEDLINE will list the names of individual group members who are authors or who are collaborators, sometimes called non-author contributors, if there is a note associated with the byline clearly stating that the individual names are elsewhere in the paper and whether those names are authors or collaborators.

3. Non-Author Contributors

Contributors who meet fewer than all 4 of the above criteria for authorship should not be listed as authors, but they should be acknowledged. Examples of activities that alone (without other contributions) do not qualify a contributor for authorship are acquisition of funding; general supervision of a research group or general administrative support; and writing assistance, technical editing, language editing, and proofreading. Those whose contributions do not justify authorship may be acknowledged individually or together as a group under a single heading (e.g., "Clinical Investigators" or "Participating Investigators"), and their contributions should be specified (e.g., "served as scientific advisors," "critically reviewed the study proposal," "collected data," "provided and cared for study patients," "participated in writing or technical editing of the manuscript").

Because acknowledgment may imply endorsement by acknowledged individuals of a study's data and conclusions, editors are advised to require that the corresponding author obtain written permission to be acknowledged from all acknowledged individuals.

B. Author Responsibilities—Conflicts of Interest

Public trust in the scientific process and the credibility of published articles depend in part on how transparently conflicts of interest are handled during the planning, implementation, writing, peer review, editing, and publication of scientific work.

A conflict of interest exists when professional judgment concerning a primary interest (such as patients' welfare or the validity of research) may be influenced by a secondary interest (such as financial gain). Perceptions of conflict of interest are as important as actual conflicts of interest.

Financial relationships (such as employment, consultancies, stock ownership or options, honoraria, patents, and paid expert testimony) are the most easily identifiable conflicts of interest and the most likely to undermine the credibility of the journal, the authors, and of science itself. However, conflicts can occur for other reasons, such as personal relationships or rivalries, academic competition, and intellectual beliefs. Authors should avoid entering in to agreements with study sponsors, both for-profit and nonprofit, that interfere with authors' access to all of the study's data or that interfere with their ability to analyze and interpret the data and to prepare and publish manuscripts independently when and where they choose.

1. Participants

All participants in the peer-review and publication process—not only authors but also peer reviewers, editors, and editorial board members of journals—must consider their conflicts of interest when fulfilling their roles in the process of article review and publication and must disclose all relationships that could be viewed as potential conflicts of interest.

a. Authors

When authors submit a manuscript of any type or format they are responsible for disclosing all financial and personal relationships that might bias or be seen to bias their work. The ICMJE has developed a Form for Disclosure of Conflicts of Interest to facilitate and standardize authors' disclosures. ICMJE member journals require that authors use this form, and ICMJE encourages other journals to adopt it.

b. Peer Reviewers

Reviewers should be asked at the time they are asked to critique a manuscript if they have conflicts of interest that could complicate their review. Reviewers must disclose to editors any conflicts of interest that could bias their opinions of the manuscript, and should recuse themselves from reviewing specific manuscripts if the potential for bias exists. Reviewers must not use knowledge of the work they're reviewing before its publication to further their own interests.

c. Editors and Journal Staff

Editors who make final decisions about manuscripts should recuse themselves from editorial decisions if they have conflicts of interest or relationships that pose potential conflicts related to articles under consideration. Other editorial staff members who participate in editorial decisions must provide editors with a current description of their financial interests or other conflicts (as they might relate to editorial judgments) and recuse themselves from any decisions in which a conflict of interest exists. Editorial staff must not use information gained through working with manuscripts for private gain. Editors should publish regular disclosure statements about potential conflicts of interests related to the commitments of journal staff. Guest editors should follow these same procedures.

2. Reporting Conflicts of Interest

Articles should be published with statements or supporting documents, such as the ICMJE conflict of interest form, declaring:

* Authors' conflicts of interest; and
* Sources of support for the work, including sponsor names along with explanations of the role of those sources if any in study design; collection, analysis, and interpretation of data; writing of the report; the decision to submit the report for publication; or a statement declaring that the supporting source had no such involvement; and
* Whether the authors had access to the study data, with an explanation of the nature and extent of access, including whether access is on-going.

To support the above statements, editors may request that authors of a study sponsored by a funder with a proprietary or financial interest in the outcome sign a statement, such as "I had full access to all of the data in this study and I take complete responsibility for the integrity of the data and the accuracy of the data analysis."

C. Responsibilities in the Submission and Peer-Review Process

1. Authors

Authors should abide by all principles of authorship and declaration of conflicts of interest detailed in section IIA and B of this document.

2. Journals

a. Confidentiality

Manuscripts submitted to journals are privileged communications that are authors' private, confidential property, and authors may be harmed by premature disclosure of any or all of a manuscript's details.

Editors therefore must not share information about manuscripts, including whether they have been received and are under review, their content and status in the review process, criticism by reviewers, and their ultimate fate, to anyone other than the authors and reviewers. Requests from third parties to use manuscripts and reviews for legal proceedings should be politely refused, and editors should do their best not to provide such confidential material should it be subpoenaed.

Editors must also make clear that reviewers should keep manuscripts, associated material, and the information they contain strictly confidential. Reviewers and editorial staff members must not publicly discuss the authors' work, and reviewers must not appropriate authors' ideas before the manuscript is published. Reviewers must not retain the manuscript for their personal use and should destroy paper copies of manuscripts and delete electronic copies after submitting their reviews.

When a manuscript is rejected, it is best practice for journals to delete copies of it from their editorial systems unless retention is required by local regulations. Journals that retain copies of rejected manuscripts should disclose this practice in their Information for Authors.

When a manuscript is published, journals should keep copies of the original submission, reviews, revisions, and correspondence for at least three years and possibly in perpetuity, depending on local regulations, to help answer future questions about the work should they arise.

Editors should not publish or publicize peer reviewers' comments without permission of the reviewer and author. If journal policy is to blind authors to reviewer identity and comments are not signed, that identity must not be revealed to the author or anyone else without the reviewers' expressed written permission.

Confidentiality may have to be breached if dishonesty or fraud is alleged, but editors should notify authors or reviewers if they intend to do so and confidentiality must otherwise be honored.

b. Timeliness

Editors should do all they can to ensure timely processing of manuscripts with the resources available to them. If editors intend to publish a manuscript, they should attempt to do so in a timely manner and any planned delays should be negotiated with the authors. If a journal has no intention of proceeding with a manuscript, editors should endeavor to reject the manuscript as soon as possible to allow authors to submit to a different journal.

c. Peer Review

Peer review is the critical assessment of manuscripts submitted to journals by experts who are usually not part of the editorial staff. Because unbiased, independent, critical assessment is an intrinsic part of all scholarly work, including scientific research, peer review is an important extension of the scientific process.

The actual value of peer review is widely debated, but the process facilitates a fair hearing for a manuscript among members of the scientific community. More practically, it helps editors decide which manuscripts are suitable for their journals. Peer review often helps authors and editors improve the quality of reporting.

It is the responsibility of the journal to ensure that systems are in place for selection of appropriate reviewers. It is the responsibility of the editor to ensure that reviewers have access to all materials that may be relevant to the evaluation of the manuscript, including supplementary material for e-only publication, and to ensure that reviewer comments are properly assessed and interpreted in the context of their declared conflicts of interest.

A peer-reviewed journal is under no obligation to send submitted manuscripts for review, and under no obligation to follow reviewer recommendations, favorable or negative. The editor of a journal is ultimately responsible for the selection of all its content, and editorial decisions may be informed by issues unrelated to the quality of a manuscript, such as suitability for the journal. An editor can reject any article at any time before publication, including after acceptance if concerns arise about the integrity of the work.

Journals may differ in the number and kinds of manuscripts they send for review, the number and types of reviewers they seek for each manuscript, whether the review process is open or blinded, and other aspects of the review process. For this reason and as a service to authors, journals should publish a description of their peer-review process.

Journals should notify reviewers of the ultimate decision to accept or reject a paper, and should acknowledge the contribution of peer reviewers to their journal. Editors are encouraged to share reviewers' comments with coreviewers of the same paper, so reviewers can learn from each other in the review process.

As part of peer review, editors are encouraged to review research protocols, plans for statistical analysis if separate from the protocol, and/or contracts associated with project-specific studies. Editors should encourage authors to make such documents publicly available at the time of or after publication, before accepting such studies for publication. Some journals may require public posting of these documents as a condition of acceptance for publication.

Journal requirements for independent data analysis and for public data availability are in flux at the time of this revision, reflecting evolving views of the importance of data availability for pre- and post-publication peer review. Some journal editors currently request a statistical analysis of trial data by an independent biostatistician before accepting studies for publication. Others ask authors to say whether the study data are available to third parties to view and/or use/reanalyze, while still others encourage or require authors to share their data with others for review or reanalysis. Each journal should establish and publish their specific requirements for data analysis and posting in a place which potential authors can easily access.

Some people believe that true scientific peer review begins only on the date a paper is published. In that spirit, medical journals should have a mechanism for readers to submit comments, questions, or criticisms about published articles, and authors have a responsibility to respond appropriately and cooperate with any requests from the journal for data or additional information should questions about the paper arise after publication (see Section III).

ICMJE believes investigators have a duty to maintain the primary data and analytic procedures underpinning the published results for at least 10 years. The ICMJE encourages the preservation of these data in a data repository to ensure their longer-term availability.

d. Integrity

Editorial decisions should be based on the relevance of a manuscript to the journal and on the manuscript's originality, quality, and contribution to evidence about important questions. Those decisions should not be influenced by commercial interests, personal relationships or agendas, or findings that are negative or that credibly challenge accepted wisdom. In addition, authors should submit for publication or otherwise make publicly available, and editors should not exclude from consideration for publication, studies with findings that are not statistically significant or that have inconclusive findings. Such studies may provide evidence that combined with that from other studies through meta-analysis might still help answer important questions, and a public record of such negative or inconclusive findings may prevent unwarranted replication of effort or otherwise be valuable for other researchers considering similar work.

Journals should clearly state their appeals process and should have a system for responding to appeals and complaints.

3. Peer Reviewers

Manuscripts submitted to journals are privileged communications that are authors' private, confidential property, and authors may be harmed by premature disclosure of any or all of a manuscript's details.

Reviewers therefore should keep manuscripts and the information they contain strictly confidential. Reviewers must not publicly discuss authors' work and must not appropriate authors' ideas before the manuscript is published.

Reviewers must not retain the manuscript for their personal use and should destroy copies of manuscripts after submitting their reviews.

Reviewers are expected to respond promptly to requests to review and to submit reviews within the time agreed. Reviewers' comments should be constructive, honest, and polite.

Reviewers should declare their conflicts of interest and recuse themselves from the peer-review process if a conflict exists.

D. Journal Owners and Editorial Freedom

1. Journal Owners

Owners and editors of medical journals share a common purpose, but they have different responsibilities, and sometimes those differences lead to conflicts.

It is the responsibility of medical journal owners to appoint and dismiss editors. Owners should provide editors at the time of their appointment with a contract that clearly states their rights and duties, authority, the general terms of their appointment, and mechanisms for resolving conflict. The editor's performance may be assessed using mutually agreed-upon measures, including but not necessarily limited to readership, manuscript submissions and handling times, and various journal metrics.

Owners should only dismiss editors for substantial reasons, such as scientific misconduct, disagreement with the long-term editorial direction of the journal, inadequate performance by agreed-upon performance metrics, or inappropriate behavior that is incompatible with a position of trust.

Appointments and dismissals should be based on evaluations by a panel of independent experts, rather than by a small number of executives of the owning organization. This is especially necessary in the case of dismissals because of the high value society places on freedom of speech within science and because it is often the responsibility of editors to challenge the status quo in ways that may conflict with the interests of the journal's owners.

A medical journal should explicitly state its governance and relationship to a journal owner (e.g., a sponsoring society).

2. Editorial Freedom

The ICMJE adopts the World Association of Medical Editors' definition of editorial freedom, which holds that editors-in-chief have full authority over the entire editorial content of their journal and the timing of publication of that content. Journal owners should not interfere in the evaluation, selection, scheduling, or editing of individual articles either directly or by creating an environment that strongly influences decisions. Editors should base editorial decisions on the validity of the work and its importance to the journal's readers, not on the commercial implications for the journal, and editors should be free to express critical but responsible views about all aspects of medicine without fear of retribution, even if these views conflict with the commercial goals of the publisher.

Editors-in-chief should also have the final say in decisions about which advertisements or sponsored content, including supplements, the journal will and will not carry, and they should have final say in use of the journal brand and in overall policy regarding commercial use of journal content.

Journals are encouraged to establish an independent editorial advisory board to help the editor establish and maintain editorial policy. Editors should seek input as needed from a broad array of advisers, such as reviewers, editorial staff, an editorial board, and readers, to support editorial decisions and potentially controversial expressions of opinion, and owners should ensure that appropriate insurance is obtained in the event of legal action against the editors, and should ensure that legal advice is available when necessary. If legal problems arise, the editor should inform their legal adviser and their owner and/or publisher as soon as possible. Editors should defend the confidentiality of authors and peer-reviewers (names and reviewer comments) in accordance with ICMJE policy (see Section II C.2.a). Editors should take all reasonable steps to check the facts in journal commentary, including that in news sections and social media postings, and should ensure that staff working for the journal adhere to best journalistic practices including contemporaneous note-taking and seeking a response from all parties when possible before publication. Such practices in support of truth and public interest may be particularly relevant in defense against legal allegations of libel.

To secure editorial freedom in practice, the editor should have direct access to the highest level of ownership, not to a delegated manager or administrative officer.

Editors and editors' organizations are obliged to support the concept of editorial freedom and to draw major transgressions of such freedom to the attention of the international medical, academic, and lay communities.

E. Protection of Research Participants

When reporting research involving human data, authors should indicate whether the procedures followed have been assessed by the responsible review committee (institutional and national), or if no formal ethics committee is available, were in accordance with the Helsinki Declaration as revised in 2013 (www.wma.net/en/30publications/10policies/b3/index.html). If doubt exists whether the research was conducted in accordance with the Helsinki Declaration, the authors must explain the rationale for their approach and demonstrate that the institutional review body explicitly approved the doubtful aspects of the study. Approval by a responsible review committee does not preclude editors from forming their own judgment whether the conduct of the research was appropriate.

Patients have a right to privacy that should not be violated without informed consent. Identifying information, including names, initials, or hospital numbers, should not be published in written descriptions, photographs, or pedigrees unless the information is essential for scientific purposes and the patient (or parent or guardian) gives written informed consent for publication. Informed consent for this purpose requires that an identifiable patient be shown the manuscript to be published. Authors should disclose to these patients whether any potential identifiable material might be available via the Internet as well as in print after publication. Patient consent should be written and archived with the journal, the authors, or both, as dictated by local regulations or laws. Applicable laws vary from locale to locale, and journals should establish their own policies with legal guidance. Since a journal that archives the consent will be aware of patient identity, some journals may decide that patient confidentiality is better guarded by having the author archive the consent and instead providing the journal with a written statement that attests that they have received and archived written patient consent.

Nonessential identifying details should be omitted. Informed consent should be obtained if there is any doubt that anonymity can be maintained. For example, masking the eye region in photographs of patients is inadequate protection of anonymity. If identifying characteristics are de-identified, authors should provide assurance, and editors should so note, that such changes do not distort scientific meaning.

The requirement for informed consent should be included in the journal's instructions for authors. When informed consent has been obtained, it should be indicated in the published article.

When reporting experiments on animals, authors should indicate whether institutional and national standards for the care and use of laboratory animals were followed. Further guidance on animal research ethics is available from the International Association of Veterinary Editors' Consensus Author Guidelines on Animal Ethics and Welfare (www.veteditors.org/consensus-author-guidelines-on-animal-ethics-and-welfare-for-editors).

III. PUBLISHING AND EDITORIAL ISSUES RELATED TO PUBLICATION IN MEDICAL JOURNALS

A. Corrections and Version Control

Honest errors are a part of science and publishing and require publication of a correction when they are detected. Corrections are needed for errors of fact. Matters of debate are best handled as letters to the editor, as print or electronic correspondence, or as posts in a journal-sponsored online forum. Updates of previous publications (e.g., an updated systematic review or clinical guideline) are considered a new publication rather than a version of a previously published article.

If a correction is needed, journals should follow these minimum standards:

+ The journal should publish a correction notice as soon as possible detailing changes from and citing the original publication; the correction should be on an electronic or numbered print page that is included in an electronic or a print Table of Contents to ensure proper indexing.
+ The journal should also post a new article version with details of the changes from the original version and the date(s) on which the changes were made.
+ The journal should archive all prior versions of the article. This archive can be either directly accessible to readers or can be made available to the reader on request.
+ Previous electronic versions should prominently note that there are more recent versions of the article.
+ The citation should be to the most recent version. Errors serious enough to invalidate a paper's results and conclusions may require retraction.

B. Scientific Misconduct, Expressions of Concern, and Retraction

Scientific misconduct includes but is not necessarily limited to data fabrication; data falsification including deceptive manipulation of images; and plagiarism. Some people consider failure to publish the results of clinical trials and other human studies a form of scientific misconduct. While each of these practices is problematic, they are not equivalent. Each situation requires individual assessment by relevant stakeholders. When scientific misconduct is alleged, or concerns are otherwise raised about the conduct or integrity of work described in submitted or published papers, the editor should initiate appropriate procedures detailed by such committees such as the Committee on Publication Ethics (COPE) (publicationethics.org/resources/flowcharts) and may choose to publish an expression of concern pending the outcomes of those procedures. If the procedures involve an investigation at the authors' institution, the editor should seek to discover the outcome of that investigation, notify readers of the outcome if appropriate, and if the investigation proves scientific misconduct, publish a retraction of the article. There may be circumstances in which no misconduct is proven, but an exchange of letters to the editor could be published to highlight matters of debate to readers.

Expressions of concern and retractions should not simply be a letter to the editor. Rather, they should be prominently labelled, appear on an electronic or numbered print page that is included in an electronic or a print Table of Contents to ensure proper indexing, and include in their heading the title of the original article. Online, the retraction and original article should be linked in both directions and the retracted article should be clearly labelled as retracted in all its forms (Abstract, full text, PDF). Ideally, the authors of the retraction should be the same as those of the article, but if they are unwilling or unable the editor may under certain circumstances accept retractions by other responsible persons, or the editor may be the sole author of the retraction or expression of concern. The text of the retraction should explain why the article is being retracted and include a complete citation reference to that article. Retracted articles should remain in the public domain and be clearly labelled as retracted.

The validity of previous work by the author of a fraudulent paper cannot be assumed. Editors may ask the author's institution to assure them of the validity of other work published in their journals, or they may retract it. If this is not done, editors may choose to publish an announcement expressing concern that the validity of previously published work is uncertain.

The integrity of research may also be compromised by inappropriate methodology that could lead to retraction.

See COPE flowcharts for further guidance on retractions and expressions of concern. See Section IV.3.g.i. for guidance about avoiding referencing retracted articles.

C. Copyright

Journals should make clear the type of copyright under which work will be published, and if the journal retains copyright, should detail the journal's position on the transfer of copyright for all types of content, including audio, video, protocols, and data sets. Medical journals may ask authors to transfer copyright to the journal. Some journals require transfer of a publication license. Some journals do not require transfer of copyright and rely on such vehicles as Creative Commons licenses. The copyright status of articles in a given journal can vary: Some content cannot be copyrighted (for example, articles written by employees of some governments in the course of their work). Editors may waive copyright on other content, and some content may be protected under other agreements.

D. Overlapping Publications

1. Duplicate Submission

Authors should not submit the same manuscript, in the same or different languages, simultaneously to more than one journal. The rationale for this standard is the potential for disagreement when two (or more) journals claim the right to publish a manuscript that has been submitted simultaneously to more than one journal, and the possibility that two or more journals will unknowingly and unnecessarily undertake the work of peer review, edit the same manuscript, and publish the same article.

2. Duplicate Publication

Duplicate publication is publication of a paper that overlaps substantially with one already published, without clear, visible reference to the previous publication.

Readers of medical journals deserve to be able to trust that what they are reading is original unless there is a clear statement that the author and editor are intentionally republishing an article (which might be considered for historic or landmark papers, for example). The bases of this position are international copyright laws, ethical conduct, and cost-effective use of resources. Duplicate publication of original research is particularly problematic because it can result in inadvertent double-counting of data or inappropriate weighting of the results of a single study, which distorts the available evidence.

When authors submit a manuscript reporting work that has already been reported in large part in a published article or is contained in or closely related to another paper that has been submitted or accepted for publication elsewhere, the letter of submission should clearly say so and the authors should provide copies of the related material to help the editor decide how to handle the submission. See also Section IV.B.

This recommendation does not prevent a journal from considering a complete report that follows publication of a preliminary report, such as a letter to the editor or an abstract or poster displayed at a scientific meeting. It also does not prevent journals from considering a paper that has been presented at a scientific meeting but was not published in full, or that is being considered for publication in proceedings or similar format. Press reports of scheduled meetings are not usually regarded as breaches of this rule, but they may be if additional data tables or figures enrich such reports. Authors should also consider how dissemination of their findings outside of scientific presentations at meetings may diminish the priority journal editors assign to their work. An exception to this principle may occur when information that has immediate implications for public health needs to be disseminated, but when possible, early distribution of findings before publication should be discussed with and agreed upon by the editor in advance.

Sharing with public media, government agencies, or manufacturers the scientific information described in a paper or a letter to the editor that has been accepted but not yet published violates the policies of many journals. Such reporting may be warranted when the paper or letter describes major therapeutic advances; reportable diseases; or public health hazards, such as serious adverse effects of drugs, vaccines, other biological products, medical devices. This reporting, whether in print or online, should not jeopardize publication, but should be discussed with and agreed upon by the editor in advance when possible.

The ICMJE will not consider as prior publication the posting of trial results in any registry that meets the criteria noted in Section III.L. if results are limited to a brief (500 word) structured abstract or tables (to include patients enrolled, key outcomes, and adverse events). The ICMJE encourages authors to include a statement with the registration that indicates that the results have not yet been published in a peer-reviewed journal, and to update the results registry with the full journal citation when the results are published.

Editors of different journals may together decide to simultaneously or jointly publish an article if they believe that doing so would be in the best interest of public health. However, the National Library of Medicine (NLM) indexes all such simultaneously published joint publications separately, so editors should include a statement making the simultaneous publication clear to readers.

Authors who attempt duplicate publication without such notification should expect at least prompt rejection of the submitted manuscript. If the editor was not aware of the violations and the article has already been published, then the article might warrant retraction with or without the author's explanation or approval.

See COPE flowcharts for further guidance on handling duplicate publication.

3. Acceptable Secondary Publication

Secondary publication of material published in other journals or online may be justifiable and beneficial, especially when intended to disseminate important information to the widest possible audience (e.g., guidelines produced by government agencies and professional organizations in the same or a different language). Secondary publication for various other reasons may also be justifiable provided the following conditions are met:

1. The authors have received approval from the editors of both journals (the editor concerned with secondary publication must have access to the primary version).
2. The priority of the primary publication is respected by a publication interval negotiated by both editors with the authors.
3. The paper for secondary publication is intended for a different group of readers; an abbreviated version could be sufficient.
4. The secondary version faithfully reflects the data and interpretations of the primary version.
5. The secondary version informs readers, peers, and documenting agencies that the paper has been published in whole or in part elsewhere—for example, with a note that might read, "This article is based on a study first reported in the [journal title, with full reference]"—and the secondary version cites the primary reference.
6. The title of the secondary publication should indicate that it is a secondary publication (complete or abridged republication or translation) of a primary publication. Of note, the NLM does not consider translations to be "republications" and does not cite or index them when the original article was published in a journal that is indexed in MEDLINE.

When the same journal simultaneously publishes an article in multiple languages, the MEDLINE citation will note the multiple languages (for example, Angelo M. Journal networking in nursing: a challenge to be shared. Rev Esc Enferm USP. 2011 Dec 45[6]:1281-2,1279-80,1283-4. Article in English, Portuguese, and Spanish. No abstract available. PMID 22241182).

4. Manuscripts Based on the Same Database

If editors receive manuscripts from separate research groups or from the same group analyzing the same data set (for example, from a public database, or systematic reviews or meta-analyses of the same evidence), the manuscripts should be considered independently because they may differ in their analytic methods, conclusions, or both. If the data interpretation and conclusions are similar, it may be reasonable although not mandatory for editors to give preference to the manuscript submitted first. Editors might consider publishing more than one manuscript that overlap in this way because different analytical approaches may be complementary and equally valid, but manuscripts based upon the same dataset should add substantially to each other to warrant consideration for publication as separate papers, with appropriate citation of previous publications from the same dataset to allow for transparency.

Secondary analyses of clinical trial data should cite any primary publication, clearly state that it contains secondary analyses/results, and use the same identifying trial registration number as the primary trial.

Sometimes for large trials it is planned from the beginning to produce numerous separate publications regarding separate research questions but using the same original patient sample. In this case authors may use the original single trial registration number, if all the outcome parameters were defined in the original registration. If the authors registered several substudies as separate entries in, for example, clinicaltrials.gov, then the unique trial identifier should be given for the study in question. The main issue is transparency, so no matter what model is used it should be obvious for the reader.

E. Correspondence

Medical journals should provide readers with a mechanism for submitting comments, questions, or criticisms about published articles, usually but not necessarily always through a correspondence section or online forum. The authors of articles discussed in correspondence or an online forum have a responsibility to respond to substantial criticisms of their work using those same mechanisms and should be asked by editors to respond. Authors of correspondence should be asked to declare any competing or conflicting interests.

Correspondence may be edited for length, grammatical correctness, and journal style. Alternatively, editors may choose to make available to readers unedited correspondence, for example, via an online commenting system. Such commenting is not indexed in Medline unless it is subsequently published on a numbered electronic or print page. However the journal handles correspondence, it should make known its practice. In all instances, editors must make an effort to screen discourteous, inaccurate, or libelous comments.

Responsible debate, critique and disagreement are important features of science, and journal editors should encourage such discourse ideally within their own journals about the material they have published. Editors, however, have the prerogative to reject correspondence that is irrelevant, uninteresting, or lacking cogency, but they also have a responsibility to allow a range of opinions to be expressed and to promote debate.

In the interests of fairness and to keep correspondence within manageable proportions, journals may want to set time limits for responding to published material and for debate on a given topic.

F. Fees

Journals should be transparent about their types of revenue streams. Any fees or charges that are required for manuscript processing and/or publishing materials in the journal shall be clearly stated in a place that is easy for potential authors to find prior to submitting their manuscripts for review or explained to authors before they begin preparing their manuscript for submission (http://pub licationethics.org/files/u7140/Principles_of_Transparency_and_Best_Practice_in_Scholarly_Publishing.pdf).

G. Supplements, Theme Issues, and Special Series

Supplements are collections of papers that deal with related issues or topics, are published as a separate issue of the journal or as part of a regular issue, and may be funded by sources other than the journal's publisher. Because funding sources can bias the content of supplements through the choice of topics and viewpoints, journals should adopt the following principles, which also apply to theme issues or special series that have external funding and/or guest editors:

1. The journal editor must be given and must take full responsibility for the policies, practices, and content of supplements, including complete control of the decision to select authors, peer reviewers, and content for the supplement. Editing by the funding organization should not be permitted.
2. The journal editor has the right to appoint one or more external editors of the supplement and must take responsibility for the work of those editors.
3. The journal editor must retain the authority to send supplement manuscripts for external peer review and to reject manuscripts submitted for the supplement with or without external review.

These conditions should be made known to authors and any external editors of the supplement before beginning editorial work on it.

4. The source of the idea for the supplement, sources of funding for the supplement's research and publication, and products of the funding source related to content considered in the supplement should be clearly stated in the introductory material.

5. Advertising in supplements should follow the same policies as those of the primary journal.

6. Journal editors must enable readers to distinguish readily between ordinary editorial pages and supplement pages.

7. Journal and supplement editors must not accept personal favors or direct remuneration from sponsors of supplements.

8. Secondary publication in supplements (republication of papers published elsewhere) should be clearly identified by the citation of the original paper and by the title.

9. The same principles of authorship and disclosure of potential conflicts of interest discussed elsewhere in this document should be applied to supplements.

H. Sponsorship or Partnership

Various entities may seek interactions with journals or editors in the form of sponsorships, partnerships, meetings, or other types of activities. To preserve editorial independence, these interactions should be governed by the same principles outlined above for Supplements, Theme Issues and Special Series (Section III.G).

I. Electronic Publishing

Most medical journals are now published in electronic as well as print versions, and some are published only in electronic form. Principles of print and electronic publishing are identical, and the recommendations of this document apply equally to both. However, electronic publishing provides opportunities for versioning and raises issues about link stability and content preservation that are addressed here.

Recommendations for corrections and versioning are detailed in Section III.A.

Electronic publishing allows linking to sites and resources beyond journals over which journal editors have no editorial control. For this reason, and because links to external sites could be perceived as implying endorsement of those sites, journals should be cautious about external linking. When a journal does link to an external site, it should state that it does not endorse or take responsibility or liability for any content, advertising, products, or other materials on the linked sites, and does not take responsibility for the sites' availability.

Permanent preservation of journal articles on a journal's website, or in an independent archive or a credible repository is essential for the historical record. Removing an article from a journal's website in its entirety is almost never justified as copies of the article may have been downloaded even if its online posting was brief. Such archives should be freely accessible or accessible to archive members. Deposition in multiple archives is encouraged. However, if necessary for legal reasons (e.g., libel action), the URL for the removed article must contain a detailed reason for the removal, and the article must be retained in the journal's internal archive.

Permanent preservation of a journal's total content is the responsibility of the journal publisher, who in the event of journal termination should be certain the journal files are transferred to a responsible third party who can make the content available.

Journal websites should post the date that nonarticle web pages, such as those listing journal staff, editorial board members, and instructions for authors, were last updated.

J. Advertising

Most medical journals carry advertising, which generates income for their publishers, but journals should not be dominated by advertisements, and advertising must not be allowed to influence editorial decisions.

Journals should have formal, explicit, written policies for advertising in both print and electronic versions. Best practice prohibits selling advertisements intended to be juxtaposed with editorial content on the same product. Advertisements should be clearly identifiable as advertisements. Editors should have full and final authority for approving print and online advertisements and for enforcing advertising policy.

Journals should not carry advertisements for products proven to be seriously harmful to health. Editors should ensure that existing regulatory or industry standards for advertisements specific to their country are enforced, or develop their own standards. The interests of organizations or agencies should not control classified and other nondisplay advertising, except where required by law. Editors should consider all criticisms of advertisements for publication.

K. Journals and the Media

Journals' interactions with media should balance competing priorities. The general public has a legitimate interest in all journal content and is entitled to important information within a reasonable amount of time, and editors have a responsibility to facilitate that. However media reports of scientific research before it has been peer-reviewed and fully vetted may lead to dissemination of inaccurate or premature conclusions, and doctors in practice need to have research reports available in full detail before they can advise patients about the reports' conclusions.

An embargo system has been established in some countries and by some journals to assist this balance, and to prevent publication of stories in the general media before publication of the original research in the journal. For the media, the embargo creates a "level playing field," which most reporters and writers appreciate since it minimizes the pressure on them to publish stories before competitors when they have not had time to prepare carefully. Consistency in the timing of public release of biomedical information is also important in minimizing economic chaos, since some articles contain information that has potential to influence financial markets. The ICMJE acknowledges criticisms of embargo systems as being self-serving of journals' interests and an impediment to rapid dissemination of scientific information, but believe the benefits of the systems outweigh their harms.

The following principles apply equally to print and electronic publishing and may be useful to editors as they seek to establish policies on interactions with the media:

+ Editors can foster the orderly transmission of medical information from researchers, through peer-reviewed journals, to the public. This can be accomplished by an agreement with authors that they will not publicize their work while their manuscript is under consideration or awaiting publication and an agreement with the media that they will not release stories before publication of the original research in the journal, in return for which the journal will cooperate with them in preparing accurate stories by issuing, for example, a press release.
+ Editors need to keep in mind that an embargo system works on the honor system—no formal enforcement or policing mechanism exists. The decision of a significant number of media outlets or biomedical journals not to respect the embargo system would lead to its rapid dissolution.
+ Notwithstanding authors' belief in their work, very little medical research has such clear and urgently important clinical implications for the public's health that the news must be released before full publication in a journal. When such exceptional circumstances occur, the appropriate authorities responsible for public health should decide whether to disseminate information to physicians and the media in advance and should be responsible for this decision. If the author and the appropriate authorities wish to have a manuscript considered by a particular journal, the editor should be consulted before any public release. If editors acknowledge the need for immediate release, they should waive their policies limiting prepublication publicity.
+ Policies designed to limit prepublication publicity should not apply to accounts in the media of presentations at scientific meetings or to the abstracts from these meetings (see Duplicate Publication). Researchers who present their work at a scientific meeting should feel free to discuss their presentations with reporters but should be discouraged from offering more detail about their study than was

presented in the talk, or should consider how giving such detail might diminish the priority journal editors assign to their work (see Duplicate Publication).

+ When an article is close to being published, editors or journal staff should help the media prepare accurate reports by providing news releases, answering questions, supplying advance copies of the article, or referring reporters to appropriate experts. This assistance should be contingent on the media's cooperation in timing the release of a story to coincide with publication of the article.

L. Clinical Trial Registration

The ICMJE's clinical trial registration policy is detailed in a series of editorials (see Updates and Editorials [www.icmje.org/update.html] and FAQs [www.icmje.org/faq_clinical.html]).

Briefly, the ICMJE requires, and recommends that all medical journal editors require, registration of clinical trials in a public trials registry at or before the time of first patient enrollment as a condition of consideration for publication. Editors requesting inclusion of their journal on the ICMJE website list of publications that follow ICMJE guidance [icmje.org/journals.html] should recognize that the listing implies enforcement by the journal of ICMJE's trial registration policy.

The ICMJE defines a clinical trial as any research project that prospectively assigns people or a group of people to an intervention, with or without concurrent comparison or control groups, to study the cause-and-effect relationship between a health-related intervention and a health outcome.

Health-related interventions are those used to modify a biomedical or health-related outcome; examples include drugs, surgical procedures, devices, behavioural treatments, educational programs, dietary interventions, quality improvement interventions, and process-of-care changes. Health outcomes are any biomedical or health-related measures obtained in patients or participants, including pharmacokinetic measures and adverse events. The ICMJE does not define the timing of first patient enrollment, but best practice dictates registration by the time of first patient consent.

The ICMJE accepts registration in any registry that is a primary register of the WHO International Clinical Trials Registry Platform (ICTRP) (www.who.int/ictrp/network/primary/en/index .html) or in ClinicalTrials.gov, which is a data provider to the WHO ICTRP. The ICMJE endorses these registries because they meet several criteria. They are accessible to the public at no charge, open to all prospective registrants, managed by a not-for-profit organization, have a mechanism to ensure the validity of the registration data, and are electronically searchable. An acceptable registry must include the minimum 20-item trial registration dataset (http://prsinfo.clinicaltrials.gov/trainTrainer /WHO-ICMJE-ClinTrialsgov-Cross-Ref.pdf or www.who.int/ictrp/network/trds/en/index.html) at the time of registration and before enrollment of the first participant.

The ICMJE considers inadequate trial registrations missing any of the 20 data fields or those that have fields that contain uninformative information. Although not a required item, the ICMJE encourages authors to include a statement that indicates that the results have not yet been published in a peer-reviewed journal, and to update the registration with the full journal citation when the results are published.

The purpose of clinical trial registration is to prevent selective publication and selective reporting of research outcomes, to prevent unnecessary duplication of research effort, to help patients and the public know what trials are planned or ongoing into which they might want to enroll, and to help give ethics review boards considering approval of new studies a view of similar work and data relevant to the research they are considering. Retrospective registration, for example at the time of manuscript submission, meets none of these purposes. Those purposes apply also to research with alternative designs, for example observational studies. For that reason, the ICMJE encourages registration of research with non-trial designs, but because the exposure or intervention in non-trial research is not dictated by the researchers, the ICMJE does not require it.

Secondary data analyses of primary (parent) clinical trials should not be registered as separate clinical trials, but instead should reference the trial registration number of the primary trial.

The ICMJE encourages posting of clinical trial results in clinical trial registries but does not require it. The ICMJE will not consider as prior publication the posting of trial results in any registry that meets the above criteria if results are limited to a brief (500 word) structured abstract or tables (to include patients enrolled, key outcomes, and adverse events).

The ICMJE recommends that journals publish the trial registration number at the end of the abstract. The ICMJE also recommends that, whenever a registration number is available, authors list this number the first time they use a trial acronym to refer either to the trial they are reporting or to other trials that they mention in the manuscript.

Editors may consider whether the circumstances involved in a failure to appropriately register a clinical trial were likely to have been intended to or resulted in biased reporting. If an exception to prospective registration is made, trials must be registered and the authors should indicate in the publication when registration was completed and why it was delayed. Editors should publish a statement indicating why an exception was allowed. The ICMJE emphasizes that such exceptions should be rare, and that authors failing to prospectively register a trial risk its inadmissibility to our journals.

IV. MANUSCRIPT PREPARATION AND SUBMISSION

A. Preparing a Manuscript for Submission to a Medical Journal

1. General Principles

The text of articles reporting original research is usually divided into Introduction, Methods, Results, and Discussion sections. This so-called "IMRAD" structure is not an arbitrary publication format but a reflection of the process of scientific discovery. Articles often need subheadings within these sections to further organize their content. Other types of articles, such as meta-analyses, may require different formats, while case reports, narrative reviews, and editorials may have less structured or unstructured formats.

Electronic formats have created opportunities for adding details or sections, layering information, cross-linking, or extracting portions of articles in electronic versions. Supplementary electronic-only material should be submitted and sent for peer review simultaneously with the primary manuscript.

2. Reporting Guidelines

Reporting guidelines have been developed for different study designs; examples include CONSORT (www.consort-statement.org) for randomized trials, STROBE for observational studies (http://strobe-statement.org/), PRISMA for systematic reviews and meta-analyses (http://prisma-statement.org/), and STARD for studies of diagnostic accuracy (www.stard-statement.org/). Journals are encouraged to ask authors to follow these guidelines because they help authors describe the study in enough detail for it to be evaluated by editors, reviewers, readers, and other researchers evaluating the medical literature. Authors of review manuscripts are encouraged to describe the methods used for locating, selecting, extracting, and synthesizing data; this is mandatory for systematic reviews. Good sources for reporting guidelines are the EQUATOR Network (www.equator-network.org/home/) and the NLM's Research Reporting Guidelines and Initiatives (www.nlm.nih.gov/services/research_report_guide.html).

3. Manuscript Sections

The following are general requirements for reporting within sections of all study designs and manuscript formats.

a. Title Page

General information about an article and its authors is presented on a manuscript title page and usually includes the article title, author information, any disclaimers, sources of support, word count, and sometimes the number of tables and figures.

Article title. The title provides a distilled description of the complete article and should include information that, along with the Abstract, will make electronic retrieval of the article sensitive and specific. Reporting guidelines recommend and some journals require that information about the study design be a part of the title (particularly important for randomized trials and systematic reviews and meta-analyses). Some journals require a short title, usually no more than 40 characters (including letters and spaces) on the title page or as a separate entry in an electronic submission system. Electronic submission systems may restrict the number of characters in the title.

Author information. Each author's highest academic degrees should be listed, although some journals do not publish these. The name of the department(s) and institution(s) or organizations where the work should be attributed should be specified. Most electronic submission systems require that authors provide full contact information, including land mail and e-mail addresses, but the title page should list the corresponding authors' telephone and fax numbers and e-mail address.

Disclaimers. An example of a disclaimer is an author's statement that the views expressed in the submitted article are his or her own and not an official position of the institution or funder.

Source(s) of support. These include grants, equipment, drugs, and/or other support that facilitated conduct of the work described in the article or the writing of the article itself.

Word count. A word count for the paper's text, excluding its abstract, acknowledgments, tables, figure legends, and references, allows editors and reviewers to assess whether the information contained in the paper warrants the paper's length, and whether the submitted manuscript fits within the journal's formats and word limits. A separate word count for the Abstract is useful for the same reason.

Number of figures and tables. Some submission systems require specification of the number of Figures and Tables before uploading the relevant files. These numbers allow editorial staff and reviewers to confirm that all figures and tables were actually included with the manuscript and, because Tables and Figures occupy space, to assess if the information provided by the figures and tables warrants the paper's length and if the manuscript fits within the journal's space limits.

Conflict of Interest declaration. Conflict of interest information for each author needs to be part of the manuscript; each journal should develop standards with regard to the form the information should take and where it will be posted. The ICMJE has developed a uniform conflict of interest disclosure form for use by ICMJE member journals (www.icmje.org/coi_disclosure.pdf) and the ICMJE encourages other journals to adopt it. Despite availability of the form, editors may require conflict of interest declarations on the manuscript title page to save the work of collecting forms from each author prior to making an editorial decision or to save reviewers and readers the work of reading each author's form.

b. Abstract

Original research, systematic reviews, and meta-analyses require structured abstracts. The abstract should provide the context or background for the study and should state the study's purpose, basic procedures (selection of study participants, settings, measurements, analytical methods), main findings (giving specific effect sizes and their statistical and clinical significance, if possible), and principal conclusions. It should emphasize new and important aspects of the study or observations, note important limitations, and not overinterpret findings. Clinical trial abstracts should include items that the CONSORT group has identified as essential (www.consort-statement.org/resources/downloads/extensions /consort-extension-for-abstracts-2008pdf/). Funding sources should be listed separately after the Abstract to facilitate proper display and indexing for search retrieval by MEDLINE.

Because abstracts are the only substantive portion of the article indexed in many electronic databases, and the only portion many readers read, authors need to ensure that they accurately reflect the content of the article. Unfortunately, information in abstracts often differs from that in the text. Authors and editors should work in the process of revision and review to ensure that information is consistent in both places. The format required for structured abstracts differs from journal to journal, and some journals use more than one format; authors need to prepare their abstracts in the format specified by the journal they have chosen.

The ICMJE recommends that journals publish the clinical trial registration number at the end of the abstract. The ICMJE also recommends that, when a registration number is available, authors list that number the first time they use a trial acronym to refer to the trial they are reporting or to other trials that they mention in the manuscript. If the data have been deposited in a public repository, authors should state at the end of the abstract the data set name, repository name and number.

c. Introduction

Provide a context or background for the study (that is, the nature of the problem and its significance). State the specific purpose or research objective of, or hypothesis tested by, the study or observation. Cite only directly pertinent references, and do not include data or conclusions from the work being reported.

d. Methods

The guiding principle of the Methods section should be clarity about how and why a study was done in a particular way. The Methods section should aim to be sufficiently detailed such that others with access to the data would be able to reproduce the results. In general, the section should include only information that was available at the time the plan or protocol for the study was being written; all information obtained during the study belongs in the Results section. If an organization was paid or otherwise contracted to help conduct the research (examples include data collection and management), then this should be detailed in the methods.

The Methods section should include a statement indicating that the research was approved or exempted from the need for review by the responsible review committee (institutional or national). If no formal ethics committee is available, a statement indicating that the research was conducted according to the principles of the Declaration of Helsinki should be included.

i. Selection and Description of Participants

Clearly describe the selection of observational or experimental participants (healthy individuals or patients, including controls), including eligibility and exclusion criteria and a description of the source population. Because the relevance of such variables as age, sex, or ethnicity is not always known at the time of study design, researchers should aim for inclusion of representative populations into all study types and at a minimum provide descriptive data for these and other relevant demographic variables. If the study was done involving an exclusive population, for example in only one sex, authors should justify why, except in obvious cases (e.g., prostate cancer)." Authors should define how they measured race or ethnicity and justify their relevance.

ii. Technical Information

Specify the study's main and secondary objectives—usually identified as primary and secondary outcomes. Identify methods, equipment (give the manufacturer's name and address in parentheses), and procedures in sufficient detail to allow others to reproduce the results. Give references to established methods, including statistical methods (see below); provide references and brief descriptions for methods that have been published but are not well-known; describe new or substantially modified methods, give the reasons for using them, and evaluate their limitations. Identify precisely all drugs and chemicals used, including generic name(s), dose(s), and route(s) of administration. Identify appropriate scientific names and gene names.

iii. Statistics

Describe statistical methods with enough detail to enable a knowledgeable reader with access to the original data to judge its appropriateness for the study and to verify the reported results. When possible, quantify findings and present them with appropriate indicators of measurement error or uncertainty (such as confidence intervals). Avoid relying solely on statistical hypothesis testing, such as P values, which fail to convey important information about effect size and precision of estimates. References for the design of the study and statistical methods should be to standard works when possible (with pages stated). Define statistical terms, abbreviations, and most symbols. Specify the statistical software package(s) and versions used. Distinguish prespecified from exploratory analyses, including subgroup analyses.

e. Results

Present your results in logical sequence in the text, tables, and figures, giving the main or most important findings first. Do not repeat all the data in the tables or figures in the text; emphasize or summarize only the most important observations. Provide data on all primary and secondary outcomes identified in the Methods Section. Extra or supplementary materials and technical details can be placed in an appendix where they will be accessible but will not interrupt the flow of the text, or they can be published solely in the electronic version of the journal.

Give numeric results not only as derivatives (for example, percentages) but also as the absolute numbers from which the derivatives were calculated, and specify the statistical significance attached to them, if any. Restrict tables and figures to those needed to explain the argument of the paper and to assess supporting data. Use graphs as an alternative to tables with many entries; do not duplicate data in graphs and tables. Avoid nontechnical uses of technical terms in statistics, such as "random" (which implies a randomizing device), "normal," "significant," "correlations," and "sample."

Separate reporting of data by demographic variables, such as age and sex, facilitate pooling of data for subgroups across studies and should be routine, unless there are compelling reasons not to stratify reporting, which should be explained.

f. Discussion

Emphasize the new and important aspects of the study and the conclusions that follow from them in the context of the totality of the best available evidence. Do not repeat in detail data or other information given in other parts of the manuscript, such as in the Introduction or the Results section. For experimental studies, it is useful to begin the discussion by briefly summarizing the main findings, then explore possible mechanisms or explanations for these findings, compare and contrast the results with other relevant studies, state the limitations of the study, and explore the implications of the findings for future research and for clinical practice.

Link the conclusions with the goals of the study but avoid unqualified statements and conclusions not adequately supported by the data. In particular, distinguish between clinical and statistical significance, and avoid making statements on economic benefits and costs unless the manuscript includes the appropriate economic data and analyses. Avoid claiming priority or alluding to work that has not been completed. State new hypotheses when warranted, but label them clearly.

g. References

i. General Considerations

Authors should provide direct references to original research sources whenever possible. References should not be used by authors, editors, or peer reviewers to promote self-interests. Although references to review articles can be an efficient way to guide readers to a body of literature, review articles do not always reflect original work accurately. On the other hand, extensive lists of references to original work on a topic can use excessive space. Fewer references to key original papers often serve as well as more exhaustive lists, particularly since references can now be added to the electronic version of published papers, and since electronic literature searching allows readers to retrieve published literature efficiently.

Do not use conference abstracts as references: they can be cited in the text, in parentheses, but not as page footnotes. References to papers accepted but not yet published should be designated as "in press" or "forthcoming." Information from manuscripts submitted but not accepted should be cited in the text as "unpublished observations" with written permission from the source.

Avoid citing a "personal communication" unless it provides essential information not available from a public source, in which case the name of the person and date of communication should be cited in parentheses in the text. For scientific articles, obtain written permission and confirmation of accuracy from the source of a personal communication.

Some but not all journals check the accuracy of all reference citations; thus, citation errors sometimes appear in the published version of articles. To minimize such errors, references should be verified using either an electronic bibliographic source, such as PubMed, or print copies from original sources. Authors are responsible for checking that none of the references cite retracted articles except in the context of referring to the retraction. For articles published in journals indexed in MEDLINE, the ICMJE considers PubMed the authoritative source for information about retractions. Authors can identify retracted articles in MEDLINE by searching PubMed for "Retracted publication [pt]," where the term "pt" in square brackets stands for publication type, or by going directly to the PubMed's list of retracted publications (www.ncbi.nlm.nih.gov/pubmed?term_retracted_publication_[pt]).

References should be numbered consecutively in the order in which they are first mentioned in the text. Identify references in text, tables, and legends by Arabic numerals in parentheses.

References cited only in tables or figure legends should be numbered in accordance with the sequence established by the first identification in the text of the particular table or figure. The titles of journals should be abbreviated according to the style used for MEDLINE (www.ncbi.nlm.nih.gov /nlmcatalog/journals). Journals vary on whether they ask authors to cite electronic references within parentheses in the text or in numbered references following the text. Authors should consult with the journal to which they plan to submit their work.

ii. Style and Format

References should follow the standards summarized in the NLM's International Committee of Medical Journal Editors (ICMJE) Recommendations for the Conduct, Reporting, Editing and Publication of Scholarly Work in Medical Journals: Sample References (www.nlm.nih.gov/bsd /uniform_requirements.html) webpage and detailed in the NLM's Citing Medicine, 2nd edition (www.ncbi.nlm.nih.gov/books/NBK7256/). These resources are regularly updated as new media develop, and currently include guidance for print documents; unpublished material; audio and visual media; material on CD-ROM, DVD, or disk; and material on the Internet.

h. Tables

Tables capture information concisely and display it efficiently; they also provide information at any desired level of detail and precision. Including data in tables rather than text frequently makes it possible to reduce the length of the text.

Prepare tables according to the specific journal's requirements; to avoid errors it is best if tables can be directly imported into the journal's publication software. Number tables consecutively in the order of their first citation in the text and supply a title for each. Titles in tables should be short but self-explanatory, containing information that allows readers to understand the table's content without having to go back to the text. Be sure that each table is cited in the text.

Give each column a short or an abbreviated heading. Authors should place explanatory matter in footnotes, not in the heading. Explain all nonstandard abbreviations in footnotes, and use symbols to explain information if needed. Symbols may vary from journal to journal (alphabet letter or such symbols as *, †, ‡, §), so check each journal's instructions for authors for required practice. Identify statistical measures of variations, such as standard deviation and standard error of the mean.

If you use data from another published or unpublished source, obtain permission and acknowledge that source fully.

Additional tables containing backup data too extensive to publish in print may be appropriate for publication in the electronic version of the journal, deposited with an archival service, or made available to readers directly by the authors. An appropriate statement should be added to the text to inform readers that this additional information is available and where it is located. Submit such tables for consideration with the paper so that they will be available to the peer reviewers.

i. Illustrations (Figures)

Digital images of manuscript illustrations should be submitted in a suitable format for print publication. Most submission systems have detailed instructions on the quality of images and check them after manuscript upload. For print submissions, figures should be either professionally drawn and photographed, or submitted as photographic quality digital prints.

For X-ray films, scans, and other diagnostic images, as well as pictures of pathology specimens or photomicrographs, send high-resolution photographic image files. Since blots are used as primary evidence in many scientific articles, editors may require deposition of the original photographs of blots on the journal's website.

Although some journals redraw figures, many do not. Letters, numbers, and symbols on figures should therefore be clear and consistent throughout, and large enough to remain legible when the figure is reduced for publication. Figures should be made as self-explanatory as possible, since many will be used directly in slide presentations. Titles and detailed explanations belong in the legends—not on the illustrations themselves.

Photomicrographs should have internal scale markers. Symbols, arrows, or letters used in photomicrographs should contrast with the background. Explain the internal scale and identify the method of staining in photomicrographs.

Figures should be numbered consecutively according to the order in which they have been cited in the text. If a figure has been published previously, acknowledge the original source and submit written permission from the copyright holder to reproduce it. Permission is required irrespective of authorship or publisher except for documents in the public domain.

In the manuscript, legends for illustrations should be on a separate page, with Arabic numerals corresponding to the illustrations. When symbols, arrows, numbers, or letters are used to identify parts of the illustrations, identify and explain each one clearly in the legend.

j. Units of Measurement

Measurements of length, height, weight, and volume should be reported in metric units (meter, kilogram, or liter) or their decimal multiples.

Temperatures should be in degrees Celsius. Blood pressures should be in millimeters of mercury, unless other units are specifically required by the journal.

Journals vary in the units they use for reporting hematologic, clinical chemistry, and other measurements. Authors must consult the Information for Authors of the particular journal and should report laboratory information in both local and International System of Units (SI).

Editors may request that authors add alternative or non-SI units, since SI units are not universally used. Drug concentrations may be reported in either SI or mass units, but the alternative should be provided in parentheses where appropriate.

k. Abbreviations and Symbols

Use only standard abbreviations; use of nonstandard abbreviations can be confusing to readers. Avoid abbreviations in the title of the manuscript. The spelled-out abbreviation followed by the abbreviation in parenthesis should be used on first mention unless the abbreviation is a standard unit of measurement.

B. Sending the Manuscript to the Journal

Manuscripts should be accompanied by a cover letter or a completed journal submission form, which should include the following information:

A full statement to the editor about all submissions and previous reports that might be regarded as redundant publication of the same or very similar work. Any such work should be referred to specifically and referenced in the new paper. Copies of such material should be included with the submitted paper to help the editor address the situation. See also Section III.D.2.

A statement of financial or other relationships that might lead to a conflict of interest, if that information is not included in the manuscript itself or in an authors' form. See also Section II.B.

A statement on authorship. Journals that do not use contribution declarations for all authors may require that the submission letter includes a statement that the manuscript has been read and approved by all the authors, that the requirements for authorship as stated earlier in this document have been met, and that each author believes that the manuscript represents honest work if that information is not provided in another form. See also Section II.A.

Contact information for the author responsible for communicating with other authors about revisions and final approval of the proofs, if that information is not included in the manuscript itself.

The letter or form should inform editors if concerns have been raised (e.g., via institutional and/or regulatory bodies) regarding the conduct of the research or if corrective action has been recommended. The letter or form should give any additional information that may be helpful to the editor, such as the type or format of article in the particular journal that the manuscript represents. If the manuscript has been submitted previously to another journal, it is helpful to include the previous editor's and reviewers' comments with the submitted manuscript, along with the authors' responses to those comments. Editors encourage authors to submit these previous communications. Doing so may expedite the review process and encourages transparency and sharing of expertise.

Many journals provide a presubmission checklist to help the author ensure that all the components of the submission have been included. Some journals also require that authors complete checklists for reports of certain study types (for example, the CONSORT checklist for reports of randomized controlled trials). Authors should look to see if the journal uses such checklists, and send them with the manuscript if they are requested.

The manuscript must be accompanied by permission to reproduce previously published material, use previously published illustrations, report information about identifiable persons, or to acknowledge people for their contributions.

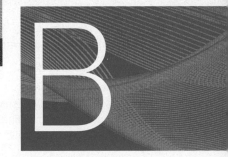

I. Peer Review Questionnaire

Please print.

1. Regarding the scientific manuscripts that you have peer-reviewed, what are your three most common criticisms?

1	
2	
3	

2. What are the three most common mistakes that clinicians make in analyzing medical research data?

1	
2	
3	

Problematic Sections

Please circle one number for each question.	1— Introduction	2— Methods	3— Results	4— Discussion
3. Which section usually contains the most flaws?	1	2	3	4
4. Which section is most often responsible for outright rejection?	1	2	3	4
5. Which section is usually too short?	1	2	3	4
6. Which section is usually too long?	1	2	3	4

7. What is the single most common type of flaw that results in outright rejection of a manuscript?

   Please circle one number.

   1—Design of the study
   2—Presentation of the results
   3—Interpretation of the findings
   4—Importance of the topic

Interpretation

8. How frequently do you encounter the following deficiencies?

Please circle one number for each row	Never 0%	Seldom 1%–25%	Occasionally 26%–75%	Frequently 76%–99%	Always 100%
1—Data too preliminary	0	1	2	3	4
2—Data inconclusive	0	1	2	3	4
3—Conclusions unsupported by data	0	1	2	3	4
4—Unconvincing evidence of cause and effect	0	1	2	3	4
5—Results not generalizable	0	1	2	3	4
6—Excessive bias in interpretation	0	1	2	3	4
7—Insufficient recognition of previous research	0	1	2	3	4
8—Economic consequences ignored or overinterpreted	0	1	2	3	4

9. Of the eight problems listed above, which is most often responsible for outright rejection?

   [   ]   Enter a number from 1 to 8.

Importance of the Research

10. How frequently do you encounter the following deficiencies?

Please circle one number for each row.	Never 0%	Seldom 1%–25%	Occasionally 26%–75%	Frequently 76%–99%	Always 100%
1—Results unoriginal, predictable, or trivial	0	1	2	3	4
2—Issue outdated or no longer relevant	0	1	2	3	4
3—Results of narrow interest or highly specialized	0	1	2	3	4
4—Few or no clinical implications	0	1	2	3	4

11. Of the four problems listed above, which is most often responsible for outright rejection?

[   ]   Enter a number from 1 to 4.

Presentation

12. How frequently do you encounter the following deficiencies?

Please circle one number for each row.	Never 0%	Seldom 1%–25%	Occasionally 26%–75%	Frequently 76%–99%	Always 100%
1—Rationale confused or contradictory	0	1	2	3	4
2—Important work by others ignored	0	1	2	3	4
3—Failure to give a detailed explanation of the experimental design	0	1	2	3	4
4—Inadequate or inappropriate presentation of data	0	1	2	3	4
5—Essential data omitted or ignored	0	1	2	3	4
6—Poorly written; excessive jargon	0	1	2	3	4
7—Excessive zeal and self-promotion	0	1	2	3	4
8—Boring	0	1	2	3	4

13. Of the eight problems listed above, which is most often responsible for outright rejection?

[ ]　Enter a number from 1 to 8.

14. What are the most important lessons that you have learned about how to write and publish a medical research paper that you wish you had been taught in medical school?

1 | |
2 | |
3 | |

Design

15. How frequently do you encounter the following deficiencies?

Please circle one number for each row.	Never 0%	Seldom 1%–25%	Occasionally 26%–75%	Frequently 76%–99%	Always 100%
1—Weak discussion	0	1	2	3	4
2—Weak conclusions	0	1	2	3	4
3—Poor presentation	0	1	2	3	4
4—Poor methods	0	1	2	3	4
5—Inadequate results	0	1	2	3	4
6—Lack of originality	0	1	2	3	4
7—Failure to adhere to journal format and policy	0	1	2	3	4
8—Inappropriate statistical analysis	0	1	2	3	4

16. Of the eight problems listed above, which is most often responsible for outright rejection?

[ ]　Enter a number from 1 to 8.

17. What is the single most common type of flaw that results in outright rejection of a manuscript?

| |

18. What is the most common form of bias that leads to rejection?

| |

19. How frequently do you encounter the following deficiencies?

Please circle one number for each row.	Never 0%	Seldom 1%–25%	Occasionally 26%–75%	Frequently 76%–99%	Always 100%
1—Inadequate control of variables	0	1	2	3	4
2—Deficiency in methodology	0	1	2	3	4
3—Research design problems	0	1	2	3	4
4—Poor conceptualiza-tion of problem or approach	0	1	2	3	4
5—Inappropriate statistical analysis	0	1	2	3	4
6—Duplication of previous work	0	1	2	3	4
7—Lack of medical supervision	0	1	2	3	4
8—Poor literature review	0	1	2	3	4
9—Inadequate protection of human subjects	0	1	2	3	4

20. Of the nine problems listed above, which is most often responsible for outright rejection?

    [   ]   Enter a number from 1 to 9.

21. Do you feel that you have adequate skills to evaluate the statistical aspects of most medical manuscripts that you are asked to review?

    0—No
    1—Yes

22. Which statistical techniques do you wish you knew more about?

    1 |
    2 |
    3 |

Statistics

23. How frequently do you encounter the following deficiencies?

Please circle one number for each row.	Never 0%	Seldom 1%–25%	Occasionally 26%–75%	Frequently 76%–99%	Always 100%
1—Insufficient information about the patient population	0	1	2	3	4
2—Inadequate sample size	0	1	2	3	4
3—Biased sample that reduced the representatives of the population studied	0	1	2	3	4
4—Confounding factors that were not taken into account	0	1	2	3	4
5—Vague end points, such as "much improved," without explanation	0	1	2	3	4
6—Straying from the hypothesis or changing the objective	0	1	2	3	4
7—Poor control of numbers (errors or inconsistencies)	0	1	2	3	4

24. Of the seven problems listed above, which is the most often responsible for outright rejection?

[ ]   Enter a number from 1 to 7.

25. How frequently do you encounter the following deficiencies?

Please circle one number for each row.	Never 0%	Seldom 1%–25%	Occasionally 26%–75%	Frequently 76%–99%	Always 100%
1—Failure to collect data on variables that could influence the interpretation of results	0	1	2	3	4
2—Poor response rates in surveys	0	1	2	3	4
3—Subjects lost to follow-up or inadequate duration of follow-up in long-term studies	0	1	2	3	4
4—Extensive missing data and quality control problems	0	1	2	3	4

26. Of the four problems listed above, which is most often responsible for outright rejection?

    ☐   Enter a number from 1 to 4.

Writing

27. How frequently do you encounter the following deficiencies?

Please circle one number for each row.	Never 0%	Seldom 1%–25%	Occasionally 26%–75%	Frequently 76%–99%	Always 100%
1—Poor flow of ideas	0	1	2	3	4
2—Verbiage, wordiness	0	1	2	3	4
3—Redundancy	0	1	2	3	4
4—Wrong words	0	1	2	3	4
5—Poor syntax, poor grammar	0	1	2	3	4
6—Excessive abstraction	0	1	2	3	4
7—Unnecessary complexity	0	1	2	3	4
8—Excessive compression	0	1	2	3	4
9—Unnecessary qualification	0	1	2	3	4

28. Of the nine writing problems listed above, which is most common?

    ☐   Enter a number from 1 to 9.

29. When you receive a manuscript, what do you find most annoying?

Advice

30. What is your definition of a good article?

31. What advice would you give to prospective authors submitting papers to your journal?

32. Can you cite an example of what you consider the ideal paper?

33. What statistical techniques do you think will be more important in the future?

34. How could this survey have been improved?

The End
Thank you.

II. Peer Review Questionnaire

1. Regarding the scientific manuscripts that you have peer reviewed, what are your three most common criticisms?

2. What are the three most common mistakes that clinicians make in analyzing medical research data?

Problematic Sections

3. Which section usually contains the most flaws?
   ○ Introduction ○ Methods ○ Results ○ Discussion

4. Which section is most often responsible for outright rejection?
   ○ Introduction ○ Methods ○ Results ○ Discussion

5. Which section is usually too short?
   ○ Introduction ○ Methods ○ Results ○ Discussion

6. Which section is usually too long?
   ○ Introduction ○ Methods ○ Results ○ Discussion

7. What is the single most common type of flaw that results in outright rejection of a manuscript?
   ○ Design of the study
   ○ Presentation of the results
   ○ Interpretation of the findings
   ○ Importance of the topic

Interpretation
How frequently do you encounter the following deficiencies?

8.1. Data too preliminary
   Never   Occasionally   Always
   (Place a mark on the scale above)

8.2. Data inconclusive
   Never   Occasionally   Always
   (Place a mark on the scale above)

8.3. Conclusions unsupported by data
   Never   Occasionally   Always
   (Place a mark on the scale above)

8.4. Unconvincing evidence of cause and effect
   Never   Occasionally   Always
   (Place a mark on the scale above)

8.5. Results not generalizable

Never   Occasionally   Always

(Place a mark on the scale above)

8.6. Excessive bias in interpretation

Never   Occasionally   Always

(Place a mark on the scale above)

8.7. Insufficient recognition of previous research

Never   Occasionally   Always

(Place a mark on the scale above)

8.8. Economic consequences ignored or overinterpreted

Never   Occasionally   Always

(Place a mark on the scale above)

9.   Of the eight problems listed above, which is most often responsible for outright rejection?

○ Data too preliminary
○ Data inconclusive
○ Conclusions unsupported by data
○ Unconvincing evidence of cause and effect
○ Results not generalizable
○ Excessive bias in interpretation
○ Insufficient recognition of previous research
○ Economic consequences ignored or overinterpreted

Importance of the Research
How frequently do you encounter the following deficiencies?

10.1. Results unoriginal, predictable, or trivial

Never   Occasionally   Always

(Place a mark on the scale above)

10.2. Issue outdated or no longer relevant

Never   Occasionally   Always

(Place a mark on the scale above)

10.3. Results of narrow interest or highly specialized

Never   Occasionally   Always

(Place a mark on the scale above)

10.4. Few or no clinical implications

Never   Occasionally   Always

(Place a mark on the scale above)

11. Of the four problems listed above, which is most often responsible for outright rejection?
    ○ Results unoriginal, predictable, or trivial
    ○ Issue outdated or no longer relevant
    ○ Results of narrow interest or highly specialized
    ○ Few or no clinical implications

Presentation
How frequently do you encounter the following deficiencies?

12.1. Rationale confused or contradictory

| Never | Occasionally | Always |

(Place a mark on the scale above)

12.2. Important work by others ignored

| Never | Occasionally | Always |

(Place a mark on the scale above)

12.3. Failure to give a detailed explanation of the experimental design

| Never | Occasionally | Always |

(Place a mark on the scale above)

12.4. Inadequate or inappropriate presentation of data

| Never | Occasionally | Always |

(Place a mark on the scale above)

12.5. Essential data omitted or ignored

| Never | Occasionally | Always |

(Place a mark on the scale above)

12.6. Poorly written; excessive jargon

| Never | Occasionally | Always |

(Place a mark on the scale above)

12.7. Excessive zeal and self-promotion

| Never | Occasionally | Always |

(Place a mark on the scale above)

12.8. Boring

| Never | Occasionally | Always |

(Place a mark on the scale above)

13.   Of the eight problems listed above, which is most often responsible for outright rejection?

○ Rationale confused or contradictory
○ Important work by others ignored
○ Failure to give a detailed explanation of the experimental design
○ Inadequate or inappropriate presentation of data
○ Essential data omitted or ignored
○ Poorly written; excessive jargon
○ Excessive zeal and self-promotion
○ Boring

14.   What are the most important lessons that you have learned about how to write and publish a medical research paper that you wish you had been taught in medical/graduate school?

Design
How frequently do you encounter the following deficiencies?

15.1. Weak discussion

Never   Occasionally   Always

(Place a mark on the scale above)

15.2. Weak conclusions

Never   Occasionally   Always

(Place a mark on the scale above)

15.3. Poor presentation

Never   Occasionally   Always

(Place a mark on the scale above)

15.4. Poor methods

Never   Occasionally   Always

(Place a mark on the scale above)

15.5. Inadequate results

Never   Occasionally   Always

(Place a mark on the scale above)

15.6. Lack of originality

Never   Occasionally   Always

(Place a mark on the scale above)

15.7. Failure to adhere to journal format and policy

Never   Occasionally   Always

(Place a mark on the scale above)

15.8. Inappropriate statistical analysis

      Never   Occasionally   Always

(Place a mark on the scale above)

16.   Of the eight problems listed above, which is most often responsible for outright rejection?

    ○ Weak discussion
    ○ Weak conclusions
    ○ Poor presentation
    ○ Poor methods
    ○ Inadequate results
    ○ Lack of originality
    ○ Failure to adhere to journal format and policy
    ○ Inappropriate statistical analysis

How frequently do you encounter the following deficiencies?

19.1. Inadequate control of variables

      Never   Occasionally   Always

(Place a mark on the scale above)

19.2. Deficiency in methodology

      Never   Occasionally   Always

(Place a mark on the scale above)

19.3. Research design problems

      Never   Occasionally   Always

(Place a mark on the scale above)

19.4. Poor conceptualization of problem or approach

      Never   Occasionally   Always

(Place a mark on the scale above)

19.5. Inappropriate statistical analysis

      Never   Occasionally   Always

(Place a mark on the scale above)

19.6. Duplication of previous work

      Never   Occasionally   Always

(Place a mark on the scale above)

19.7. Lack of medical supervision

      Never   Occasionally   Always

(Place a mark on the scale above)

19.8. Poor literature review

Never   Occasionally   Always

<!-- scale -->

(Place a mark on the scale above)

19.9. Inadequate protection of human subjects

Never   Occasionally   Always

<!-- scale -->

(Place a mark on the scale above)

20.   Of the nine problems listed above, which is most often responsible for outright rejection?

- ◯ Inadequate control of variables
- ◯ Deficiency in methodology
- ◯ Research design problems
- ◯ Poor conceptualization of problem or approach
- ◯ Inappropriate statistical analysis
- ◯ Duplication of previous work
- ◯ Lack of medical supervision
- ◯ Poor literature review
- ◯ Inadequate protection of human subjects

21.   Do you feel that you have adequate skills to evaluate the statistical aspects of most medical manuscripts that you are asked to review?

◯ Yes   ◯ No

22.   Which statistical techniques do you wish you knew more about?

Statistics
How frequently do you encounter the following deficiencies?

23.1. Insufficient information about the patient population

Never   Occasionally   Always

<!-- scale -->

(Place a mark on the scale above)

23.2. Inadequate sample size

Never   Occasionally   Always

<!-- scale -->

(Place a mark on the scale above)

23.3. Biased sample that reduced the representativeness of the population studied

Never   Occasionally   Always

<!-- scale -->

(Place a mark on the scale above)

23.4. Confounding factors that were not taken into account

Never   Occasionally   Always

<!-- scale -->

(Place a mark on the scale above)

23.5. Vague end points, such as "much improved," without explanation

Never   Occasionally   Always

(Place a mark on the scale above)

23.6. Straying from the hypothesis or changing the objective

Never   Occasionally   Always

(Place a mark on the scale above)

23.7. Poor control of numbers (errors or inconsistencies)

Never   Occasionally   Always

(Place a mark on the scale above)

24.   Of the seven problems listed above, which is the most often responsible for outright rejection?

○ Insufficient information about the patient population
○ Inadequate sample size
○ Biased sample that reduced the representativeness of the population studied
○ Confounding factors that were not taken into account
○ Vague end points, such as, "much improved," without explanation
○ Straying from the hypothesis or changing the objective
○ Poor control of numbers (errors or inconsistencies)

How frequently do you encounter the following deficiencies?

25.1. Failure to collect data on variables that could influence the interpretation of results

Never   Occasionally   Always

(Place a mark on the scale above)

25.2. Poor response rates in surveys

Never   Occasionally   Always

(Place a mark on the scale above)

25.3. Subjects lost to follow-up or inadequate duration of follow-up in long-term studies

Never   Occasionally   Always

(Place a mark on the scale above)

25.4. Extensive missing data and quality control problems

Never   Occasionally   Always

(Place a mark on the scale above)

26.   Of the four problems listed above, which is most often responsible for outright rejection?

○ Failure to collect data on variables that could influence the interpretation of results
○ Poor response rates in surveys
○ Subjects lost to follow-up or inadequate duration of follow-up in long-term studies
○ Extensive missing data and quality control problems

Writing
How frequently do you encounter the following deficiencies?

27.1. Poor flow of ideas

Never   Occasionally   Always

(Place a mark on the scale above)

27.2. Verbiage, wordiness

Never   Occasionally   Always

(Place a mark on the scale above)

27.3. Redundancy

Never   Occasionally   Always

(Place a mark on the scale above)

27.4. Wrong words

Never   Occasionally   Always

(Place a mark on the scale above)

27.5. Poor syntax, poor grammar

Never   Occasionally   Always

(Place a mark on the scale above)

27.6. Excessive abstraction

Never   Occasionally   Always

(Place a mark on the scale above)

27.7. Unnecessary complexity

Never   Occasionally   Always

(Place a mark on the scale above)

27.8. Excessive compression

Never   Occasionally   Always

(Place a mark on the scale above)

27.9. Unnecessary qualification

Never   Occasionally   Always

(Place a mark on the scale above)

28. Of the nine writing problems listed above, which is most common?
    - ○ Poor flow of ideas
    - ○ Verbiage, wordiness
    - ○ Redundancy
    - ○ Wrong words
    - ○ Poor syntax, poor grammar
    - ○ Excessive abstraction
    - ○ Unnecessary complexity
    - ○ Excessive compression
    - ○ Unnecessary qualification

29. When you receive a manuscript, what do you find most annoying?

30. What is your definition of a good article?

31. What advice would you give to prospective authors submitting papers to your journal?

32. Can you cite an example of what you consider the ideal paper?

33. What statistical techniques do you think will be more important in the future?

34. Which group do you belong to?
    - ○ Nobel Laureate
    - ○ Editor of a medical journal
    - ○ JAMA reviewer
    - ○ Other

35. Specify other _____

36. Comments.

_____
_____
_____

(Thank you!)

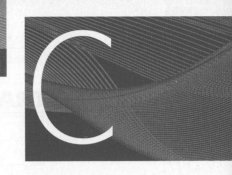

Sample Data
Collection Form

Institute for Trauma and Emergency Care
New York Medical College

Logged __/__/__

ITEC TRAUMA SYSTEMS STUDY

1. (Last name)

2. (First name)

3. (Medical record no.)

4. Age

5. Date of birth

6. Case no.

7. Sex   1 ☐ Male   2 ☐ Female

8. Admission date

9. Street

10. City

11. State

12. Zip

13. Patient arrived
   1 ☐ Directly from scene
   2 ☐ Transferred from another hospital
   3 ☐ Other

14. Hospital transferred from

16. Race   1 ☐ White   2 ☐ Black
         3 ☐ Hispanic   4 ☐ Asian   9 ☐ Other

15. Type of insurance
   1 ☐ No fault
   2 ☐ Worker's compensation
   3 ☐ Medicaid
   4 ☐ Medicare
   5 ☐ BC/BS
   6 ☐ Major Medical
   7 ☐ Self
   9 ☐ Other
   0 ☐ None

17. Location injury occurred
   1 ☐ Home   2 ☐ Travel   3 ☐ Work
   4 ☐ School   9 ☐ Other

18. Date of injury

19. Day of the week injured
        M   T   W   Th   F   Sat   Sun
        1   2   3   4   5   6   7

20. Cause of injury
   1 ☐ MVA (driver)
   2 ☐ MVA (passenger)
   3 ☐ Motorcycle
   4 ☐ ATV, 3 or 4 wheel
   5 ☐ Moped
   6 ☐ Bicycle
   7 ☐ Airplane
   8 ☐ Pedestrian hit in MVA
   9 ☐ Gunshot wound
   10 ☐ Shotgun wound
   11 ☐ Stab wound
   12 ☐ Fall
   13 ☐ Machinery
   14 ☐ Athletic
   15 ☐ Boating
   16 ☐ Assault
   17 ☐ Animal bite
   18 ☐ Human bite
   19 ☐ Other

21. Mode of arrival
   1 ☐ Private ambulance
   2 ☐ Volunteer ambulance
   3 ☐ Public ambulance
   4 ☐ Police
   5 ☐ Helicopter
   6 ☐ Fire
   7 ☐ Self
   9 ☐ Other

22. Level of care
   1 ☐ BLS   2 ☐ ALS   3 ☐ ALS & BLS
   4 ☐ Untrained   9 ☐ Other   0 ☐ None

23. Care rendered
   1 ☐ IV fluids [_____] cc   5 ☐ Immobilization
   2 ☐ MAST   6 ☐ CPR
   3 ☐ MAST not inflated   9 ☐ Other
   4 ☐ Intubation   0 ☐ None

25. If MVA, was patient wearing seat belt?
   If motorcycle, was helmet worn?
         1 ☐ No   2 ☐ Yes

24. Was it a suicide attempt?
   1 ☐ No   2 ☐ Yes   3 ☐ Suspected

26. Does patient have a history of alcohol or drug abuse?
           1 ☐ No   2 ☐ Yes
   Was patient under the influence of drugs or ETOH at injury time?
           1 ☐ No   2 ☐ Yes   3 ☐ Suspected

   BAC [_____]   Toxic screen   1 ☐ Pos   2 ☐ Neg   3 ☐ None

ADDRESS WHERE INJURY OCCURRED

27. Street	28. City	29. State
30. Cross street	31. County	32. Zip

33. Actual military time		34. Elapsed time	
a. Time of injury		a. Response time	
b. Time call was received		b. Time at scene	
c. Time of dispatch		c. Transport time	
d. Time arrived at scene		d. Time in ER	
e. Time of departure from scene		e. Time from injury to OR	
f. Time arrived at ER		f. Time from injury to 1st ER	
g. Time of triage		g. Time from injury to 2nd ER	
h. Time of departure from ER		h. Time call rec'd to OR	
i. Time arrived at 2nd ER		i. Time call rec'd to 1st ER	
j. Time arrived at OR		j. Time call rec'd to 2nd ER	
k. Time arrived at floor			

35. Trauma scoring (Value/Score)	At scene	Worst prehosp	First ER	Worst 1 hr	During transfer	Second ER
Pulse rate						
BP systolic						
Respirations per minute						
Eye opening						
Verbal response						
Motor response						
Total Glasgow score						

INITIAL HOSPITAL

36. Did patient receive	37. Units of blood	
1 ☐ CAT scan of head 2 ☐ CAT scan of abdomen 3 ☐ Swan-Ganz catheter 4 ☐ Abdominal tap 5 ☐ Angiogram 6 ☐ NMR test 7 ☐ Intubation	In first 24 hours	
	In first 48 hours	
	During hospital stay	

38. Prior to transfer: Procedure at transferring hospital	ICD-9
1	
2	
3	
4	
5	
6	

RECEIVING HOSPITAL

39. Did patient receive	40. Units of blood given
1 ☐ CAT scan of head 2 ☐ CAT scan of abdomen 3 ☐ Swan-Ganz catheter 4 ☐ Abdominal tap 5 ☐ Angiogram 6 ☐ NMR test 7 ☐ Intubation	In first 24 hours In first 48 hours During hospital stay

41. Performed in this hospital: Procedure or treatment	ICD-9
1	
2	
3	
4	
5	
6	
7	
8	

42. Complications		Day	Describe	ICD-9
☐ 0—None ☐ 1—Pulmonary	1			
☐ 2—Cardiovascular ☐ 3—Hematologic	2			
☐ 4—Renal ☐ 5—Hepatic	3			
☐ 6—Infection/sepsis ☐ 7—Hemorrhage	4			
☐ 8—Neurologic ☐ 9—Other	5			
43. Total no. of complications			44. Days in ICU	

DISCHARGE INFORMATION

45. Final confirmed diagnosis	ICD-9	AIS/Code
1		
2		
3		
4		
5		
6		

(continued)

7			
8			
9			
10			

46. External cause of injury (ICD-9 E Code)

47. Date discharged

48. Disposition
    ☐ 1—Home
    ☐ 2—Rehabilitation facility
    ☐ 3—Other hospital
    ☐ 4—Morgue

49. Days in hospital

50. ISS

51.

DIAGNOSIS RELATED GROUPS

DRG code   DRG days allowed   Was patient an outlier?
                                                         1 ☐ No   2 ☐ Yes

52. Extent of disability at discharge

INFORMATION ON DEATHS

53. Date expired

54. Time expired

55. Hours from injury to death

56. Was an autopsy performed?
    1 ☐ No   2 ☐ Yes

57. Where did the patient die?
    1 ☐ At scene   2 ☐ In transit   3 ☐ ER   4 ☐ Hospital floor
    5 ☐ ICU   6 ☐ OR   7 ☐ Recovery room   9 ☐ Other

58. Was an organ donated from this patient?   1 ☐ No   2 ☐ Yes

59. If yes, list organs donated:

Cause of death

60. First

61. Second

62. Third

63. Fourth

64. Reviewed by (Code no.)

65. Comments:

Reprinted by permission of New York Medical College Institute for Trauma and Emergency Care, Valhalla, New York.

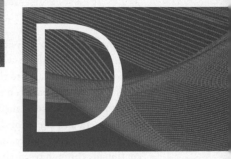

APPENDIX

WMA Declaration of Helsinki–Ethical Principles for Medical Research Involving Human Subjects[1]

Adopted by the 18th WMA General Assembly, Helsinki, Finland, June 1964 and amended by the:

29th WMA General Assembly, Tokyo, Japan, October 1975
35th WMA General Assembly, Venice, Italy, October 1983
41st WMA General Assembly, Hong Kong, September 1989
48th WMA General Assembly, Somerset West, Republic of South Africa, October 1996
52nd WMA General Assembly, Edinburgh, Scotland, October 2000
53rd WMA General Assembly, Washington DC, USA, October 2002 (Note of Clarification added)
55th WMA General Assembly, Tokyo, Japan, October 2004 (Note of Clarification added)
59th WMA General Assembly, Seoul, Republic of Korea, October 2008
64th WMA General Assembly, Fortaleza, Brazil, October 2013

Preamble

1. The World Medical Association (WMA) has developed the Declaration of Helsinki as a statement of ethical principles for medical research involving human subjects, including research on identifiable human material and data.

   The Declaration is intended to be read as a whole and each of its constituent paragraphs should be applied with consideration of all other relevant paragraphs.
2. Consistent with the mandate of the WMA, the Declaration is addressed primarily to physicians. The WMA encourages others who are involved in medical research involving human subjects to adopt these principles.

General Principles

3. The Declaration of Geneva of the WMA binds the physician with the words, "The health of my patient will be my first consideration," and the International Code of Medical Ethics declares that, "A physician shall act in the patient's best interest when providing medical care."

---

[1]Reprinted with permission from the World Medical Association.

4. It is the duty of the physician to promote and safeguard the health, well-being and rights of patients, including those who are involved in medical research. The physician's knowledge and conscience are dedicated to the fulfilment of this duty.

5. Medical progress is based on research that ultimately must include studies involving human subjects.

6. The primary purpose of medical research involving human subjects is to understand the causes, development and effects of diseases and improve preventive, diagnostic and therapeutic interventions (methods, procedures and treatments). Even the best proven interventions must be evaluated continually through research for their safety, effectiveness, efficiency, accessibility and quality.

7. Medical research is subject to ethical standards that promote and ensure respect for all human subjects and protect their health and rights.

8. While the primary purpose of medical research is to generate new knowledge, this goal can never take precedence over the rights and interests of individual research subjects.

9. It is the duty of physicians who are involved in medical research to protect the life, health, dignity, integrity, right to self-determination, privacy, and confidentiality of personal information of research subjects. The responsibility for the protection of research subjects must always rest with the physician or other health care professionals and never with the research subjects, even though they have given consent.

10. Physicians must consider the ethical, legal and regulatory norms and standards for research involving human subjects in their own countries as well as applicable international norms and standards. No national or international ethical, legal or regulatory requirement should reduce or eliminate any of the protections for research subjects set forth in this Declaration.

11. Medical research should be conducted in a manner that minimises possible harm to the environment.

12. Medical research involving human subjects must be conducted only by individuals with the appropriate ethics and scientific education, training and qualifications. Research on patients or healthy volunteers requires the supervision of a competent and appropriately qualified physician or other health care professional.

13. Groups that are underrepresented in medical research should be provided appropriate access to participation in research.

14. Physicians who combine medical research with medical care should involve their patients in research only to the extent that this is justified by its potential preventive, diagnostic or therapeutic value and if the physician has good reason to believe that participation in the research study will not adversely affect the health of the patients who serve as research subjects.

15. Appropriate compensation and treatment for subjects who are harmed as a result of participating in research must be ensured.

Risks, Burdens and Benefits

16. In medical practice and in medical research, most interventions involve risks and burdens.

   Medical research involving human subjects may only be conducted if the importance of the objective outweighs the risks and burdens to the research subjects.

17. All medical research involving human subjects must be preceded by careful assessment of predictable risks and burdens to the individuals and groups involved in the research in comparison with foreseeable benefits to them and to other individuals or groups affected by the condition under investigation.

   Measures to minimise the risks must be implemented. The risks must be continuously monitored, assessed and documented by the researcher.

18. Physicians may not be involved in a research study involving human subjects unless they are confident that the risks have been adequately assessed and can be satisfactorily managed.

   When the risks are found to outweigh the potential benefits or when there is conclusive proof of definitive outcomes, physicians must assess whether to continue, modify or immediately stop the study.

Vulnerable Groups and Individuals

19. Some groups and individuals are particularly vulnerable and may have an increased likelihood of being wronged or of incurring additional harm.

   All vulnerable groups and individuals should receive specifically considered protection.

20. Medical research with a vulnerable group is only justified if the research is responsive to the health needs or priorities of this group and the research cannot be carried out in a non-vulnerable group. In addition, this group should stand to benefit from the knowledge, practices or interventions that result from the research.

Scientific Requirements and Research Protocols

21. Medical research involving human subjects must conform to generally accepted scientific principles, be based on a thorough knowledge of the scientific literature, other relevant sources of information, and adequate laboratory and, as appropriate, animal experimentation. The welfare of animals used for research must be respected.

22. The design and performance of each research study involving human subjects must be clearly described and justified in a research protocol.

   The protocol should contain a statement of the ethical considerations involved and should indicate how the principles in this Declaration have been addressed. The protocol should include information regarding funding, sponsors, institutional affiliations, potential conflicts of interest, incentives for subjects and information regarding provisions for treating and/or compensating subjects who are harmed as a consequence of participation in the research study.

   In clinical trials, the protocol must also describe appropriate arrangements for post-trial provisions.

Research Ethics Committees

23. The research protocol must be submitted for consideration, comment, guidance and approval to the concerned research ethics committee before the study begins. This committee must be transparent in its functioning, must be independent of the researcher, the sponsor and any other undue influence and must be duly qualified. It must take into consideration the laws and regulations of the country or countries in which the research is to be performed as well as applicable international norms and standards but these must not be allowed to reduce or eliminate any of the protections for research subjects set forth in this Declaration.

   The committee must have the right to monitor ongoing studies. The researcher must provide monitoring information to the committee, especially information about any serious adverse events. No amendment to the protocol may be made without consideration and approval by the committee. After the end of the study, the researchers must submit a final report to the committee containing a summary of the study's findings and conclusions.

Privacy and Confidentiality

24. Every precaution must be taken to protect the privacy of research subjects and the confidentiality of their personal information.

Informed Consent

25. Participation by individuals capable of giving informed consent as subjects in medical research must be voluntary. Although it may be appropriate to consult family members or community leaders, no individual capable of giving informed consent may be enrolled in a research study unless he or she freely agrees.

26. In medical research involving human subjects capable of giving informed consent, each potential subject must be adequately informed of the aims, methods, sources of funding, any possible conflicts of interest, institutional affiliations of the researcher, the anticipated benefits and potential risks of the study and the discomfort it may entail, post-study provisions and any other relevant aspects of the study. The potential subject must be informed of the right to refuse to participate in the study or to withdraw consent to participate at any time without reprisal. Special attention should be given to the specific information needs of individual potential subjects as well as to the methods used to deliver the information.

    After ensuring that the potential subject has understood the information, the physician or another appropriately qualified individual must then seek the potential subject's freely-given informed consent, preferably in writing. If the consent cannot be expressed in writing, the non-written consent must be formally documented and witnessed.

    All medical research subjects should be given the option of being informed about the general outcome and results of the study.

27. When seeking informed consent for participation in a research study the physician must be particularly cautious if the potential subject is in a dependent relationship with the physician or may consent under duress. In such situations the informed consent must be sought by an appropriately qualified individual who is completely independent of this relationship.

28. For a potential research subject who is incapable of giving informed consent, the physician must seek informed consent from the legally authorised representative. These individuals must not be included in a research study that has no likelihood of benefit for them unless it is intended to promote the health of the group represented by the potential subject, the research cannot instead be performed with persons capable of providing informed consent, and the research entails only minimal risk and minimal burden.

29. When a potential research subject who is deemed incapable of giving informed consent is able to give assent to decisions about participation in research, the physician must seek that assent in addition to the consent of the legally authorised representative. The potential subject's dissent should be respected.

30. Research involving subjects who are physically or mentally incapable of giving consent, for example, unconscious patients, may be done only if the physical or mental condition that prevents giving informed consent is a necessary characteristic of the research group. In such circumstances the physician must seek informed consent from the legally authorised representative. If no such representative is available and if the research cannot be delayed, the study may proceed without informed consent provided that the specific reasons for involving subjects with a condition that renders them unable to give informed consent have been stated in the research protocol and the study has been approved by a research ethics committee. Consent to remain in the research must be obtained as soon as possible from the subject or a legally authorised representative.

31. The physician must fully inform the patient which aspects of their care are related to the research. The refusal of a patient to participate in a study or the patient's decision to withdraw from the study must never adversely affect the patient-physician relationship.

32. For medical research using identifiable human material or data, such as research on material or data contained in biobanks or similar repositories, physicians must seek informed consent for its collection, storage and/or reuse. There may be exceptional situations where consent would be impossible or impracticable to obtain for such research. In such situations the research may be done only after consideration and approval of a research ethics committee.

Use of Placebo

33. The benefits, risks, burdens and effectiveness of a new intervention must be tested against those of the best proven intervention(s), except in the following circumstances:

    Where no proven intervention exists, the use of placebo, or no intervention, is acceptable; or

    Where for compelling and scientifically sound methodological reasons the use of any intervention less effective than the best proven one, the use of placebo, or no intervention is necessary to determine the efficacy or safety of an intervention and the patients who receive any intervention less effective than the best proven one, placebo, or no intervention will not be subject to additional risks of serious or irreversible harm as a result of not receiving the best proven intervention.

    Extreme care must be taken to avoid abuse of this option.

Post-Trial Provisions

34. In advance of a clinical trial, sponsors, researchers and host country governments should make provisions for post-trial access for all participants who still need an intervention identified as beneficial in the trial. This information must also be disclosed to participants during the informed consent process.

Research Registration and Publication and Dissemination of Results

35. Every research study involving human subjects must be registered in a publicly accessible database before recruitment of the first subject.
36. Researchers, authors, sponsors, editors and publishers all have ethical obligations with regard to the publication and dissemination of the results of research. Researchers have a duty to make publicly available the results of their research on human subjects and are accountable for the completeness and accuracy of their reports. All parties should adhere to accepted guidelines for ethical reporting. Negative and inconclusive as well as positive results must be published or otherwise made publicly available. Sources of funding, institutional affiliations and conflicts of interest must be declared in the publication. Reports of research not in accordance with the principles of this Declaration should not be accepted for publication.

Unproven Interventions in Clinical Practice

37. In the treatment of an individual patient, where proven interventions do not exist or other known interventions have been ineffective, the physician, after seeking expert advice, with informed consent from the patient or a legally authorised representative, may use an unproven intervention if in the physician's judgement it offers hope of saving life, re-establishing health or alleviating suffering. This intervention should subsequently be made the object of research, designed to evaluate its safety and efficacy. In all cases, new information must be recorded and, where appropriate, made publicly available.

Ode to Multiauthorship: A Multicentre, Prospective Random Poem

All cases complete, the study was over
the data were entered, lost once, and recovered.
Results were greeted with considerable glee
p value (two-tailed) equalling 0.0493.
The severity of illness, oh what a discovery,
was inversely proportional to the chance of recovery.
When the paper's first draft had only begun
the wannabe authors lined up one by one.
To jockey for their eternal positions
(for who would be first, second, and third)
and whom "et aled" in all further citations.
Each centre had seniors, each senior ten bees,
the bees had technicians and nurses to please.
The list it grew longer and longer each day,
as new authors appeared to enter the fray.
Each fought with such fury to stake his or her place
being just a "participant" would be a disgrace.
For the appendix is piled with hundreds of others
and seen by no one but spouses and mothers.
If to "publish or perish" is how academics are bred
then to miss the masthead is near to be dead.
As the number of authors continued to grow
they outnumbered the patients by two to one or so.
While PIs faxed memos to company headquarters
the bees and the nurses took care of the orders.
They'd signed up the patients, and followed them weekly
heard their complaints, and kept casebooks so neatly.
There were seniors from centres that enrolled two or three
who threatened "foul play" if not on the marquee.
But the juniors and helpers who worked into the night
were simply "acknowledged" or left off outright.
"Calm down" cried the seniors to the quivering drones
there's place for you all on the RPU clones.
When the paper was finished and sent for review
six authors didn't know that the study was through.
Oh the work was so hard, and the fights oh so bitter
for the glory of publishing and grabbing the glitter.
Imagine the wars when in six months or better
The Editor's response, "please make it a letter."

The order of the authors is not necessarily related to specific contributions, but to the order in which each made their acquaintance with the first author. However, all have made significant contributions to the poem. The authors acknowledge their debt to Theodore Geisel. This letter was originally submitted to The Lancet *as an article.*

RPU = repeating publishable unit; PI = principle investigator

Howard W. Horowitz,[a] Nicholas H. Fiebach,[b] Stuart M. Levitz,[c] Jo Seibel,[d] Edwin H. Small,[c] Edward E. Telzak,[e] Gary P. Wormser,[a] Robert B. Nadelman,[a] Marisa Montecalvo,[a] John Nowakowski,[a] and John Raffali.[a]

[a]Departments of Medicine, New York Medical College, Valhalla, NY.
[b]Yale University School of Medicine, New Haven, CT.
[c]Boston University School of Medicine, Boston, MA.
[d]MetroWest Medical Center, Framingham, MA.
[e]Albert Einstein School of Medicine, Bronx, NY.

Originally printed in The Lancet. *1996;348:1746.*

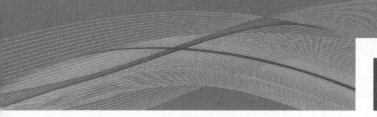
Bibliography

Abby M, Massey MD, Galandiuk S, et al. Peer review is an effective screening process to evaluate medical manuscripts. *JAMA*. 1994;272(2):105–107.

Albert T. *Winning the Publications Game: How to Write a Scientific Paper without Neglecting Your Patients*. 3rd ed. Boca Raton, FL: CRC Press; 2011.

Alpha-Tocopherol, Beta Carotene Cancer Prevention Study Group. The effect of vitamin E and beta carotene on the incidence of lung cancer and other cancers in male smokers. *N Engl J Med*. 1994;330(15):1029–1035.

Altman DG. *Practical Statistics for Medical Research*. London, United Kingdom: Chapman & Hall; 1991.

Altman DG. The scandal of poor medical research. *BMJ*. 1994;308:283–284.

Altman DG, Goodman SN, Schroter S. How statistical expertise is used in medical research. *JAMA*. 2002;287 (21):2817–2820.

Altman DG, Goodman SN. Transfer of technology from statistical journals to the biomedical literature: past trends and future predictions. *JAMA*. 1994;272(2):129–132.

Altman DG, Machin D, Bryant T, et al. *Statistics with Confidence: Confidence Intervals and Statistical Guidelines*. London, United Kingdom: British Medical Journal; 2000.

The American Heritage Dictionary of the English Language. 5th ed. Boston, MA: Houghton Mifflin Harcourt; 2012.

American Medical Association. *AMA Manual of Style: A Guide for Authors and Editors*. 10th ed. New York, NY: Oxford University Press; 2007.

American Psychological Association. *Publication Manual of the American Psychological Association*. 6th ed. Washington, DC: American Psychological Association; 2010.

American Psychological Association. Summary report of journal operations, 1995. *American Psychologists*. 1996;51:876–877.

Andersen B. *Methodological Errors in Medical Research: An Incomplete Catalogue*. Oxford, United Kingdom: Blackwell Scientific Publications; 1990.

Armitage P, Berry G, Matthews JNS. *Statistical Methods in Medical Research*. 4th ed. Oxford, United Kingdom: Wiley-Blackwell; 2001.

Armitage P, Colton T, eds. *Encyclopedia of Biostatistics: 8-Volume Set*. 2nd ed. New York, NY: Wiley; 2005.

Austin PC. An introduction to propensity score methods for reducing the effects of confounding in observational studies. *Multivariate Behav Res*. 2011;46(3):399–424.

Babbie ER. *The Practice of Social Research*. 14th ed. Boston, MA: Cengage Learning; 2015.

Bailar JC III, Hoaglin DC, eds. *Medical Uses of Statistics*. 3rd ed. Hoboken, NJ: Wiley; 2009.

Baker SS. *Writing Nonfiction that Sells*. Cincinnati, OH: Writer's Digest Books; 1986.

Barnett AG, van der Pols JC, Dobson AJ. Regression to the mean: what it is and how to deal with it. *Int J Epidemiol*. 2005;34(1):215–220.

Barnum BS. *Writing and Getting Published: A Primer for Nurses*. New York, NY: Springer; 1995.

Bartko JJ. Rationale for reporting standard deviations rather than standard errors of the mean. *Am J Psychiatry*. 1985;142(9):1060.

Berry DA. Comment: ethics and ECMO. *Stat Sci*. 1989;4(4):306–310.

Bertin J. *Graphics and Graphic Information Processing*. Berg WJ, Scott P, trans. Boston, MA: Walter De Gruyter Inc; 1981.

Bertin J. *Semiology of Graphics: Diagrams, Networks, Maps*. Redlands, CA: Esri Press; 2010.

Berwick DM. Quality of health care. Part 5: payment by capitation and the quality of care. *N Engl J Med*. 1996; 335(16):1227–1231.

Bland JM, Altman DG. Statistical methods for assessing agreement between two methods of clinical measurement. *Lancet*. 1986;1(8476):307–310.

Blumenthal D. Part 1: quality of care—what is it? *N Engl J Med*. 1996;335(12):891–894.

Blumenthal D. Quality of health care. Part 4: the origins of the quality-of-care debate. *N Engl J Med*. 1996;335 (15):1146–1149.

Blumenthal D, Epstein AM. Quality of health care. Part 6: the role of physicians in the future of quality management. *N Engl J Med*. 1996;335(17):1328–1331.

Brallier JM. *Medical Wit and Wisdom: The Best Medical Quotations from Hippocrates to Groucho Marx.* Philadelphia, PA: Running Press; 1993.

Breslow NE, Day NE. *Statistical Methods in Cancer Research. Volume 1—The Analysis of Case-Control Studies.* Lyon, France: International Agency for Research on Cancer; 1980. IARC Scientific Publications No. 32.

Breslow NE, Day NE. *Statistical Methods in Cancer Research. Volume 2—The Design and Analysis of Cohort Studies.* Lyon, France: International Agency for Research in Cancer; 1987. IARC Scientific Publications No. 82.

Briscoe MH. *Preparing Scientific Illustrations: A Guide to Better Posters, Presentations, and Publications.* 2nd ed. New York, NY: Springer-Verlag; 2013.

Brook RH, McGlynn EA, Cleary PD. Quality of health care. Part 2: measuring quality of care. *N Engl J Med.* 1996;335(13):966–970.

Browner WS. *Publishing and Presenting Clinical Research.* 3rd ed. Philadelphia, PA: Wolters Kluwer; 2012.

Bulpitt CJ. *Randomised Controlled Clinical Trials.* 2nd ed. New York, NY: Springer; 2013.

Burgess S, Thompson SG. *Mendelian Randomization: Methods for Using Genetic Variants in Causal Estimation.* Boca Raton, FL: Chapman & Hall/CRC; 2015.

Byrne DW. Common reasons for rejecting manuscripts at medical journals: a survey of editors and peer reviewers. *Science Editor.* 2000;23(2):39–44.

Byrne DW, Biaggioni I, Bernard GR, et al. Clinical and translational research studios: a multidisciplinary internal support program. *Acad Med.* 2012;87(8):1052–1059.

Byrne DW, Goetzel RZ, McGown PW, et al. Seven-year trends in employee health habits from a comprehensive workplace health promotion program at Vanderbilt University. *J Occup Environ Med.* 2011;53(12):1372–1381.

Calvert M, Blazeby J, Altman DG, et al. Reporting of patient-reported outcomes in randomized trials: the CONSORT PRO extension. *JAMA.* 2013;309(8):814–822.

Chassin MR. Quality of health care. Part 3: improving the quality of care. *N Engl J Med.* 1996;335(14):1060–1063.

Chicago Manual of Style. 16th ed. Chicago, IL: University of Chicago Press; 2010.

Clark S. *Taming the Marketing Jungle: Marketing When Your Creativity Is High and Your Budget Is Low.* Seattle, WA: Hara; 1994.

Collett D. *Modelling Survival Data in Medical Research.* 3rd ed. Boca Raton, FL: Chapman & Hall/CRC; 2014.

Colton T. The 'power' of sound statistics. *JAMA.* 1990;263(2):281.

Conover WJ. Some reasons for not using the Yates continuity correction on 2 × 2 contingency tables. *J Am Stat Assoc.* 1974;69:374–376.

Council of Science Editors. *Scientific Style and Format: The CSE Manual for Authors, Editors, and Publishers.* 8th ed. New York, NY: Cambridge University Press; 2014.

Cox DR. Regression models and life-tables. *J R Stat Soc B.* 1972;34:187–220.

Crichton M. Sounding board: medical obfuscation: structure and function. *N Engl J Med.* 1975;293:1257–1259.

Daintith J, Isaacs A, eds. *Medical Quotes: A Thematic Dictionary.* Oxford, United Kingdom: Market House Books; 1989.

Dawson B, Trapp RG. *Basic & Clinical Biostatistics.* 4th ed. Norwalk, CT: Lange Medical Books/McGraw-Hill; 2005.

Day RA, Gastel B. *How to Write and Publish a Scientific Paper.* 7th ed. Santa Barbara, CA: Greenwood; 2011.

Donders AR, van der Heijden GJ, Stijnen T, et al. Review: a gentle introduction to imputation of missing values. *J Clin Epidemiol.* 2006;59(10):1087–1091.

Dorland's Illustrated Medical Dictionary. 32nd ed. Philadelphia, PA: Saunders; 2011.

Dupont WD. *Statistical Modeling for Biomedical Researchers: A Simple Introduction to the Analysis of Complex Data.* Cambridge, United Kingdom: Cambridge University Press; 2009.

Ewigman BG, Crane JP, Frigoletto FD, et al. Effect of prenatal ultrasound screening on perinatal outcome. *N Engl J Med.* 1993;329(12):821–827.

Falco FJ, Hennessey WJ, Goldberg G, et al. Standardized nerve conduction studies in the lower limb of the healthy elderly. *Am J Phys Med Rehabil.* 1994;73(3):168–174.

Fayers PM, Machin D. *Quality of Life: The Assessment, Analysis and Reporting of Patient-reported Outcomes.* 3rd ed. West Sussex, United Kingdom: Wiley-Blackwell. 2016.

Fiske RH. *Thesaurus of Alternatives to Worn-Out Words and Phrases.* Cincinnati, OH: Writer's Digest Books; 1994.

Fleiss JL, Levin B, Paik MC. *Statistical Methods for Rates and Proportions.* 3rd ed. New York, NY: Wiley-Interscience; 2003.

Fleiss JL, Tytun A, Ury HK. A simple approximation for calculating sample sizes for comparing independent proportions. *Biometrics.* 1980;36(2):343–346.

Fletcher RH, Fletcher SW, Fletcher GS. *Clinical Epidemiology: The Essentials.* 5th ed. Philadelphia, PA: Lippincott Williams & Wilkins; 2012.

Fondiller SH, Nerone BJ. *Health Professionals Style Manual.* New York, NY: Springer; 2006.

Fox RJ, Crask MR, Kim J. Mail survey response rate: a meta-analysis of selected techniques for inducing response. *Public Opin.* 1988;52:467–491.

Fried C. The practice of experimentation. In: Bearn AG, Black DAK, Hiatt HH, eds. *Medical Experimentation: Personal Integrity and Social Policy.* New York, NY: American Elsevier; 1974:158.

Friedman GD. *Primer of Epidemiology.* 5th ed. New York, NY: McGraw-Hill Medical; 2003.

Friedman LM, Furberg CD, DeMets D, et al. *Fundamentals of Clinical Trials.* 5th ed. New York, NY: Springer; 2015.

Gabor A. *The Man Who Discovered Quality: How W. Edwards Deming Brought the Quality Revolution to America— The Stories of FORD, XEROX, and GM.* New York, NY: Penguin Books; 1992.

Garfield E. *SCI Journal Citation Reports: A Bibliographic Analysis of Science Journals in the ISI Database.* Philadelphia, PA: Institute for Scientific Information. http://thomsonreuters.com/journal-citation-reports/. Accessed June 17, 2016.

Garland J. In: Strauss MB, ed. *Familiar Medical Quotations.* Boston, MA: Little Brown; 1968;672.

Gilmore E. "Call me Jim": James Thurber speaking. In: Fensch T, ed. *Conversations with James Thurber.* Jackson, MI: University Press of Mississippi; 1989:50.

Glass DJ. *Experimental Design for Biologists.* 2nd ed. Cold Spring Harbor, NY: Cold Spring Harbor Laboratory Press; 2014.

Gordis L. *Epidemiology.* 5th ed. Philadelphia, PA: Saunders; 2013.

Greenland S. Basic methods for sensitivity analysis of biases. *Int J Epidemiol.* 1996;25:1107–1116.

Hackam DG, Redelmeier DA. Translation of research evidence from animals to humans. *JAMA.* 2006;296(14):1731–1732.

Hall GM, ed. *How to Write a Paper.* 5th ed. Malden, MA: Blackwell; 2012.

Halsey MJ. References. In: Hall GM, ed. *How to Write a Paper.* 5th ed. Malden, MA: Blackwell; 2012.

Hansen LO, Young RS, Hinami K, et al. Interventions to reduce 30-day rehospitalization: a systematic review. *Ann Intern Med.* 2011;155(8):520–528.

Harris PA, Scott KW, Lebo L, et al. ResearchMatch: a national registry to recruit volunteers for clinical research. *Acad Med.* 2012;87(1):66–73.

Harris PA, Taylor R, Thielke R, et al. Research electronic data capture (REDCap)—a metadata-driven methodology and workflow process for providing translational research informatics support. *J Biomed Inform.* 2009;42(2):377–381.

Haynes RB, Sackett DL, Guyatt GH, et al. *Clinical Epidemiology: How to Do Clinical Practice Research.* 3rd ed. Philadelphia, PA: Lippincott Williams & Wilkins; 2011.

He W, Pinheiro J, Kuznetsova OM. *Practical Considerations for Adaptive Trial Design and Implementation.* New York, NY: Springer; 2014.

Hebel JR, McCarter RJ. *A Study Guide to Epidemiology and Biostatistics.* 7th ed. London, United Kingdom: Jones & Bartlett Learning; 2011.

Hill AB. The environment and disease: association or causation? *Proc R Soc Med.* 1965;58(5):295–300.

Hosmer DW Jr, Lemeshow S, Sturdivant RX. *Applied Logistic Regression.* 3rd ed. New York, NY: John Wiley & Sons; 2012.

Hulley SB, Cummings SR, Browner WS, et al. *Designing Clinical Research.* 4th ed. Philadelphia, PA: Lippincott Williams & Wilkins; 2013.

Huth EJ. *Writing and Publishing in Medicine.* 3rd ed. Baltimore, MD: Lippincott Williams & Wilkins; 1999.

Ingelfinger JA, Mosteller R, Thibodeau LA, et al. *Biostatistics in Clinical Medicine.* 3rd ed. New York, NY: McGraw-Hill; 1994.

International Committee of Medical Journal Editors. Uniform requirements for manuscripts submitted to biomedical journals. *N Engl J Med.* 1997;336(4):309–315. http://www.icmje.org/. Accessed June 17, 2016.

International Conference on Harmonisation. Guidelines on structure and content of clinical study reports. *Fed Regist.* 1996;61:37319–37343.

ISIS-2 (Second International Study of Infarct Survival) Collaborative Group. Randomised trial of intravenous streptokinase, oral aspirin, both, or neither among 17,187 cases of suspected acute myocardial infarction: ISIS-2. *Lancet.* 1988;2(8607):349–360.

James KE. Regression toward the mean in uncontrolled clinical studies. *Biometrics.* 1973;29(1):121–130.

Kahneman D. *Thinking, Fast and Slow.* New York, NY: Farrar, Straus and Giroux; 2013.

Kaplan EL, Meier P. Nonparametric estimation from incomplete observations. *J Am Stat Assoc.* 1958;53:457–481.

Kassirer JP, Angell M. Redundant publication: a reminder. *N Engl J Med.* 1995;333(7):449–450.

Kassirer JP, Campion EW. Peer review: crude and understudied, but indispensable. *JAMA*. 1994;272(2):96–97.

Katz MH. *Evaluating Clinical and Public Health Interventions: A Practical Guide to Study Design and Statistics*. Cambridge, United Kingdom: Cambridge University Press; 2010.

Katz MH. *Multivariable Analysis: A Practical Guide for Clinicians and Public Health Researchers*. Cambridge, NY: Cambridge University Press; 2011.

Katz MH. *Study Design and Statistical Analysis: A Practical Guide for Clinicians*. Cambridge, NY: Cambridge University Press; 2006.

Kent DM, Rothwell PM, Ioannidis JP, et al. Assessing and reporting heterogeneity in treatment effects in clinical trials: a proposal. *Trials*. 2010;11:85.

Kirkwood B, Sterne J. *Essential Medical Statistics*. 2nd ed. Malden, MA: Blackwell; 2003.

Kleinbaum DG, Klein M. *Logistic Regression: A Self-Learning Text*. 3rd ed. New York, NY: Springer; 2010.

Kleinbaum DG, Kupper LL, Nizam A, et al. *Applied Regression Analysis and Other Multivariable Methods*. 5th ed. Boston, MA: Cengage Learning; 2013.

Kleinbaum DG, Kupper LL, Morgenstern H. *Epidemiologic Research: Principles and Quantitative Methods*. New York, NY: Van Nostrand; 1982.

Knol MJ, Groenwold RH, Grobbee DE. P-values in baseline tables of randomised controlled trials are inappropriate but still common in high impact journals. *Eur J Prev Cardiol*. 2012;19(2):231–232.

Kuzma JW, Bohnenblust SE. *Basic Statistics for the Health Sciences*. 5th ed. New York, NY: McGraw-Hill; 2004.

Lang TA. *How to Write, Publish, and Present in the Health Sciences: A Guide for Clinicians and Laboratory Researchers*. Philadelphia, PA: American College of Physicians; 2009.

Lang TA, Secic M. *How to Report Statistics in Medicine: Annotated Guidelines for Authors, Editors, and Reviewers*. 2nd ed. Philadelphia, PA: American College of Physicians; 2006.

Last JM, Spasoff RA, Harris SS, eds. *A Dictionary of Epidemiology*. 4th ed. New York, NY: Oxford University Press; 2000.

Lee ET, Wang JW. *Statistical Methods for Survival Data Analysis*. 4th ed. New York, NY: John Wiley & Sons; 2013.

Lehmann EL. Nonparametric confidence intervals for a shift parameter. *Ann Math Stat*. 1963;34:1507–1512.

Leibson T, Koren G. Informed consent in pediatric research. *Paediatr Drugs*. 2015;17(1):5–11.

Lenth RV. Some practical guidelines for effective sample size determination. *The American Statistician*. 2001;55:187–193.

Lenth RV. Statistical power calculations. *J Anim Sci*. 2007;85(13 Suppl):E24–E29.

Liggins GC, Howie RN. A controlled trial of antepartum glucocorticoid treatment for prevention of the respiratory distress syndrome in premature infants. *Pediatrics*. 1972;50:515–525.

Lipsitz SR, Fitzmaurice GM, Orav EJ, et al. Performance of generalized estimating equations in practical situations. *Biometrics*. 1994;50(1):270–278.

Little RJ, D'Agostino R, Cohen ML, et al. The prevention and treatment of missing data in clinical trials. *N Engl J Med*. 2012;367(14):1355–1360.

Lock SP. *The Future of Medical Journals: In Commemoration of 150 Years of the British Medical Journal*. London, United Kingdom: British Medical Journal; 1991.

Lorch U, Berelowitz K, Ozen C, et al. The practical application of adaptive study design in early phase clinical trials: a retrospective analysis of time savings. *Eur J Clin Pharmacol*. 2012;68(5):543–551.

Mann HB, Whitney DR. On a test of whether one of two random variables is stochastically larger than the other. *Ann Math Stat*. 1947;18:50–60.

Mantel N, Haenszel W. Statistical aspects of the analysis of data from retrospective studies of disease. *J Natl Cancer Inst*. 1959;22(4):719–748.

Marantz PR. Beta carotene, vitamin E, and lung cancer. *N Engl J Med*. 1994;331(9):611–614.

Maron DJ, Stone GW, Berman DS, et al. Is cardiac catheterization necessary before initial management of patients with stable ischemic heart disease? Results from a Web-based survey of cardiologists. *Am Heart J*. 2011;162(6):1034–1043.

Mausner JS, Kramer S. *Mausner & Bahn Epidemiology: An Introductory Text*. 2nd ed. Philadelphia, PA: WB Saunders; 1985.

Mehta CR, Patel NR, Gray R. Computing an exact confidence interval for the common odds ratio in several 2×2 contingency tables. *J Am Stat Assoc*. 1985;80:969–973.

Merriam-Webster's Dictionary. Springfield, MA: Merriam-Webster; 2016.

Mitjà O, Houinei W, Moses P, et al. Mass treatment with single-dose azithromycin for yaws. *N Engl J Med*. 2015; 372(8):703–710.

Morton RF, Hebel JR, McCarter RJ. *A Study Guide to Epidemiology and Biostatistics*. 5th ed. New York, NY: Aspen; 2001.

Moses LE, Emerson JD, Hosseini H. Analyzing data from ordered categories. *N Engl J Med*. 1984;311(7):442–448.

Naber SP, Tsutsumi Y, Yin S, et al. Strategies for the analysis of oncogene overexpression: studies of the neu oncogene in breast carcinoma. *Am J Clin Pathol*. 1990;94:125–136.

National Center for Health Statistics. *User's Manual: The National Death Index*. Washington, DC: US Government Printing Office; 1981. DHHS publication PHS 81–1148.

Noto MJ, Domenico HJ, Byrne DW, et al. Chlorhexidine bathing and health care-associated infections: a randomized clinical trial. *JAMA*. 2015;313(4):369–378.

Norris M. *Between You & Me: Confession of a Comma Queen*. New York, NY: W. W. Norton & Company; 2015.

O'Connor M. *Writing Successfully in Science*. London, United Kingdom: Routledge; 1992.

Olson CM. Peer review of the biomedical literature. *Am J Emerg Med*. 1990;8(4):356–358.

Oppenheimer DM. Consequences of erudite vernacular utilized irrespective of necessity: problems with using long words needlessly. *Appl Cognit Psychol*. 2006;20:139–156.

Orwell G. Politics and the English language. In: Orwell G, ed. *A Collection of Essays*. Mariner Books; 1970:162–176.

Payne LV. *The Lively Art of Writing*. Upper Saddle River, NJ: Prentice Hall; 1987.

Piwowar HA, Day RS, Fridsma DB. Sharing detailed research data is associated with increased citation rate. *PLoS One*. 2007;2(3):e308.

Polit DF, Beck CT. *Nursing Research: Generating and Assessing Evidence for Nursing Practice*. 9th ed. Philadelphia, PA: Lippincott Williams & Wilkins; 2011.

Protection of human subjects, 45 C.F.R. §46 (2009). *Fed Regist*. 2009;56:28003–28032. http://www.hhs.gov/ohrp/policy/ohrpregulations.pdf. Accessed June 17, 2016.

Pruitt BA, Mason AD Jr, Moncrief JA. Hemodynamic changes in the early postburn patient: the influence of fluid administration and of a vasodilator (hydralazine). *J Trauma*. 1971;11(1):36–46.

Robertson D, Williams GH. *Clinical and Translational Science: Principles of Human Research*. London, United Kingdom: Academic Press; 2008.

Roe A. *The Making of a Scientist*. Santa Barbara, CA: Praeger; 1974.

Rosenbaum PR. *Design of Observational Studies*. New York, NY: Springer; 2010.

Ross PE. Lies, damned lies and medical statistics. *Forbes*. August 14, 1995:130–135.

Rothman KJ, Greenland S, Lash TL. *Modern Epidemiology*. 3rd ed. Philadelphia, PA: Lippincott Williams & Wilkins; 2012.

Royall RM, Bartlett RH, Cornell RG, et al. Ethics and statistics in randomized clinical trials. *Stat Sci*. 1991;6:52–88.

Ruxton GD, Colegrave N. *Experimental Design for the Life Sciences*. 3rd ed. Oxford, United Kingdom: Oxford University Press; 2010.

Sabin WA. *The Gregg Reference Manual*. 11th ed. New York, NY: McGraw-Hill/Irwin; 2010.

Sackett DL. Bias in analytic research. *J Chronic Dis*. 1979;32:51–63.

Salsburg DS. The religion of statistics as practiced in medical journals. *Am Stat*. 1985;39:220–223.

Salzberg CA, Byrne DW, Cayten CG, et al. A new pressure ulcer risk assessment scale for individuals with spinal cord injury. *Am J Phys Med Rehabil*. 1996;75(2):96–104.

Sandve GK, Nekrutenko A, Taylor J, et al. Ten simple rules for reproducible computational research. *PLoS Comput Biol*. 2013;9(10):e1003285.

Seeff LB, Buskell-Bales Z, Wright EC, et al. Long-term mortality after transfusion-associated non-A, non-B hepatitis. *N Engl J Med*. 1992;327(27):1906–1911.

Senn SS. *Dicing with Death: Chance, Risk and Health*. Cambridge, United Kingdom: Cambridge University Press; 2003.

Senn SS. *Statistical Issues in Drug Development*. 2nd ed. New York, NY: Wiley-Interscience; 2008.

Sheridan DR, Dowdney DL. *How to Write and Publish Articles in Nursing*. New York, NY: Springer; 1997.

Silvia PJ. *How to Write a Lot: A Practical Guide to Productive Academic Writing*. Washington, DC: American Psychological Association; 2007.

Snedecor GW, Cochran WG. *Statistical Methods*. 8th ed. Ames, IA: Iowa State University Press; 1989.

Spilker B. *Guide to Clinical Trials*. New York, NY: Raven Press; 1991.

Spilker B, Schoenfelder J. *Data Collection Forms in Clinical Trials*. New York, NY: Raven Press; 1991.

Sprinthall RC. *Basic Statistical Analysis*. 9th ed. Upper Saddle River, NJ: Pearson; 2011.

Standards of Reporting Trials Group. A proposal for structured reporting of randomized controlled trials. *JAMA*. 1994;272(24):1926–1931.

Stedman's Medical Dictionary. 28th ed. Baltimore, MD: Lippincott Williams & Wilkins; 2005.

Stein J, Flexner SB, eds. *Random House College Thesaurus*. New York, NY: Random House; 2005.

Steyerberg EW. *Clinical Prediction Models: A Practical Approach to Development, Validation, and Updating*. New York, NY: Springer; 2010.

Strunk W Jr, White EB. *The Elements of Style*. New York, NY: Longman; 2009.

Sun GW, Shook TL, Kay GL. Inappropriate use of bivariable analysis to screen risk factors for use in multivariable analysis. *J Clin Epidemiol*. 1996;49(8):907–916.

Testa MA, Simonson DC. Assessment of quality-of-life outcomes. *N Engl J Med*. 1996;334(13):835–840.

Truog RD. Randomized controlled trials: lessons from ECMO. *Clin Res*. 1992;40(3):519–527.

Tufte ER. *The Visual Display of Quantitative Information*. 2nd ed. Cheshire, CT: Graphics Press; 2001.

Tufte ER. *Beautiful Evidence*. Cheshire, CT: Graphics Press; 2006.

US Department of Health and Human Services. Federal policy for the protection of human subjects: notices and rules. *Fed Regist*. 1991;46:28001–28032.

US Department of Health and Human Services. *Healthy People 2000*. Washington, DC: US Government Printing Office; 1991. DHHS publication PHS 91–50212.

Virchow R. Quoted by Garrison FH in Bulletin of the New York Academy of Medicine 1928;4:94. In: Strauss MB, ed. *Familiar Medical Quotations*. Boston, MA: Little Brown; 1968.

Wang R, Lagakos SW, Ware JH, et al. Statistics in medicine—reporting of subgroup analyses in clinical trials. *N Engl J Med*. 2007;357(21):2189–2194.

Ware JH, Mosteller F, Ingelfinger JA. P values. In: Bailar JC III, Hoaglin DC, eds. *Medical Uses of Statistics*. 3rd ed. Boston, MA: Massachusetts Medical Society; 2009.

Ware JH, Harrington DH, Hunter DJ, et al. Missing data. *N Engl J Med*. 2012;367:1353–1354.

Wickham H. *ggplot2: Elegant Graphics for Data Analysis (Use R!)*. New York, NY: Springer; 2010.

Wilcoxon F. Individual comparisons by ranking methods. *Biomed Bull*. 1945;1(6):80–83.

Williams JM. *Style: Lessons in Clarity and Grace*. 11th ed. Harlow, United Kingdom: Longman; 2013.

World Medical Association. Declaration of Helsinki: recommendations guiding physicians in biomedical research involving human subjects. *JAMA*. 1997;227(11):925–926. http://www.wma.net/en/20activities/10ethics/10helsinki/. Accessed June 17, 2016.

Yancey JM. Ten rules for reading clinical research reports. *Am J Surg*. 1990;159(6):533–539.

Zeger SL, Liang KY. Longitudinal data analysis for discrete and continuous outcomes. *Biometrics*. 1986;42(1):121–130.

Zeiger M. *Essentials of Writing Biomedical Research Papers*. 2nd ed. New York, NY: McGraw-Hill; 1999.

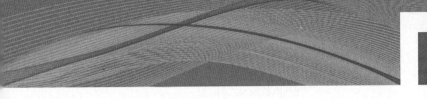

Index

Note: Page numbers in *italics* indicate illustrations; page numbers followed by t indicate tables.